MANUAL OF BLOOD PLATELETS
Morphology, Physiology and Pharmacology

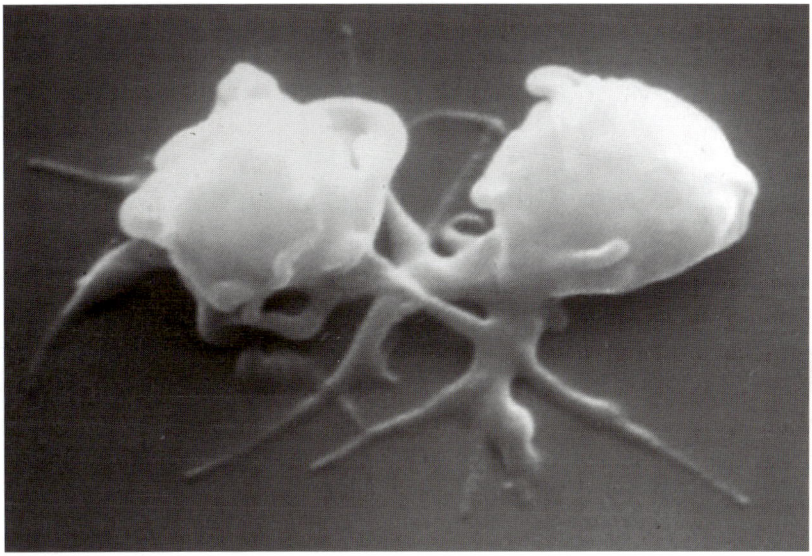

Sponsored by

South Asian Society on Atherosclerosis and Thrombosis (SASAT)
Division of Clinical and Preventive Cardiology, Medanta Hospital
Gurugram, Haryana, India

MANUAL OF BLOOD PLATELETS
Morphology, Physiology and Pharmacology

Editor

Gundu HR Rao PhD
Emeritus Professor
Laboratory Medicine and Pathology
Director
Thrombosis Research
Lillehei Heart Institute
Academic Health Center
University of Minnesota
Minneapolis, Minnesota, USA

Foreword

Jawed Fareed PhD DSc FAHA

JAYPEE

JAYPEE BROTHERS MEDICAL PUBLISHERS
The Health Sciences Publisher
New Delhi | London | Panama

Jaypee Brothers Medical Publishers (P) Ltd

Headquarters

Jaypee Brothers Medical Publishers (P) Ltd
4838/24, Ansari Road, Daryaganj
New Delhi 110 002, India
Phone: +91-11-43574357
Fax: +91-11-43574314
E-mail: jaypee@jaypeebrothers.com

Overseas Offices

J P Medical Ltd
83 Victoria Street, London
SW1H 0HW (UK)
Phone: +44 20 3170 8910
Fax: +44 (0)20 3008 6180
E-mail: info@jpmedpub.com

Jaypee-Highlights Medical Publishers Inc
City of Knowledge, Bld. 235, 2nd Floor, Clayton
Panama City, Panama
Phone: +1 507-301-0496
Fax: +1 507-301-0499
E-mail: cservice@jphmedical.com

Jaypee Brothers Medical Publishers (P) Ltd
Bhotahity, Kathmandu, Nepal
Phone: +977-9741283608
Email: kathmandu@jaypeebrothers.com

Website: www.jaypeebrothers.com
Website: www.jaypeedigital.com

Manual of Blood Platelets: Morphology, Physiology and Pharmacology

First Edition: **2019**

ISBN: 978-93-5270-202-2

Printed at Sanat Printers

Dedication

I dedicate this monograph to my mentor and associate
Regents Professor of Pediatrics and Pathology
(Late) James G White, MD

Foreword

This comprehensive book represents a detailed description of platelet biology highlighting the detailed structural and functional aspects of these anuclear cells. The illustrations and material included in this book represent a descriptive account of cutting edge work carried out during a 45-year period (1970–2015) and portray some of the lead discoveries on platelet structure and function. These discoveries have impacted the understanding of platelet-related diseases and the development of newer antiplatelet drugs, adding a new dimension to the treatment of cardiovascular diseases. Platelets were discovered accidentally by Professor Bizzozero in 1865 and since then have been a subject of focused basic and clinical research by experts from different disciplines. However, the work carried out at the University of Minnesota scientists led by Professor James White represents a major cornerstone in the overall development of platelet sciences. This book is a portrayal of the outstanding basic and clinical research on the structure and function of platelets and their interactions with the endothelium and other blood cells.

Of particular note, this book is a result of a very strong professional relationship between the author, Dr Rao and then lead hematologist at the University of Minnesota Professor James White, who was truly a pioneer in platelet related sciences. Dr Rao's recognition of the importance of compiling a complete account of the outstanding work carried out by Professor White is not only timely but is an inspirational tribute to a great mentor, Professor White. The compilation of this book and recognition of the pioneering work in nearly all aspects of platelet biology with a strong focus on the ultra-structure is the most appropriate way to acknowledge a mentor for which Dr Rao is to be commended. Professor White had dedicated most of his life to the study of platelets and related disorders. He himself was a 1955 graduate of the University of Minnesota Medical School, Minnesota, USA. After his initial training, he spent over 50 years at the same institution practicing hematology and overseeing a group of clinicians and scientists working on platelets. He is and will continue to be recognized as a lead investigator who applied great scientific vision and an integrated approach to identify the role of platelets in health and disease. His work on the fine structural details of platelets as they relate to the function of these anuclear cells revolutionized our understanding of the physiology and pharmacology of platelets. This book, illustrating the different aspects of platelet structure and function and a progressive evolution of innovative approaches resulting in various discoveries truly identifies him as a great mentor and leader. His interest in electron microscopy and its application to the study of platelets and blood cells encouraged the entire University of Minnesota team to advance this technique to its heights which resulted in the production of so many interesting images included some of which are included in the book. The photo micrographs and images generated at the University of Minnesota's hematology laboratories adorn the pages of the best hematology books all over the world and some of the lead publications carry these images and their references. Dr Rao has expertly summarized the complex fields of platelet morphology, physiology, pathology and pharmacology in this monograph in a masterly fashion which is easy to read and will be of major value for the students and scholars working in the field of platelets.

This monograph is comprised of 16 chapters which are dexterously prepared with beautiful illustrations wherever applicable. The first chapter provides a very clear account of platelet morphology with specific reference to different structural components. The discussion on the structure is so well written that it can be understood by those with minimal background in hematology. The second chapter, dealing with platelet morphology and function, contains beautiful illustrations and a description of various techniques used to characterize functional morphology of platelets. Complimentary to this, the 3rd chapter interfaces platelet morphology with functional alterations in various diseases highlighting the structural components involved in some of these disorders. From an evolutionary stand point platelet dysfunction in animals is referenced to highlight some points. The 4th chapter deals with platelet physiology including the progressive changes in platelet regulatory actions. Once again the emphasis is on functional changes and the impact of structural alterations is highlighted. The 5th chapter deals with biochemical pathways involved in the platelet activation mechanism. For students working in signal transduction and other areas this will be important reading. Chapter 6 illustrates the role of calcium in platelet activation. Special emphasis is placed on modulation of ionized calcium by agonists and antagonists. The platelet activation and deactivation mechanisms are illustrated. Chapter 7 deals with the role of prostaglandins in platelet function whereas Chapter 8 discusses the calcium modulation by cyclic nucleotides.

The author has great expertise in the modulation of platelets by drugs and has masterfully described the pharmacology of antiplatelet drugs in Chapter 9. The mechanism of action of these drugs and their potential impact on treatment of diseases is also illustrated. Complimentary to this, Chapter 10 provides a comprehensive account of antiplatelet drugs in clinical trials. Of note, the work of the scientists at the University of Minnesota to develop point of care instrumentation to measure platelet response to antiplatelet drugs is highlighted. Once again stating the impact of physician/scientist collaboration at the University of Minnesota. Platelets have complex physiological processes and drug resistance is a major problem. Chapter 11 deals with aspirin resistance, a subject in which the author is an expert, and provides valuable guidelines to deal with this complication. Diabetes mellitus is associated with major platelet dysfunctions and this is beautifully illustrated in Chapter 12 in terms of the role of platelets in diabetes.

Professor Rao has a strong interest in acute coronary syndrome and is a great scholar of the pathophysiology and the pharmacologic management of this syndrome. In a very concise and masterful fashion, he has compiled Chapter 13 on platelet hyper-function as a risk factor for acute coronary events. In addition, the contribution of platelet activation of circulating blood cells and activation leading to vascular dysfunction is detailed. To address the monitoring of acute coronary events, the need for a point of care assay for monitoring antiplatelet and antithrombotic therapies is also discussed. Professor Rao rightly pointed to the fact that South Asians have a very high incidence of coronary artery disease suggesting the genetic components involved in this process. The membrane modulation concept was coined at the University of Minnesota where epinephrine mediated events were implicated. This led to the understanding of the initial mechanisms involved in the activation of platelets in health and disease. The role of alpha-adrenergic receptor antagonists and beta blockers in the modulation of this process was proposed. Chapter 15 discusses the platelet vessel wall interaction which plays an important role in the progression of hemostatic plug and atherosclerotic plaque. The interplay between endothelial cells and platelets is illustrated. To investigate these interactions experimental approaches using the annular chamber profusion system are described. This chapter also contains some beautiful illustrations on the interactions of platelets and endothelial cells. Platelet reaction time (PRT) monitoring device to monitor sheer force mediated platelet activation and clot formation was also highlighted. The final chapter is dedicated to the discussion of blood biocompatibility studies with a focused reference to the contributions of the blood biocompatibility laboratory (BBL) at the medical school of the University of Minnesota. In this chapter, integrated approaches involving various groups including the faculty at the Lillehei Heart Institute are highlighted. This provided a strong academia-industry platform and the BBL offered the opportunity for medical device companies to work together to advance stroke research and other various scientific approaches to understand blood compatibility with surfaces, in particular the role of platelets in blood biomaterial interactions. Platelet physiology and function utilizing simple instruments as a Chandler loop coupled with electron-microscopic illustration of cellular activation validated blood biomaterial interactions. Other techniques dealing with blood cells under flow conditions, exposure of blood cells to fully assembled heart walls, and platelet adhesion to biomaterials were detailed. As the field of nano-microparticles emerged, this group also worked on cardiovascular drug delivery and targeting processes.

It can be easily seen that the evolution of platelet function with reference to morphometric alterations laid the foundation for a most comprehensive, multidisciplinary research approach including nearly all basic sciences. This would not have been possible without the intimate mentor trainee relationship which was initiated by Professor Jim White over 50 years ago. Dr Rao's recognition of Professor White's unparalleled drive and leadership resulted in a very productive group which continued to advance in the field of vascular medicine, the diagnosis of bleeding and thrombotic disorders related to platelets. Platelets are now considered to be an integral component of the vascular system. There is so much more to be learned. Advances in cellular and molecular biology have transformed platelet biology and have led us to recognize these cells in health and disease. This would not have been possible without the great vision of Professor White and his ability to recruit outstanding trainees, transforming them to lead physicians and scientists who will continue to impact this area for years to come. Professor Rao worked under Professor White and, like his mentor, has trained many younger scientists in the most integrated fashion bridging basic science and clinical medicine as portrayed in this book. While this book is a true tribute to Professor White at the Lillehei Heart Institute of the University of Minnesota which will remain a pioneering institution in cardiovascular research for years to come, its publication in India has a major significance including the outstanding talents in teaching and research and the pursuit for excellence. The information has direct relevance on the public health impact, in particular, the cardiovascular disease care in South Asian countries.

Jawed Fareed PhD DSc FAHA
Professor of Pharmacology and Pathology
Loyola University School of Medicine
Maywood, Illinois, USA

Preface

Blood platelets play a very important role in the pathogenesis of atherosclerosis, thrombosis and stroke. In 1998, Kluwer Academic Publishers of Boston, USA contacted me and asked me to put together a Handbook on Platelet Physiology and Pharmacology. I recruited well-known national and international researchers, working in the area of atherosclerosis, thrombosis and stroke, to contribute articles for this book. I made a special request to all the contributors, to make an all-out effort to describe platelet morphology, biochemistry, physiology and pharmacology as it relates to function. When elite group of researchers develop a multidisciplinary project, by and large, they stick to their expertise and will not develop a cohesive, comprehensive story to summarize their collective experience. Our monograph was a collection of state-of-the-art topics, but failed to tell a story that summarizes what is known of platelets and how they work. Since then, I have discussed this issue many a times with my mentor, Prof James G White. We both were fascinated with the mechanisms involved in platelet activation and function. We discussed the topic, "How Platelet Works" many a times, in our long-working relationship. I wanted to put together a book on this subject with his help. However, I was not able to do it for various reasons, which are not worth discussing here. I came to know about his passing way, when I was vacationing in India this summer (www.startribune.com/obituaries/detail/145854/?). His obituary mentions, that he had over 700 articles to his credit. It made me feel bad, thinking about the missed opportunity for a collective description of our work, which lasted for forty years. Since the time, I received the news of his (Dr White's) deteriorating health from our close friend and associate Dr Gines Escolar from Barcelona, Spain (Currently resides in New Jersey, USA), I have been thinking nothing but to find a way to put together a monograph, that covers our four decades of work on Platelets. With these thoughts in mind, I approached our longtime friend (Mr Jitendar P Vij) at the Jaypee Brothers Medical Publishers (P) Ltd, New Delhi, India. They have published four of our books from 2001 to 2007, under the aegis of South Asian Society on Atherosclerosis and Thrombosis (SASAT). In spite of the fact that this is too specialized a subject and may attract only selected group of readers, they graciously accepted my request and agreed to publish this book. Electron photomicrographs that I have used in this book to illustrate platelet morphology and function, were gifted to me by late James G White. His long-term associate Ms Marlys Krumweide willingly prepared a set of slides for my use at various scientific conferences. I acknowledge my sincere thanks to them and dedicate this monograph to my mentor and associate, Regents Professor of Pediatrics and Pathology, James G White, MD. Many other illustrations were prepared for us for our presentations by the professional art and graphics department, at the University of Minnesota. Some of the illustrations, I have taken the liberty of borrowing from public domain (Internet). I also have taken liberty of using significant information from our previously published articles. The author assures the readers that the major part of the work presented in this book comes from the four decades of work done by Prof James G White, Prof Gundu HR Rao, and associates at the Thrombosis Research Laboratory, Lillehei Heart Institute, University of Minnesota, Minneapolis, Minnesota. In each chapter, author has provided references to published work of their own group as well as relevant references from other experts. At the end of the book, author has provided a complete bibliography of their work on platelets, for those who are interested in additional reference material to the source of information. We take this opportunity to sincerely thank all those who have contributed to our collective knowledge base.

One may wonder, why I am putting together a monograph on Blood Platelets? Recently I read a historical review on Platelets, which had over 400 references. I found only one reference to our work of 40 years and over 1000 articles collectively. This shows that either the reviewer has ignored completely our contribution to this collective knowledge or has no idea of their existence in the platelet literature. Either way, we feel that it is important to present our collective thoughts on this subject for the readers, who may be interested in looking at this topic from a different perspective. In addition to this reasoning, after reading several of these reviews, I found out, that they are like viewing a rain forest from sky. You see a canopy not individual tress. In this monograph, I will not try to catalogue all that is published on this subject. I will try to write more about how platelets work (read Platelet Story) rather than minute details, which may or may not make any sense to a beginner or for someone, who wants to get to know as to how platelet works. The monograph is compiled for the beginners, and for those who are new to this area and not for experts in this field of investigation.

Gundu HR Rao PhD

Acknowledgments

I would like to acknowledge significant contributions of Dr Jonathan Gerrard of Winnipeg, Canada, as well as Dr Gines Escolar of Barcelona, Spain, for our understanding of morphology, physiology and function of blood platelets. I have included references to the work of other researchers on this topic, so that those interested in learning more about specific pathways, mechanisms, will be able to access them. I express my sincere thanks to my father-in-law, Dr TN Ramachandra Rao, a pioneer scientist in our family, for his continued encouragement of my international activities. One of his wishes was, that I should put together a "single author" book on Platelets. I am glad that his wish is being fulfilled by the publication of this monograph. I express my sincere thanks to my wife, Dr Yashoda T Rao for her patience, cooperation and encouragement. I also would like to thank our grandson, Master Akshay R Tate, for his technical support in the preparation of this manuscript. I thank Mr Jitendar P Vij (Group Chairman), Mr Ankit Vij (Group President), Ms Chetna Malhotra Vohra (Associate Director—Content Strategy) and the team at Jaypee Brothers Medical Publishers (P) Ltd, New Delhi, India, for taking the responsibility of publishing this book for our professional society, South Asian Society on Atherosclerosis and Thrombosis (SASAT), Division of Clinical and Preventive Cardiology, Medanta Hospital, Gurugram, Haryana, India.

In a book, that is dedicated to the memory of my mentor and associate, (Late) Prof James G White, I would be failing in my duty and responsibilities, if I do not mention the names of the other four mentors who shaped my professional career. First and the foremost, my PhD thesis adviser, (Late) Donald A Wilbur, Professor, Department of Entomology, Kansas State University, Manhattan, Kansas, Dr (Late) Neville Crawford, Professor and Head, Department of Biochemistry, Royal College of Surgeons, Lincoln Inn Fields, London, Dr (Late) Sir Vijay V Kakkar, Founder-Director, Thrombosis Research Institute, Emeritus Professor of Surgery, King's College, Denmark Hill Road, London and Dr (Late) MG Doni, Professor, Instituto di Fisiologia Umana (Institute of Human Physiology), University of Padova, Padova, Italy.

Contents

Four Decades of Global Collaborative Studies

Principal collaborator for these studies was Late James G White, mentor, and associate for over four decades. I will not be able to list all the collaborators by name. Hence, I humbly request all those who worked with us, if they do not see their names mentioned under this chapter, to excuse me. I do thank each and every one of them, for their valuable contributions. Dr Jonathan M Gerrard, a Canadian clinician joined us in the early 70s as a research fellow to do his PhD. He introduced us to eicosanoids. Prof John W Eaton, a molecular anthropologist in our department, introduced us to the free radical chemistry and their role in oxidation-reduction mechanisms. Dr Douglas Peterson, who was a freelance researcher worked with us for a short period and made significant contribution to our understanding of arachidonic acid-heme interactions as well as the role of epinephrine modulation of some of the steps in (Peterson DA, et al. Science. 1982;215:71-73) agonist-mediated signal transduction events. Dr Maurie J Stuart, a Professor from Children's Hospital, Thomas Jefferson University, Philadelphia, joined us a research fellow and worked with Dr Gerrard and our research group. For the first time, she demonstrated in a drug induced animal model, that the balance between prostaglandins from platelets and vessel wall is altered in hyperglycemic animals. Furthermore, she showed that islet cell transplantation in these animals restored the prostaglandin synthesis to normal levels. Chadwick A Cox, a Biochemist from Oklahoma University Health Center, Oklahoma, joined us as an honorary faculty and worked on topics related to platelet cytoskeletal rearrangements and phosphorylation of proteins associated with activation and inactivation processes (Cox AC, et al. J Cell Biol. 1984;98:8-15). Dr Douglas Weiss, a Professor in the Veterinary College, University of Minnesota, Minnesota and Gerhard J Johnson, an Adjunct faculty, Department of Medicine, University of Minnesota, Minnesota and a staff at the Veterans Administration Hospitals, collaborated with us on studies, which used various animal models.

In the areas of clinical studies, (Late) Prof Carl J Witkop, a pioneer and expert in studies on Albinism associated disorders, shared with us an National Institutes of Health (NIH) program project research grant on this topic and helped us work on patients with Albinism (Hermansky-Pudlak syndrome) from all over the world. We also shared an NIH program project with Prof Mark Nesbit, a pediatric oncologist, on bone marrow transplantation. In the cardiovascular research area, we shared an NIH program project with Prof Robert Vernier. In the basic sciences field, we shared an NIH program project grant with Prof Ellis Benson and Prof Andreas Rosenberg on Hemoglobinopathies. We collaborated extensively with Cardiology group (Prof Stanley Einzig, Prof Carl White, Prof Robert Wilson, Prof Gladwin Das). Professor James G White and I shared NIH research grants for well over three decades (36 years) including an NIH-Merritt Award for 10 years in the 80s.

International Collaboration was a very important part of our activities. Dr Rao obtained a National Science Foundation (NSF) travel grant to visit India, in the 80s to establish bilateral research projects between the USA and India. Prof John W Eaton and Dr Rao visited India in the 80s. They visited major Medical Institutions from Kashmir in the North, to Thiruvananthapuram in the South. They gave lectures on various topics at each of this Medical Institution. Institutions visited included, Kashmir Medical College, Srinagar; Postgraduate Medical Institute, Chandigarh; All India Institute of Medical Sciences, New Delhi, National Malaria Institute, New Delhi; Postgraduate Medical Institute, Lucknow; Indian Institute of Science, Bengaluru; Postgraduate Medical Institute, Chennai; and Christian Medical College, Vellore. Dr Rao was a visiting Professor in the Department of Surgery (Prof Sir Vijay J Kakkar) and Pharmacology, King's College, Denmark Hills, London, in 1986 and in the Biochemistry Department (Prof Neville Crawford) in the Royal College of Surgeons, London, in the summer of 1987, and in the Thrombosis Research Institute (Prof VJ Kakkar), London in 1989. He taught one summer at the Institute of Human Physiology (Prof Maria Gabriella Doni), University of Padova, Padova, Italy. The Government of India, invited Dr Rao as a Senior Consultant in the year 1990, under a United Nations (UN) program called, TOKTEN (Transfer of Knowledge by Expatriate Nationals). Dr Khalilullah, Professor of Cardiology and Director of GB Pant Hospital, New Delhi, India, sponsored the application for this fellowship. Dr Rao spent 6 weeks in India visiting major Medical Institutions. Dr Rao visited India again in 1991 and 1992 under the same UN program.

With the seed money (USD 10,000) obtained from the International Society on Thrombosis and Hemostasis (ISTH), USA. Dr Rao started a professional society, South Asian Society on Atherosclerosis and Thrombosis (SASAT) in Minnesota in1993. Under the aegis of SASAT, he organized 15 international conferences on the topics of Atherosclerosis and Thrombosis in India. Dr. Rao served as senior adviser to the Presidents of North American Thrombosis Forum (Prof. Samuel Goldhaber, Harvard University: www.natfonline.org), International Union of Angiology (IUA), France.

Platelet Story

I joined Late Professor James G White's group as an assistant scientist to establish an analytical laboratory, to conduct biochemical and functional studies, to follow his ultra-structural studies as well as to support his earlier findings with evidence-based biochemical investigations. Being new to this area, I was wondering as to how I can contribute anything more to his massive cumulative knowledge of the subject. I started off by setting up new analytical methods, to monitor various biochemical components of platelets (serotonin, adenine nucleotides, prostaglandins, cytosolic calcium), which were known to play a critical role in platelet physiology and function. Just at the beginning of my career in this department, Jonathan Gerrard a Canadian doctor joined our group to do his PhD (He is currently a Member of the Parliament in Manitoba). He spent over five years with us and was great moving force behind research into the emerging field of prostanoids.

Just at this time, we discovered that some specific fluorescent molecules (Quin-2 and Fura-2) could be used to monitor cytosolic free calcium. Using these techniques, we were for the first time, able to demonstrate the role of agonists in calcium mobilization from internal storage sites. We were able to demonstrate at the same time, that the antagonists were capable of lowering the elevated cytosolic calcium by activating adenylyl/guanylyl-cyclases and generating second messengers, cAMP and cGMP. These studies formed the basis for our simple platelet story. By this time, a young investigator from Barcelona, Spain, Dr Gines Escolar (Senior Consultant, Hemostasis Coagulation/Hemotherapy Hospital Clinic, Department of Hemotherapy and Hemostasis) joined us. He introduced us to, some newer techniques, to follow the platelet interactions with the vessel wall. Collective information that we gathered in these years formed the basis for the "Platelet Story". During the four decades, that I spent at the University of Minnesota, we also were able to discover a unique phenomenon of "Membrane Modulation", which is described in detail, in a later chapter in this book.

Investigations in our laboratory at the University of Minnesota established the existence of a novel mechanism capable of securing irreversible platelet aggregation independent of ADP secretion, prostaglandin synthesis or the generation of platelet activating factor (PAF). The new mechanism, termed membrane modulation, is associated with the platelet surface, mediated through alpha-adrenergic receptors and stimulated by exposure to epinephrine. Platelets rendered refractory to a variety of aggregating agents can be restored to a normal state of sensitivity through activation of the mechanism of membrane modulation. This included platelets treated with aspirin in vivo or in vitro. In view of the fact, that our studies demonstrated that the mechanism of platelet membrane modulation was dependent upon alpha-adrenergic receptor function, we explored the significance and nature of this dependency. Since these mechanisms seems to be critical for the restoration of the sensitivity of refractory platelets to the action of a variety of agonists, any impairment of alpha adrenergic receptor function will therefore, interfere with the mechanism of membrane modulation.

Major contributions of the Platelet Research Laboratory, Laboratory Medicine and Pathology and the Thrombosis Research Laboratory, Lillehei Heart Institute, Academic Health Center, the University of Minnesota, include; superb Electron Microscopical Studies on Platelet Ultrastructure and function of normal human platelets, platelets of patients with various hematological disorders, and platelets of various animals. In view of the fact that these were not only state-of-the-art investigations at the cellular and subcellular level, but also one-of-a-kind studies, the National Institutes of Health, USA graciously funded these studies, for well over three decades. As a part of the original investigations at the Thrombosis Research Laboratory, we did a variety of biochemical studies to explore and complement the ultrastructural findings of Prof James G White.

Our association with Prof Gines Escolar and Dr Thomas Chandy introduced us to studies on blood-vessel interaction as well as blood-biomaterial interactions. Blood compatibility studies, were supported by the Departments of Chemical Engineering (Center for Interface Engineering), and the Biomedical Research Institute, Academic Health Center, the University of Minnesota. We were able to establish a state-of-the-art device/biomaterial testing facility and serve the Institute of Engineering Medicine, University of Minnesota as well as many device material manufacturing companies in the USA. One of my close associate (Dr Daniel Ericson), who joined us as an industrial fellow from 3M company, in the late 70s, established his own research laboratory (SUBc, Inc) at Rochester, Minnesota and developed two NIH (STTR) research grants for medical device development. IBM Rochester served as a contractor for the development of this device. I was the Principal Investigator for both of these device development research proposals. Multidisciplinary experience gained at the University of Minnesota, helped me initiate collaborative programs in India in several institutions. Since our research on platelets spanned over four decades, I have included a comprehensive bibliography of our collective work for readers who want to supplement their knowledge on this subject as a separate section at the end of this book.

Introduction

As I mentioned in the preface to this monograph, Professor (Late) James G White has published over 700 articles related to platelet ultrastructure, biology, physiology, pathology and function. The last time I met him in his office, I asked him, if he is interested or planning to publish a book on this subject. He said he was not planning to publish any books on this subject. I asked him, if he had digitized and archived all his precious Electron Photomicrographs (EM). His reply was negative. I requested him (June 30th 2015) to spare me a copy of one of his historical presentations titled, "Platelet Pathology inside and out", so that I could use this information in my presentations and reviews. He generously obliged me a copy his Power Point Presentation (PPP) on the topic. I have used many illustrations from that PPP. When I wrote to the publishers my desire to publish this book, I explained to them, that passing away of Dr James G White was a great loss. All of the knowledge that he had acquired on this subject is in a way lost, unless someone can read all his 700 articles and publish a dedicated monograph. Since they agreed to publish our work as a dedicated monograph, I will try to include a small collection of his electron micrographs to illustrate our collective findings and our understanding of how platelet works. Those who have not paid attention to our collective contribution to this field may not pay any attention to this work and may not agree with our findings. However, we strongly feel, that it is important to understand that Dr White and I worked together on this topic as outsiders, trying to understand the complexities of platelet stimulus activation-contraction-secretion coupling. Every time I gave a series of lectures on this topic in Padova, Italy or in New Delhi, India, people have asked me, as to where they can find this information? I could not give any single published reference or review on this subject, which explained the activation mechanisms, as we understood it worked. At the invitation of Prof Maria Gabriella Doni of Institute of Human Physiology, University of Padova, Italy, in the late 80s, I gave a series of lectures to undergraduate students on this topic for 12 weeks. I also gave a similar series of lectures on this topic to the Clinical Chemistry faculty at the GB Pant Hospital, New Delhi, India in 1991. Following this workshop, Dr DK Srivastava (Head, Division of Clinical Chemistry, GB Pant Hospital) and I organized the First International Conference on "Platelets" at the GB Pant Hospital, New Delhi, India. In this monograph, I have tried to put together our collective findings, the way I have been presenting it in my presentations worldwide.

Historical Perspective on the Discovery of Platelets

According to Brewer (Br J Hematol, 2006), Max Shultze published the first accurate description of platelets as a part of a study devoted to the white cells in 1865. In 1865 Bizzozero a Professor at Turin University, Italy, made further comprehensive observations on platelets. He observed them microscopically in the circulating blood of living animals, and in the blood removed from the blood vessels. In well thought out studies, he demonstrated that they were the first components of the blood to adhere to damaged blood vessels in vivo and in vitro. He also demonstrated that they were the first components of the blood to adhere, to the filaments that subsequently became covered with fibrin.[1] de Gaetano writing about the first centennial of Giulio Bizzozero's death recollects, how this great researcher discovered 100 years ago and described blood platelet function in flowing conditions and the relationship between platelet adhesion to an artificial surface, aggregation and subsequent fibrin formation.[2] Steinhubl in his historical article on the discovery of platelets writes, "An understanding of the historical paths that have led to our current state of knowledge in the field of platelet studies can be both illuminating and inspiring. Considering that the existence and function of platelets were initially described barely over 100 years ago". He further states, that it is exciting to recognize how far our knowledge has advanced in such a short period of time.[3-7] Knowledge about Platelet biology, platelet function testing and antiplatelet therapies, have contributed significantly to our understanding of the pathogenesis of atherosclerosis, thrombosis, stroke and the effective management of atherothrombotic events.[7-27] Other than the earlier writings, which are really historical on this topic,[1-7] several recent articles also have described historical perspectives about various findings on platelet physiology, pathology, pharmacology and function.[27-58] Inhis relatively recent overview, Professor Coller from Rockefeller University, New York separates the eras of platelet research into the "Descriptive Period" extending from 1880–1960 and the "Mechanistic Period", encompassing the past 50 years since 1960. In view of the excellent contributions made by researchers in the last 50 years for our understanding of how platelet works, Professor Coller describes this era as Golden Age of Platelet Research.[58] I am very fortunate that I was able to work with a mentor like Professor James G White, in this Golden Age of Platelet Research, for four of the five decades. What we describe here in this book will be the "Platelet Story" of this Golden Age, when much of the discoveries were made. In most of the historical articles, reviews, books, authors have described either about their own contribution, their group's contributions or collective history of discovery on a topic of interest.[43-54] Continuing in the same line of thinking, in this book, which is dedicated to the Life and Works of Professor James White of Minnesota, work collectively done on this topic by various contributors, have been described. Having said that, I assure the readers, that it is only a small portion of the subject discussed and no attempt has been made, to present only the work that was done in Minnesota on the subject of Platelets.

REFERENCES

1. Brewer DB, Max Shultze, G Bizzozero and the discovery of the platelet. Br J Hematol. 2006;1865;1882;133(3):251-6.
2. Osler W. On certain problems in the physiology of blood corpuscles. The Medical News. 1886;48:421-5.
3. de Gaetano G, Cerietti C. Platelet adhesion and aggregation and fibrin formation in flowing blood: a historical contribution by Giulio Bizzozero. 2002.
4. Steinhubl SR. Historical observations on the discovery of platelets, platelet function testing and the first antiplatelet agent. Curr Drug Targets. 2011;12(12):1792-804.
5. Wright JH. The origin and nature of platelets. Boston Med Surg J. 1906;154:643-5.
6. Mac Kay W. The blood platelet: its clinical significance. Quart J Med. 1930;24:285-93.
7. Tocantins LM. The origin and nature of blood platelets. Blood. 1948;3:1073-82.

8. Marcus AJ, Zucker MB. The physiology of blood platelets. New York: Grune and Stratton, Inc. 1965.
9. Kowalski E, Niewiarowski S. Biochemistry of blood platelets. New York, Academic Press, 1966.
10. Robb-Smith AH. Why the platelets were discovered. Br J Hematol. 1967;13:618-37.
11. Caen J. Platelet Aggregation. Paris: Masson and Cie, 1971.
12. Brinkhous KM, Sherman RW, Mostof FK. The Platelet. Williams and Wilkinson Co. 1971.
13. Johnson SA. The circulating platelets. New York: Academic Press, 1971.
14. Weiss HJ. Platelets and their role in hemostasis. Ann Rev New York Acad Sci. 1972;201: 1-450.
15. Ciba Foundation. Biochemistry and Pharmacology of platelets. New York: Elsevier, 1975.
16. Caen JP, Chronberg S, Kubisz P. Platelet physiology and pathology. New York: Stratton International Medical Book Co. 1975.
17. de Gaetano G, Grattini S. Platelets: a multidisciplinary approach. New York Raven Press, 1877.
18. Kwan HC, Bowie EJW. Thrombosis. Philadelphia. WB Sanders, 1982.
19. Phillips DR, Shuman MA. Biochemistry of Platelets. New York Academic Press, 1986.
20. Colman RW, Hirsh J, Marders VJ, Salzman EW. Hemostasis and thrombosis: basic principles and clinical practice. Philadelphia: JB Lippincott Co. 1987.
21. Bloom AJ, Thomas DP. Haemostasis and Thrombosis. London: Churchill Livingstone, 1987.
22. Margurie G, Zwaal RFA. Biochemistry and Pathophysiology of platelet membrane. London: John Libbey, 1988.
23. Corriveau DM, Fristma GA. Hemostasis and thrombosis in the clinical laboratory. Philadelphia: JB Lippincott Co. 1988.
24. Mehta JL, Conti RC. Thrombosis and platelets in myocardial ischemia. Philadelphia. FA Davis Company, 1987.
25. Authi KS, Watson SP, Kakkar VV. Mechanisms of platelet activation. New York: Academic Press, 1993.
26. Gundu HR Rao. Handbook of Platelet Physiology and Pharmacology. Boston: Kluwer Academic Publishers, 1999.
27. Michelson AD. Platelets. Burlington, MA: Academic Press, 2007.
28. de Gaetano G. Historical overview of the role of platelets in hemostasis and thrombosis. Haematologica. 2001;86:349-56.
29. Federici AB, Bentrop E, Lee CA. The 80th anniversary of von Willebrand disease: history, management and research. Hemophilia. 2006;12:563-72.
30. Berbard J. History of congenital hemorrhagic thrombocytopathic dystrophy Blood Cells. 1983;9:179.
31. Hovig T. The early discoveries of collagen-platelet interactions and studies son its role in hemostatic plug formation. J Thromb Haemost. 2005;3:1-6.
32. Jackson CW. Megakaryocyte endomitosis: a review. Int J Cell Cloning. 1990;8:224-6.
33. Hellem A, Borchgrevink CF, Ames SB. The role of red cells in haemostasis: the relation between hematocrit, bleeding time and platelet adhesiveness. Br J Hematol. 1961;7:42-50.
34. Gaarder A, Johnson J, Laland S, et al. Adenosine diphosphate in red cells as a factor in the adhesiveness of human blood platelets. Nature. 1961;192:531-2.
35. White JG, Clawson CC. Overview article: biostructure of blood platelets Ultrastructural Pathology. 1980;1:533-58.
36. Niewiarowski S. Proteins secreted by the platelet. Thromb Haemost. 1977;38:924-38.
37. Born GV. Aggregation of blood platelets by adenosine diphosphate and its reversal Nature. 1962;194:927-9.
38. O'Brien. Platelet Aggregation 11. Some results from a new method of study. J Clin Pathol. 1962;15:452-81.
39. Sakariassen KS, Turitto VT, Baumgartner HR. Recollections of the flow devices for studying mechanisms of hemostasis and thrombosis in flowing whole blood. J Thromb Haemost. 2004;2:1681-90.
40. Marcus AJ. The role of lipids in platelet function: with particular reference to the arachidonic acid pathway. J Lipid Res. 1978;19: 793-826.
41. Wagner DD, Frenette PS. The vessel wall and its interactions. Blood. 2008;111:5270-81.
42. Rink TJ. Cytosolic calcium in platelet activation. Experientia. 1988;44:97-100.

43. Nurden AT, Phillips DR, George JN. Platelet membrane glycoproteins: historical perspectives. J Thromb Haemost. 2006;4:3-9.
44. Nurden P, Nurden AT. Congenital disorders associated with platelet dysfunction. Thromb Haemost. 2008;99:253-63.
45. Hawiger J. Adhesive interactions of platelets and their blockade. Ann NY Acad Sci. 1991;614:270-8.
46. Weiss HJ. The discovery of the antiplatelet effect of aspirin: a personal reminiscence. J Thromb Haemost. 2003;1:1869-75.
47. Jack DB. One hundred years of aspirin. 1997;350:437-9.
48. Fuster V, Sweeny JM. Aspirin: a historical and contemporary therapeutic overview. Circulation. 13:768-78.
49. Zucker MB. Platelet physiology: a personal perspective. Platelets. 1990;1:3-9.
50. Coller BS. Platelet GP11.b/111a antagonists: the first anti-integrin receptor therapeutics. J Clin Invest. 1997;92:2373-80.
51. Behnke O. Electron microscopical observations on the surface coating of human blood platelets. J Ultrasound Res. 1968;24:51-69.
52. Packham MA, Rand LM. Historical perspectives on ADP-induced platelet activation. Purinergic Signal. 2011;7(3):283-92.
53. Mustard JF, Packham MA. Factors influencing platelet function, adhesion, release, and aggregation. Pharmacol Rev. 1970;22:97-187.
54. White JG. Fine structural alterations induced by adenosine diphosphate. Blood. 1968;31:604-22.
55. Born GV. Aggregation of blood platelets. J Physiol. 1963;168:178-95.
56. Macmillan DC, Sim AK. A comparative study of platelet aggregation in man and laboratory animals. Thromb Diath Haemost. 1970;24:385-9.
57. de Gaetano G. Historical overview of the role of platelets in hemostasis and thrombosis. Haematologica. 2001;86:349-56.
58. Coller BS. Historical perspectives and future direction in platelet research. J Thromb Haemost. 2011;9(10):374-95.

CHAPTER 1

Platelet Ultrastructure Morphology

Abstract that Professor James G White wrote for his NIH Grant several decades ago best summarizes the type of work that we did at the Platelet Research Laboratory at the University of Minnesota, Medical School, Minneapolis, Minnesota.

"Investigations in this laboratory will continue to be directed toward development of knowledge on blood platelet function in normal hemostasis, its role in the pathogenesis of inherited and acquired bleeding disorders, and its contribution to vascular injury, thrombosis, and atherosclerosis. Analytical, scanning, and transmission electron microscopy, freeze-fracture, cytochemistry, and immunocytochemistry combined with cyclic nucleotide, adenine nucleotide, and prostaglandin biochemistry and advanced physiological techniques, including micropipette elastometry and lumi-aggregometry, will be used to develop new information on these problems and related areas. Particular emphasis has been placed on achievement of six specific aims. New approaches to the study of membrane ultrastructure will be used to identify physical alterations in platelet membranes and membrane systems not evident previously. Giant platelets with normal function from patients with the May-Hegglin anomaly will permit study of platelet membrane deformability before and after activation and surface receptor mobility (capping and patching) for the first time. Freeze-fracture and other sophisticated technology will be used to solve basic problems presented by inherited disorders of platelet function. A new mechanism of membrane modulation regulating platelet activation and the phenomenon of disaggregation and reaggregation of irreversibly aggregated platelets was recently discovered in this laboratory. It offers excellent opportunities to gain new knowledge of platelet biochemistry and physiology. Megakaryocytes can be concentrated and purified. We will recover them from a dog model permitting in-depth study of each stage of maturation and use of the techniques of structural physiology. Accomplishment of these aims will allow us to gain the knowledge required to control or prevent hemorrhagic and thrombotic disease." http://grantome.com/grant/NIH/R01-HL011880-17.

In the early days of thrombosis research, there was strong emphasis placed on the coagulation mechanisms in hemostatic reactions. In addition, preparation of platelets for studies posed a problem, as they were considered very fragile and very reactive. It was the appreciation that platelets were as important as coagulant proteins in the hemostasis and thrombosis processes that demanded the knowledge of their physiology, pathology, and function.[1] A new era of ultrastructural investigation began in the early 1960s. Rapid developments in biochemistry and physiology had created the need for a more critical analysis of platelet fine structure and function. Cytochemical, immunochemical, and autoradiographic techniques capable of demonstrating specific chemical constituents in thin section of fixed platelets expanded the scope of ultrastructural investigations. A new concept of platelet anatomy, structural physiology and function was developed from electron microscopic investigations. By that time, I joined Dr White, he had already studied platelet ultrastructure for over a decade and published more than 200 articles on this topic.

Dr White in his "concept paper" on platelet structure, which was his HP Smith award lecture in 1978, emphasized the need to develop knowledge of basic relationships between platelet structure, biochemistry, and function in order to define the mechanisms involved in normal hemostatic activity and pathologic behavior (Figs. 1.1 to 1.5).

The specialized approach to identify these associations has been termed platelet structural physiology and pathology.[1] Platelet in circulating blood has a "disk" or plate-like shape, with smooth convex contours (Fig. 1.5). Figure 1.2A represents a schematic diagram of a cross-section of a platelet showing internal structure and contents essential for executing physiological responses. Figure 1.2B shows cross-section of a platelet as seen in the electron microscope.

Primary purpose for the existence of circulating platelets is to keep a watch on the vessel wall, identify any injury or damage to the blood vessel, interact with the cell matrix of the injured wall, adhere, spread, cover the damaged site, and form an effective hemostatic plug. In order to emphasize this role, Professor White used to use a photograph of a "one in a million" shot of a platelet, which he used to refer as "cross-eyed platelet" (Fig. 1.4). Indeed, this photo of platelet became so famous that several commercial companies wanted to use it for promotional purposes.

I remember one company distributing small replica of "cross-eyed" sticky platelets

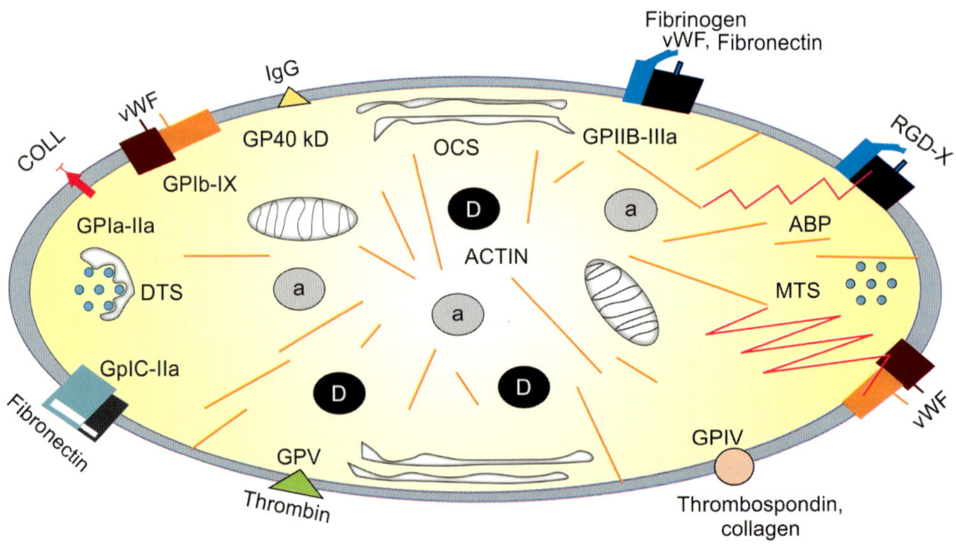

Fig. 1.1: Schematic representation of platelet ultrastructure shows platelet membrane-associated integrin (GpIIb/IIIa, GpIc/IIa), nonintegrin (GPV, vWF) glycoprotein domains, dense tubular system (DTS), open canalicular system, mitochondria, ACTIN, actin-binding protein, and microtubules. (GPV: Glycoprotein V; vWF: von Willebrand factor).

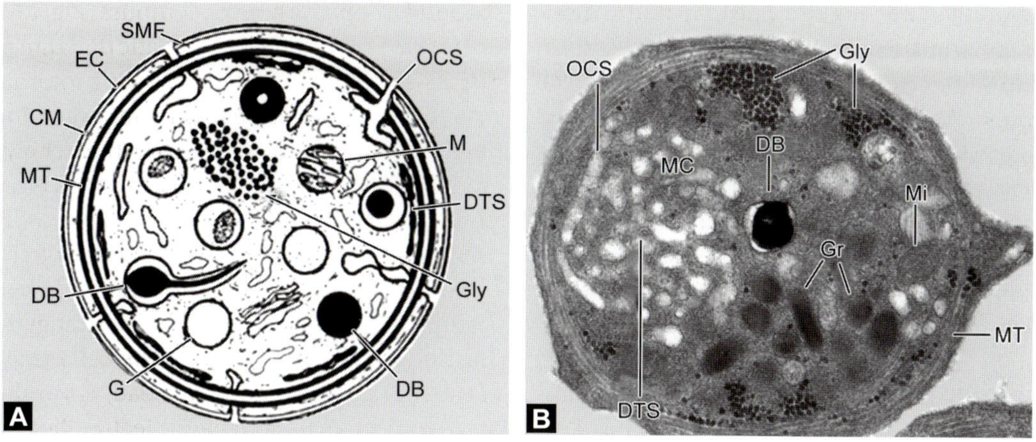

Figs. 1.2A and B: (A) Schematic representation of a platelet. (B) Cross-section of a platelet as visualized by electron microscopy. (CM: Cell membranes; DB: Dense body; DTS: Dense tubular system; EC: Exterior coat; G: Alpha granules; Gly: Glycogen; MT: Microtubules; OCS: Open canalicular system; SMF: Submembrane filaments; Mi: Mitochondria; Gr: Granules; MC: Membrane channels).

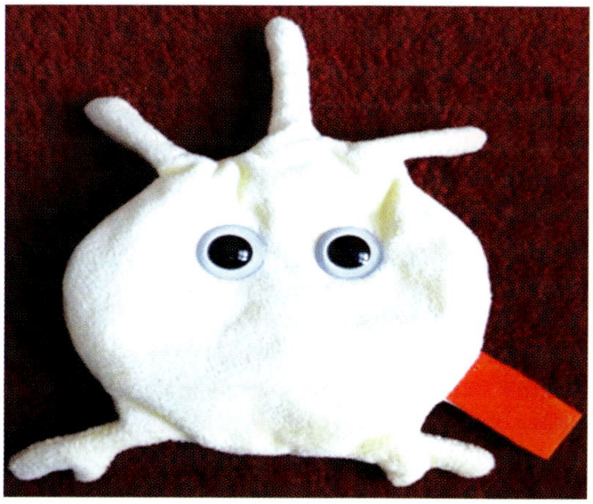

Fig. 1.3: Platelet from giant microbes.

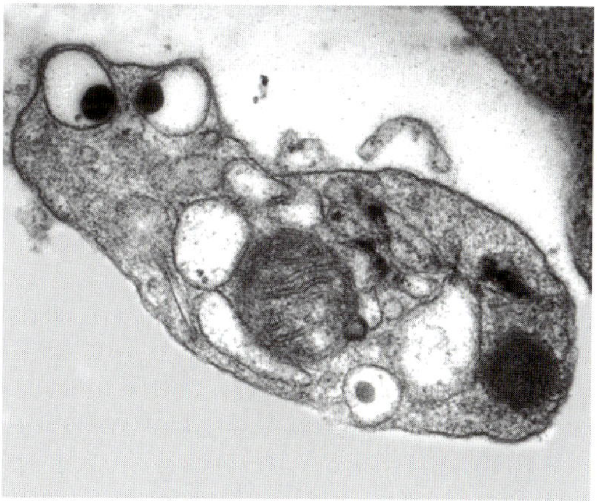

Fig. 1.4: Cross-eyed platelet.

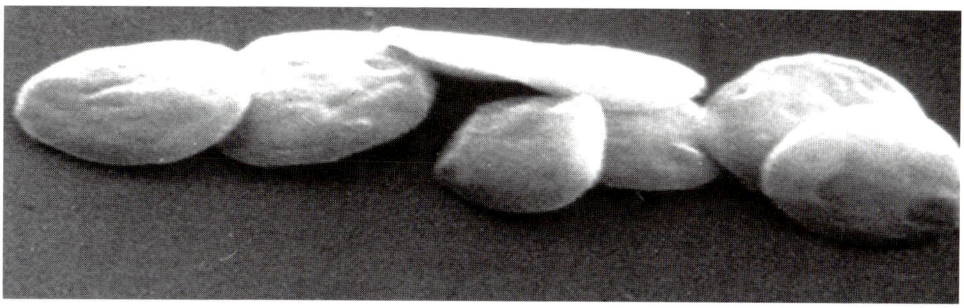

Fig. 1.5: Discoid platelets as seen by scanning electron microscopy.

made of some colored fabric to the participants at the International Society of Thrombosis and Hemostasis (ISTH) meetings. Of course, Dr White did not like the idea and requested them to stop that practice. However, the very thought of a platelet with two eyes must have encouraged or inspired Giantmicrobes, Inc. of Wilmington DE (www.giantmicrobes.com) to produce an attractive soft platelet look-alike with two eyes (Fig. 1.3).

In order to simplify the complicated structural features, internal contents, and relate them to activation mechanism, such as agonist receptor interactions, signal transduction events, biochemical and functional activities, Prof White divided the anatomy of a platelet into four major regions: *the peripheral zone, the sol-gel zone, the organelle zone,* and *the platelet membrane system.* Three basic mechanisms govern the activity of platelets in hemostasis: adhesion (aggregation), contraction, and secretion. The peripheral zone mediates all stimuli triggering the platelet response, and conversion from the nonsticky to sticky state takes place in this region.

The peripheral zone comprises the phospholipid membranes and the receptors and glycoprotein-rich domains, which play a major role in cell activation and signal transduction mechanisms. It consists of an exterior coat, or glycocalyx, rich in glycoproteins. Specific agonist receptors as well as integrin and nonintegrin domains, which are important for external stimulus coupling for platelet activation, are located at this zone. This zone is also rich in phospholipids. More than 15% of the dry weight of platelets is lipid of which 80% is phospholipid.[2,3] Major lipids include cholesterol (30.8%), phosphatidylcholine (26.3%), phosphatidylethanolamine (8.6%), phosphatidylserine (6.6%), and phosphatidylinositol (2.7%). Recent research in lipidomics revealed the existence of over 8,000 species of lipids in platelets.[4] At the time of this writing, the most prominent lipid substrates that played a major role in modulation of platelet and vessel wall functions were arachidonic acid, substrate for cyclooxygenase, thromboxane synthetase, and prostacyclin synthetase enzymes. In addition, a family of cell–cell and cell–surface receptors have been identified on platelet surface membranes.[5] The first glycoprotein receptor to be identified was the 11b-111a complex, which when activated can bind four different adhesive proteins: fibrinogen, fibronectin, von Willebrand factor (vWF), and vitronectin. All of these adhesion receptors consist of two noncovalently associated alpha subunit (GPIIb) and beta subunit (GPIIIa). This complex is one of the most abundant receptor proteins present on the platelet surface membranes (>50,000 copies). Integrin receptors are transmembrane glycoproteins with alpha and beta subunits (GPIIb-IIIa, GPIa-IIa, GPIc-IIa). In addition, there are nonintegrin (GPVI) glycoprotein domains on platelet surface membrane, capable of binding other cell matrix components such as collagen and vWF. In the activation mediated by collagen, integrin alpha-2, beta-1 (GPIIa-Ib), and nonintegrin GPVI are involved.

The sol-gel zone is the matrix of the cytoplasm. It contains fibers and filaments in various states of polymerization. This system of filamentous proteins, capable of polymerization and depolymerization supports the discoid shape in circulating platelets, and provides a contractile system for accomplishing shape change, pseudopod formation, spreading, contraction, and retraction. The contractile system constitutes 30% of the total platelet protein. Significant portion of this system is actin. Other proteins of this system include myosin, tropomyosin, actin-binding protein, alpha actinin, gelsolin, profilin, vinculin, and spectrin. In platelets, shape change, pseudopod formation, retraction, and spreading involve dissociation of existing actin structure and reformation of new ones. Thus, it is evident that these structural alterations are dynamic processes and are regulated by a large number of actin-binding proteins. In platelets, some of the proteins identified to play a role in such dynamic process are Arp2/3, cofilin, and capping protein, as well as 2E4/kaptin, gelsolin, VASP, and profilin.[6-12] Actin is a globular monomer known to assemble reversibly to form long fibers. Actin fibers, if sufficiently stiff and organized into bundles, could maintain the cell and parts of the cell in particular configurations, for instance, pseudopods of platelets. Working with myosin could generate the contractility needed for spreading, release of granule contents, and clot retraction. Actin filaments could also act as ties for parts of the cell, including its membrane. It has become increasingly clear that action of actin is influenced by enormous number of actin-binding proteins.[12-18]

The organelle zone consists of dense bodies, which are the storage sites for releasable components, such as ADP, ATP, calcium, and serotonin. Other components of this system include peroxisomes, lysosomes, mitochondria, and glycogen. This zone serves as the storage site for various enzymes, nonmetabolic adenine nucleotides, serotonin, and antioxidants such as taurine, ascorbic acid, and glutathione. On activation, platelets seem to secrete more than 300 active substances from their intracellular granules.[13] Proteomic studies have demonstrated that hundreds of bioactive proteins are released from alpha granules.[14] Though the role of these granule components was considered to play a role in thrombosis and hemostasis, recent studies have demonstrated their participation in inflammation, atherosclerosis, antimicrobial host defense, wound healing, angiogenesis, and malignancy.[14]

The membrane system plays a major role in platelet physiology, pathology, and function. The dense tubular system (DTS) has been shown to be the site where calcium, an important bioregulator, is sequestered. The DTS is also the site where enzymes involved in fatty acid metabolism and prostaglandin synthesis are localized.[15] Platelet membrane system includes not only structures similar to endoplasmic reticulum (ER), which have been described by White as dense tubular system, but also the boundary or demarcation membranes of a variety of granular organelles within the cytoplasmic matrix: mitochondria, lysosomes, alpha-granules, and dense granules.[16] Professor White has described two distinct channel systems in blood platelets.[17] The open canalicular system, with its canaliculi, which are continuous with surrounding plasma, serves as a conduit for uptake of plasma-borne substances and as a path for extrusion of endogenous chemicals secreted during the platelet-release reaction.

A series of studies by White and associates have demonstrated that canaliculi of the open canalicular system (OCS) are continuous with the surrounding plasma, particles taken up by the system can be transferred to apparently intact granules, and channels remain open before, and after physical alterations during aggregation and release of secretory products. Existence of the two distinctly different membrane systems in platelets was described first by Behnke.[19] White extended these studies to demonstrate a functional role for these membrane systems. On the basis of his extensive studies and that of other researchers working in this area, he concluded that platelets were not merely similar to muscle cells, but are muscle cells of the blood, and that contractile physiology dominated the functional activity of platelets in hemostasis.[16-18]

REFERENCES

1. White JG. Current concepts of platelet structure. Am J Clin Pathol. 1979;71:363-78.
2. Purdon D. Phospholipid metabolism in platelets. Mod Meth Pharmacol. 1987;4:229-42.
3. Marcus AJ. The role of lipids in platelet function: with particular reference to arachidonic acid pathway. J Lipid Res. 1978;19:793-826.
4. O'Donnell VB, Murphy RC, Watson SP. Platelet lipidomics: modern day perspectives on lipid discovery and characterization in platelets. Circ Res. 2014;114:1185-203.
5. Phillips DR, Charo IF, Parise LV, Fitzgerald LA. The Platelet membrane glycoprotein 11b-111a complex. Blood. 1988;71(4):831-43.
6. White JG. The submembrane filaments of blood platelets. Am J Pathol. 1969;56:267-77.
7. White JG. Arrangement of actin filaments in the cytoskeleton of human platelets Am J Pathol. 1984;117:207-17.
8. White JG, Rao GHR. Microtubule coil versus surface membrane cytoskeleton in maintenance of platelet discoid shape. Am J Pathol. 1998;152:597-609.
9. Schollmeyer JV, Rao GHR, White JG An actin-binding protein in human platelets. Interactions with alpha-actinin on gelation of actin and the influence of cytochalasin B. Am J Pathol. 1978;93(2):433-46.
10. Bearer EL, Prakash JM, Li Z. Actin dynamics in platelets. Int Rev Cytol. 2002;217:137-82.
11. Pollard TD, Cooper JA. Actin and actin-binding proteins: a critical evaluation of mechanisms and functions. Annu Rev Biochem. 1986;55:987-1035.
12. Stossel TP. Contribution of actin to the structure of the cytoplasmic matrix. J Cell Biol. 1984;99(1):S15-S21.
13. Golebiewska EM, Poole AW. Platelet secretion: from haemostasis to wound healing and beyond. Blood Rev. 2015;29(3):153-62.
14. Blair P, Flaumenhaft R. Platelet alpha-granules: basic biology and clinical correlates. Blood Rev. 2009;23(4):177-89.
15. Gerrard JM, White JG, Rao GH, Townsend D. Localization of platelet prostaglandin production in the platelet dense tubular system. Am J Pathol. 1976;83:283-98.
16. Crawford N. Structural and molecular properties of platelet membrane. In: George JN (Ed). Platelet Membrane Glycoproteins. Plenum Press: New York; 1985.
17. Cove DH, Crawford. Platelet contractile proteins: separation and characterization of the actin and myosin like components. J Mechanochem Cell Motil. 1975;3(2):123-33.
18. White JG. Interaction of membrane systems in blood platelets. Am J Pathol. 1972;66(2):295-312.
19. Behnke O. Electron microscope observations on the membrane systems of the rat blood platelet. Anat Rec. 1967;158:121-37.

CHAPTER 2

Platelet Morphology and Function

INTRODUCTION TO PLATELETS

Platelets circulate in the blood in discoid- or plate-like shape (Fig. 2.1). This shape seems to keep them at the vicinity of the vessel wall, so that they can find the damaged or injured site on the vessel, interact with the exposed extracellular matrix (ECM) components, adhere, change shape, spread, and form an effective hemostatic plug.

The ECM is the noncellular component present within the tissues and organs, providing not only scaffolding for cellular constituents, but also initiates biochemical receptor-mediated activation signaling events essential for eliciting functional response. For instance, the cell adhesion, which is critical for hemostasis, thrombosis, and wound healing events, is mediated by ECM receptors, such as integrins and nonintegrin domains. The main fibrous ECM components include collagens, elastins, fibronectins, and laminins. Proteoglycans [glycosaminoglycan (GAG)] fill the bulk of the space within the tissues in the form of a hydrated gel. GAGs are highly negatively charged structures. Collagen is the most abundant fibrous protein within the interstitial ECM and accounts for more than 30% of the total protein mass. It is associated with elastin to achieve recoil to the tissues that exist as repeated stretches. Another abundant ECM protein is fibronectin, which has a crucial role in mediating cell attachment and spreading.[1-3]

Degree of activation of platelet depends on stimulus and the information on the surface of interaction. For instance, with minimal stimuli, they become sticky, change shape, and extend pseudopods to feel the surface (Fig. 2.2). At this phase, it still is in reversible

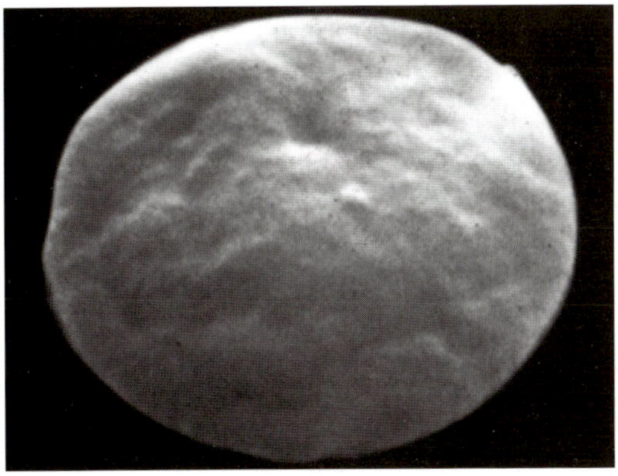

Fig. 2.1: Discoid platelet.

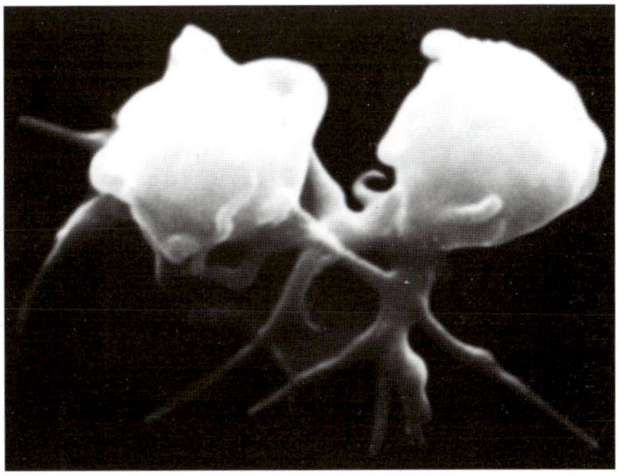

Fig. 2.2: Platelets feeling the surface.

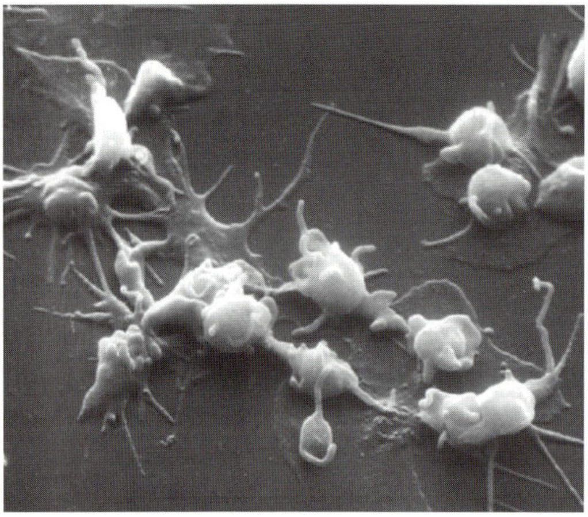

Fig. 2.3: Platelets undergoing activation on surface.

phase of activation. If the stimulus is not strong enough, they can withdraw the pseudopods and go back to the resting state. The nature of stimuli and the information on the surface on which they are adhering drive the progress and extent of platelet activation (Figs. 2.2 and 2.3). Integrin and nonintegrin receptors have recognition sites that will interact with the repeating sequence of amino acids of importance on the extracellular matrix proteins. For instance, types I and IV collagens support the adhesion of platelets but will not elicit aggregation and secretion. Only triple helical type III collagen is capable of eliciting full-activation sequences leading to aggregation and secretion of granule contents.

Platelet responses can be divided into two categories: first, the reversible responses, including shape change, development of stickiness, adhesion, aggregation; and second, spreading, contraction, and release of granule contents. Most stimuli including shear pressure cause a change in shape of platelets. Discoid cells, when stimulated, extend pseudopodia or filopodia from their peripheral zone. The fine pseudopodia, formed upon stimulation, consists mainly of bundles of actin filaments complexed with actin-binding proteins. These extensions of the peripheral zone are the feelers of the surface for information related to site of interaction. As shown in Figure 2.4, the information containing on the interactive site dictates the type of changes that follow such activation. For instance, laminin elicits just a tethering of platelets on the surface. Laminin is a large mosaic protein (900 kDa) composed of many distinct domains.[4] It is associated with type IV collagen, entactin, fibronectin, and perelecan. Some of the biological functions of laminin similar to other ECMs are associated with peptide sequences. For example, the peptide

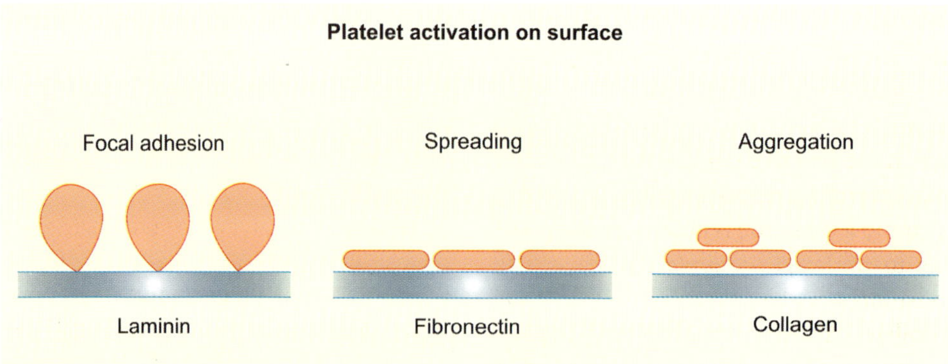

Fig. 2.4: Schematic representation of platelets spreading on surfaces.

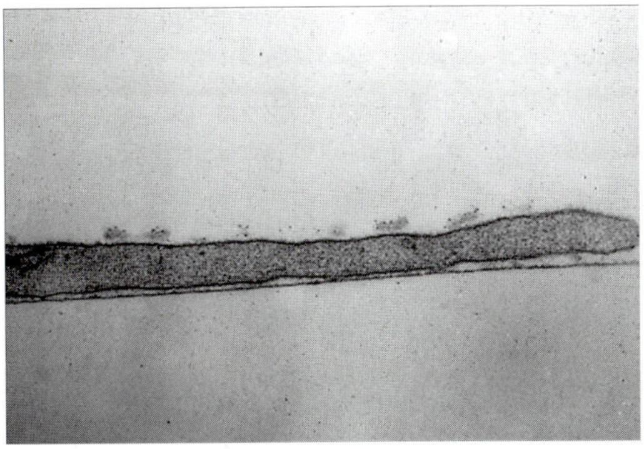

Fig. 2.5: Spreading on surface.

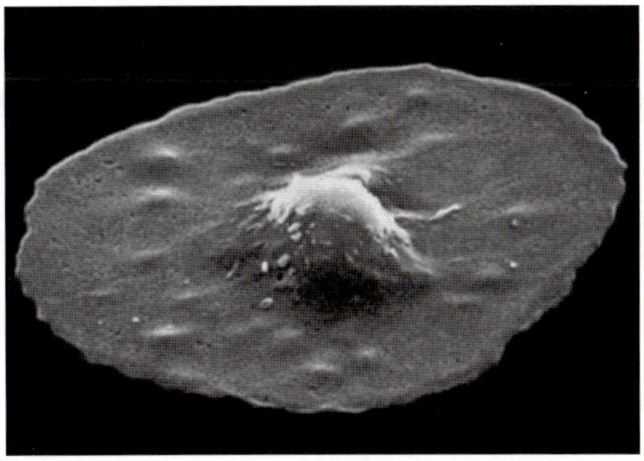

Fig. 2.6: Fully spread platelet.

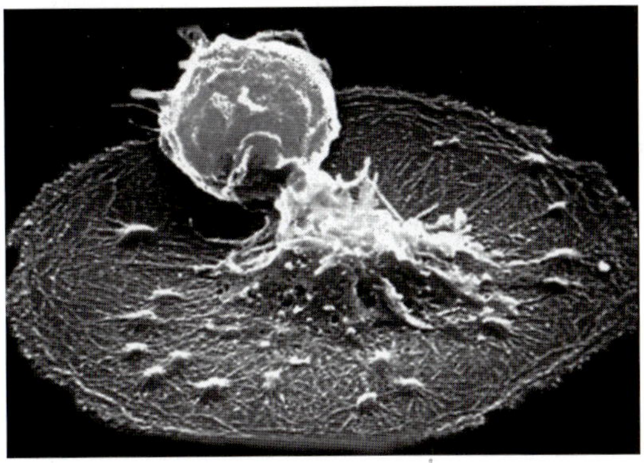

Fig. 2.7: Platelet cytoskeleton.

sequence (GTFALRGDNGDNGQ) located on α chain of laminin promotes adhesion of cells. The peptide sequence RGD seems to be common in most of the adhesive molecules (laminin, fibrinogen, fibronectin). Having said that, it is not clear as to what sequences dictate, simple tethering, adhesion, shape change, spreading, and aggregate formation.

Fibronectin (FN) elicits spreading on the surface. If the reactive surface is rich in FN, it elicits a spreading response (Figs. 2.5 to 2.7). This is quite a dynamic reaction, as the platelet has to undergo dynamic changes in its composition and cytoskeleton. The cell has to mobilize calcium, assemble filamentous actin, interact with a variety of actin-binding proteins, and spread the membrane over the injured surface rich in fibronectin. Fibronectin is involved in many cellular processes, including tissue repair, embryogenesis, blood clotting, and cell migration. It sometimes serves as general cell adhesion molecule by anchoring to collagen or proteoglycans.[1]

Proteoglycans are composed of GAG chains covalently linked to a specific protein core and are classified according to their core proteins: small leucine-rich proteoglycans, modular proteoglycans, and cell-surface proteoglycans. These are extremely hydrophilic and adopt highly extended conformations that are necessary for hydrogel formation that enables these molecules to withstand high compressive forces. FN can be a ligand for dozen members of the integrin receptor family. Large number of different integrins bind to fibronectin, including $\alpha_5\beta_1$ receptor. Studies have demonstrated the regions involved in cell adhesion along the lengthy FN molecule to several minimal integrin recognition sites, best known seems to be RGD sequences that are the binding sites in fibrinogen as well.

Collagen, on the other hand, elicits platelet response depending on its configuration. Types I and IV collagen support a monolayer of platelets. Single polypeptide chain consists of repeats of glycine, proline, and hydroxyproline molecules. The collagen (type III) triple

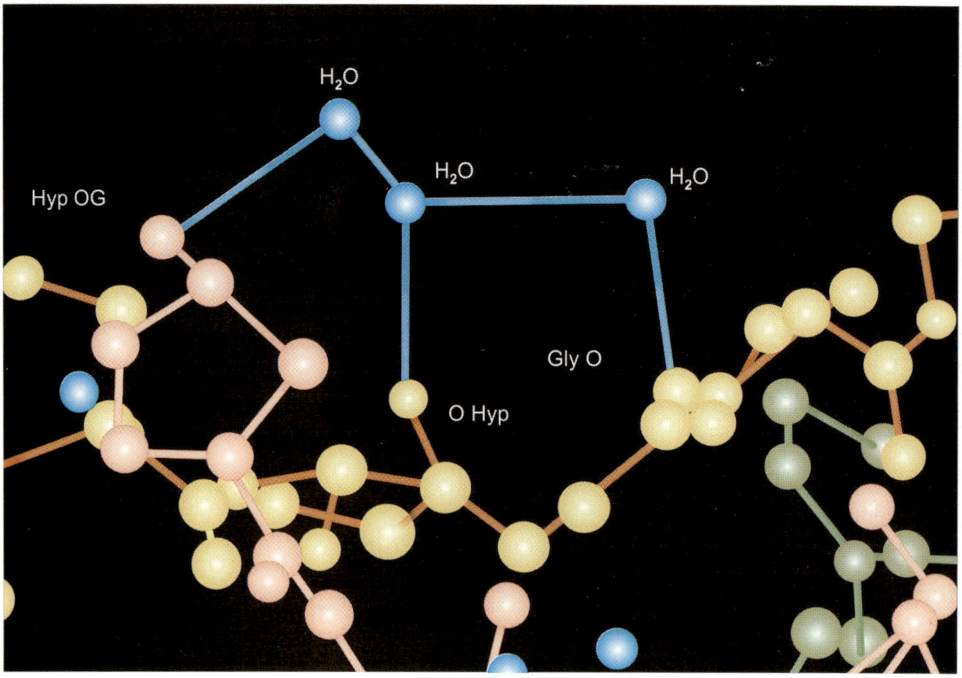

Fig. 2.8: Structure of type-III collagen.
Source: Brodsky and Shah FASEB J. 1995;15:1537-46.

helix is stabilized by an interchain hydrogen-bonding network, involving the hydroxyl group of hydroxyproline, the glycine carbonyl group, and water molecules (Fig. 2.8).

More than 19 different collagen types have been recognized. They are divided into fibril-forming and nonfibril-forming collagens. Nine different types have been reported from the vessel wall tissues: types, I, III-VI, VIII and XII through XIV.[5] Monomeric and fibrillar collagens support platelet adhesion, whereas for eliciting aggregation and secretion, the native triple-helical structure is required. Rao et al. demonstrated that a synthetic triple-helical, "mini-collagen," which had a known adhesion site; "α_1 (IV) 1263-1277" could elicit platelet adhesion, aggregation response.[6] Rao et al. used ACAS 570 interactive laser cytometer to show platelet–collagen interaction on the vessel wall as well as on surfaces.

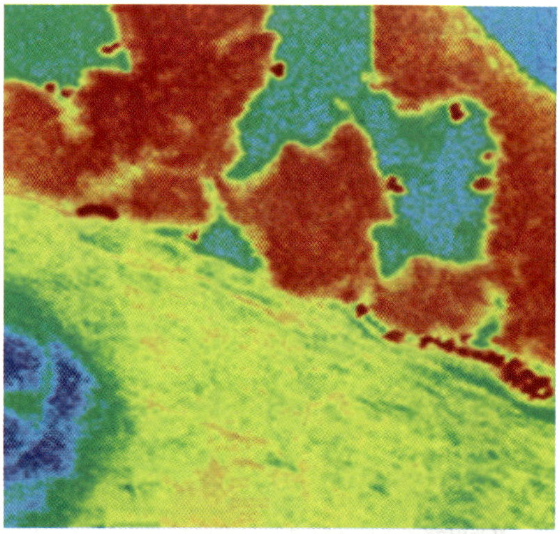

Fig. 2.9: Platelet thrombus.

Figures 2.9 and 2.10 show platelet interaction with type III collagen on denuded subendothelium, as well as on surface-coated

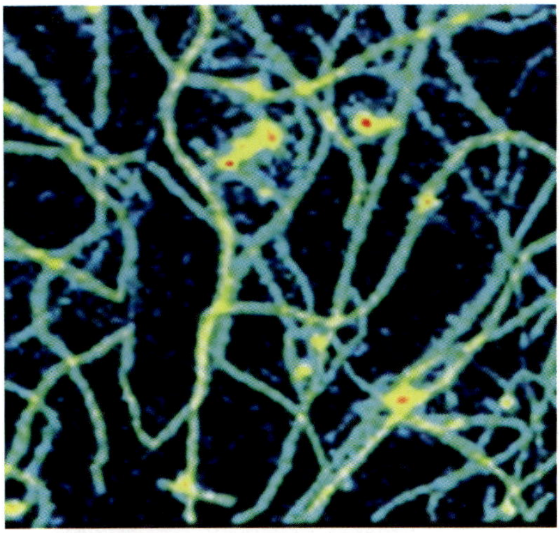

Fig. 2.10: Platelets on collagen fibrils.

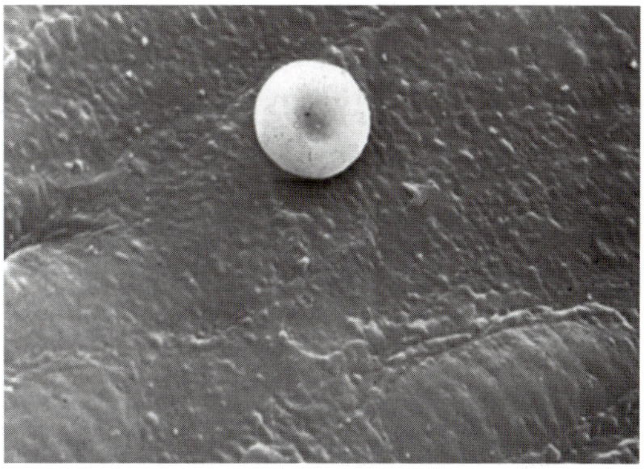

Fig. 2.11: Nonreactive endothelium.

collagen. Platelet aggregates and thrombus were visualized by staining filamentous actin.

All blood vessels are lined with a monolayer of endothelial cells (ECs), which provide a nonreactive internal surface for the flow of blood (Figs. 2.11 and 2.12). Functional and structural changes of vascular endothelium are modulated by a variety of thrombogenic as well as antithrombotic factors. Some of the vasoactive compounds released by the ECs include adenosine, ADPase, prostacyclins, and nitric oxide.

These molecules keep the endothelial cell surface free of platelets and other blood cells. However, if there is any injury to the vessel wall, the exposed cell matrix components attract platelets to the site of injury and initiate a healing response.

Figure 2.13 shows the response of blood cells to denuded rabbit aorta. Platelets are seen in various stages of interaction with the ECMs.

Having briefly discussed platelet structure and its relationship with surface interactions, it is time to review some of our early works at the Platelet Research Laboratory headed by Dr James G White and Thrombosis Research Laboratory headed by Gundu HR Rao. How did Professor White demonstrate role of platelet structural elements to the function?

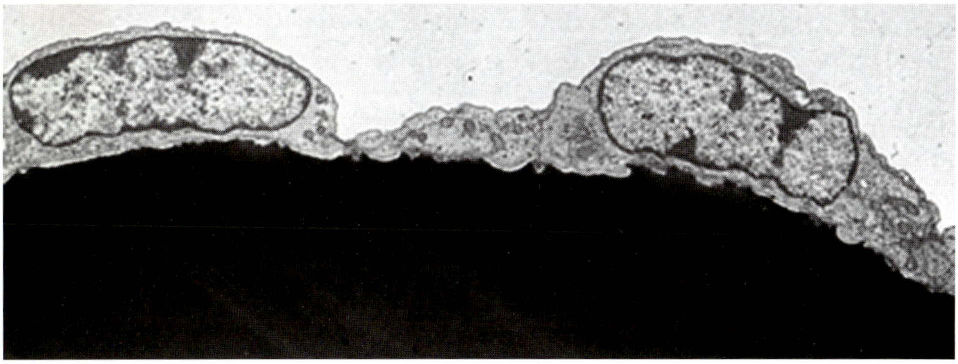

Fig. 2.12: Monolayer of endothelial cells.

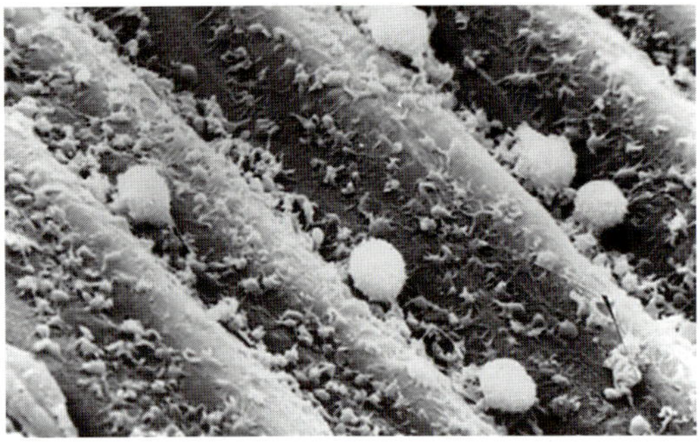

Fig. 2.13: Platelet interaction on denuded rabbit aorta.

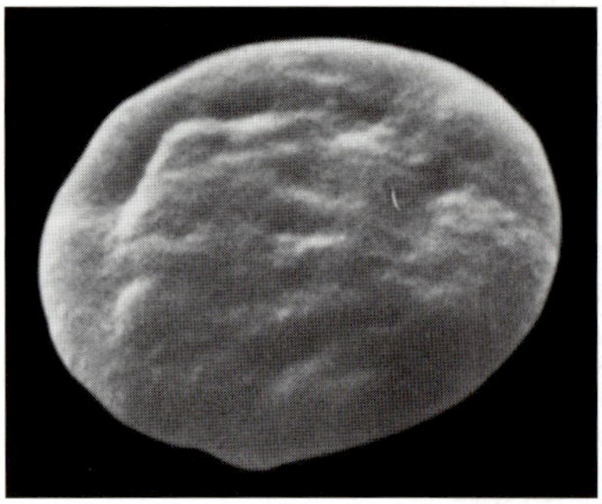

Fig 2.14: Discoid platelet by scanning electron microscopy.

James G White started working at the University of Minnesota in 1960 first in the Pediatrics Department and then in the Laboratory Medicine and Pathology. Since he was a well-known platelet ultrastructure biologist, experts all over the world collaborated with him. He used a variety of techniques to demonstrate the structure and function of platelets in various phases of activation.[7-20]

ELECTRON MICROSCOPY

Freshly obtained platelets in plasma or washed platelets in appropriate buffers (~100 μL) were fixed in approximately 100 μL of 0.1% glutaraldehyde in White's saline, and processed for conventional electron microscopy (EM). For immunoelectron microscopy (IEM), the fractions were fixed in a mixture of 2% paraformaldehyde and 0.2% glutaraldehyde in 0.1M sodium phosphate buffer (pH 7.4). After washing, samples were frozen, cryosectioned, and immunogold labeled according to established procedures. Sections were viewed in a Philips (Mahwah, NJ, United States) 301 and JEOL 1200CX electron microscope (JEOL, Tokyo, Japan). Resting platelets were obtained from freshly fixed whole blood that was collected directly from the vein into fixative containing 2.4% paraformaldehyde and 0.24% glutaraldehyde in 0.1 m sodium phosphate buffer (pH 7.4) (1:5 v/v). Resting platelets by scanning electron microscopy (SEM) at low and high resolution are shown in Figures 2.14 to 2.16.

ATOMIC FORCE MICROSCOPY

For atomic force microscopy (AFM), the specimens were fixed with cytochalasin B to prevent actin filament assembly and shape change. They were placed on polylysine-coated grids for viewing in the AFM (Nanoscope AFM, Digital Instruments Inc.). Scanning probe microscopes measure real space images of cells on flat surfaces. In brief, the AFM works by scanning a very sharp conducting tip (SiN) over the surface of a conducting biological membrane. Cantilevers used for probing were short-tipped thing legs (0.22 nm spring constant). Scanning was done with the J-size scanner (150 × 150 micron scan area). Resting platelets were treated with cytochalasin B to prevent actin filament assembly and shape change prior to being placed on polylysine-coated grid surfaces.

To obtain high-resolution as well as corrugations of plasma membrane surfaces, images were recorded with a contact mode (Nanoscope 4.1 software). AFM image of platelet

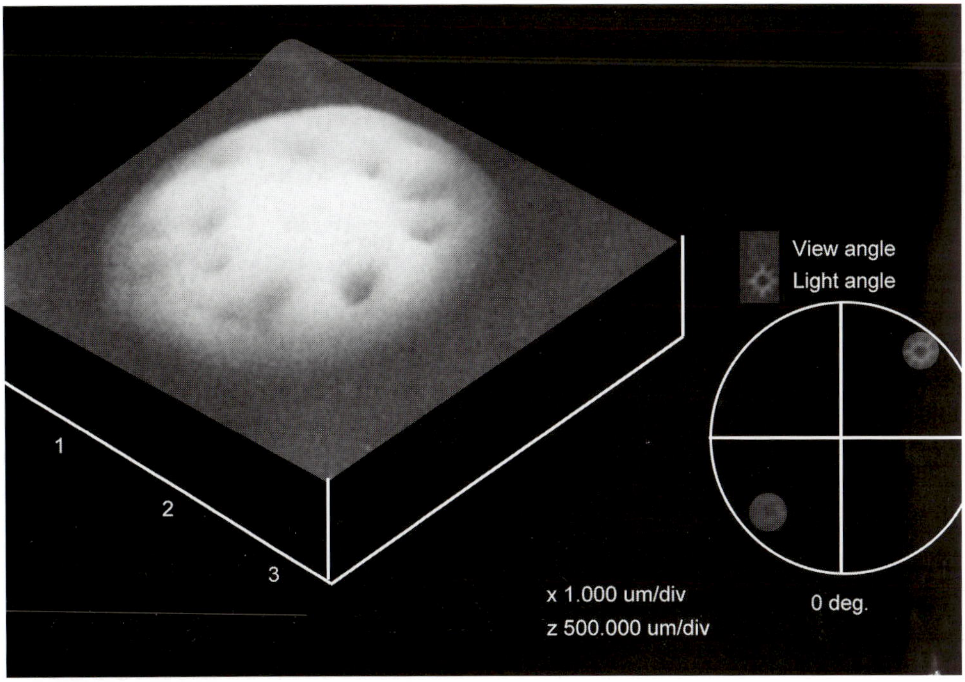

Fig. 2.15: Discoid platelet by atomic force microscopy.

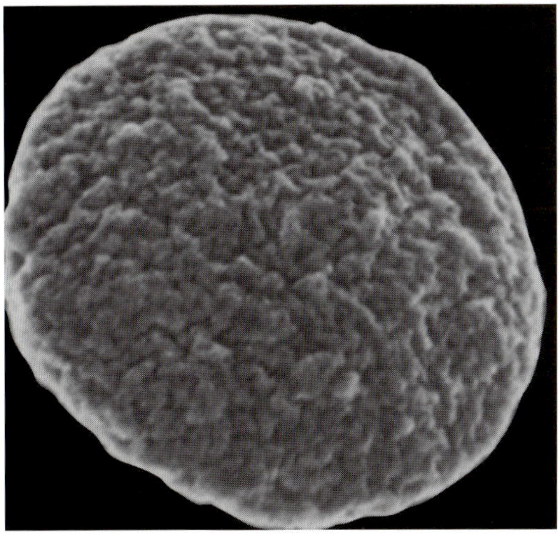

Fig. 2.16: Platelet high-resolution scanning electron microscopy.

(Fig. 2.17) reveals typical discoid-appearance characteristic of resting platelets. Higher-resolution SEM shows the corrugations of the surface membrane (Fig. 2.16). High-resolution AFM shows the openings of the open canalicular system (OCS) on the plasma membrane (Fig. 2.17).

FLUORESCENT AND CONFOCAL MICROSCOPY

Fluorescence imaging uses high-intensity illumination to excite fluorescent molecules in the sample. When a molecule absorbs photons, electrons are excited to a higher-energy level. As electrons relax back to the ground state, vibrational energy is lost; as a result, the emission spectrum will be shifted to longer wavelengths. Several instruments are available in the market for this kind of imaging work. Nikon upright, inverted polarized or stereo-microscope or Nikon's Biostation incubator imaging system could be used for these kinds

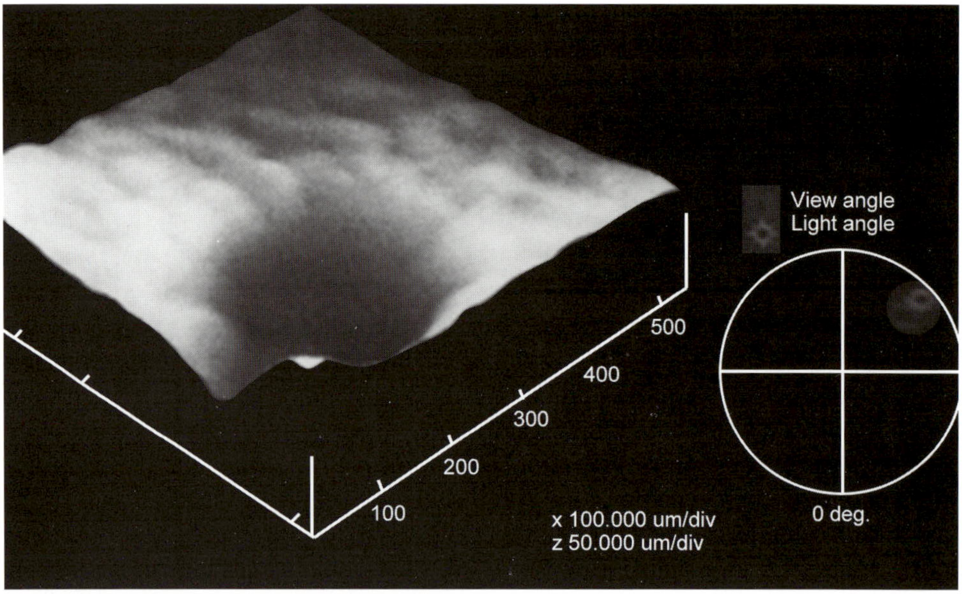

Fig. 2.17: High-resolution atomic force microscopy.

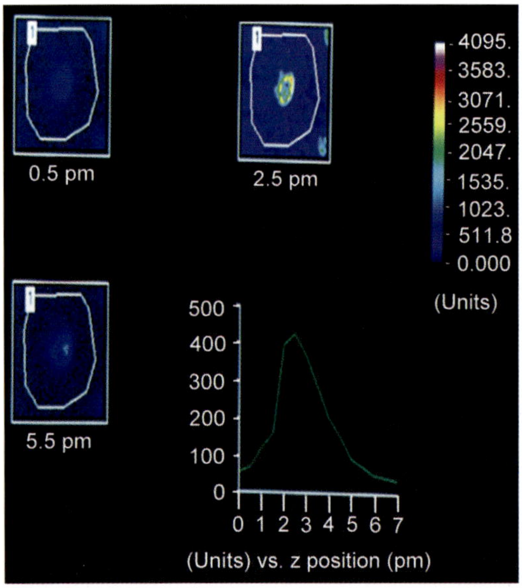

Fig. 2.18: Fluorescence microscopy.

of studies. Resolution in fluorescence imaging is improved with the use of confocal microscopy (Nikon LiveScan Swept Field Systems).

Examples for monitoring protein kinase C (PKC) activity and distribution during platelet activation are shown in Figures 2.18 to 2.20. PKC was visualized by using fluorescent-coupled phorbol myristate acetate (PMA), a specific substrate of PKC. Mobilization of the granules to the central mass can be seen both by confocal (Fig. 2.19) as well as electron micrographs (Fig. 2.20).

PLATELET AGGREGOMETRY STUDIES

Before the establishment of the biochemistry laboratory (1972), to complement his studies, White had done extensive studies using the electron microscope (both transmission as well as scanning) and platelet aggregometer. Methods followed in his laboratory for these studies have been described in most of his publications.[10-20]

Blood was drawn from adult volunteers and mixed immediately with citrate-citric acid-dextrose, pH 6.5 (citrate 0.1 M, citric acid 7 mM, dextrose 0.14 M) in a ratio of 1 part of anticoagulant to 9 parts of blood.[7]

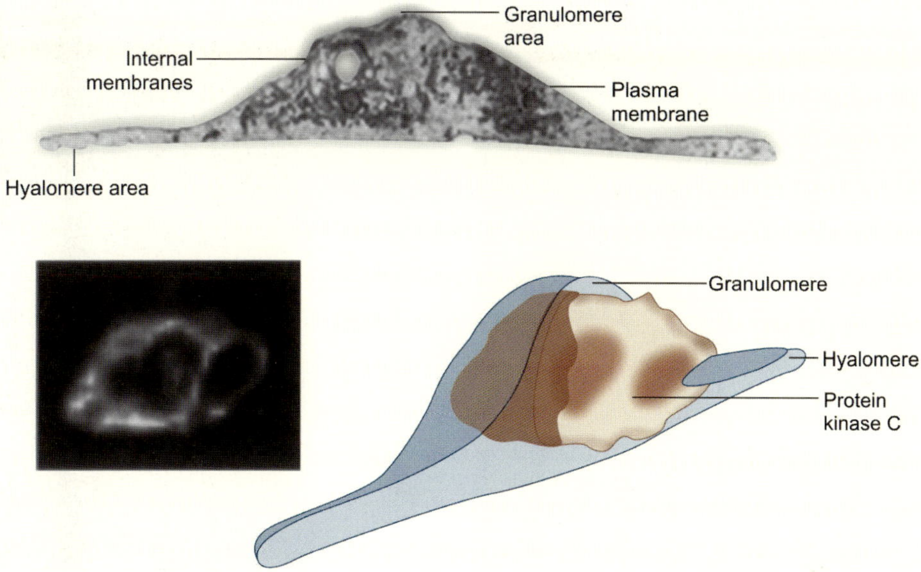

Fig. 2.19: Confocal microscopy.

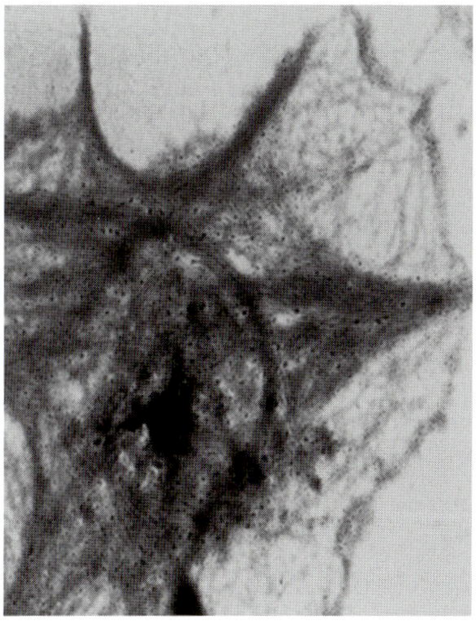

Fig. 2.20: Granule mobilization.

Platelet-rich plasma was separated by centrifugation of whole blood at room temperature for 20 minutes at 100 × g in a Sorvall swinging bucket centrifuge. Platelet aggregation studies were done in 60s using a Born aggregometer and later by Payton dual-channel aggregometer or Chrono-log aggregometer (whole blood as well as lumi-aggregometer).

Following aggregation of platelets in response to various agonists by turbidometry has been a gold standard method for testing platelet function since the time Gustav Born described this method in early 1960s.[7] Agonists usually used for activating platelets in suspension include adenosine diphosphate (ADP 3 uM), bovine thrombin (0.2 U/mL), serotonin (5HT 10 uM), vasopressin (100 mU/mL), epinephrine (5 uM), arachidonic acid (0.4–0.6 uM), platelet-activating factor (PAF, 2 uM), and collagen (2 ug/mL). For additional information on platelet function testing, refer recent reviews.[7,8] Using firefly luciferase and luciferin, we followed the release of ATP as a marker for release reaction (Fig. 2.21). Agonist-induced aggregation of platelets is modulated by the activation of GPIIb/IIIa receptor fibrinogen binding (Fig. 2.22) and release of granule contents, such as serotonin and ATP.[21-31]

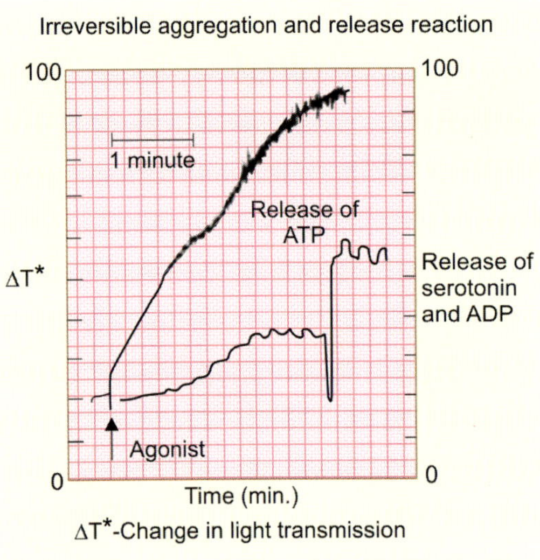

Fig. 2.21: Aggregation and release reaction.

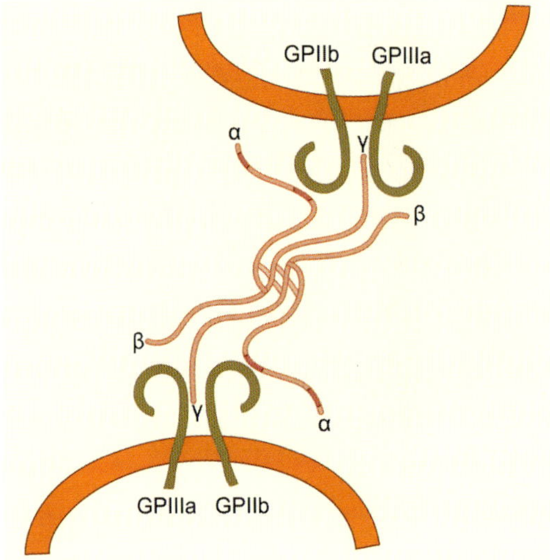

Fig. 2.22: Schematics of F-binding.

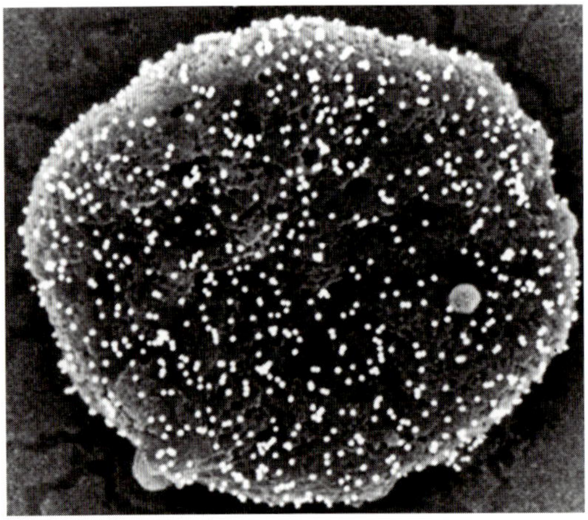

Fig. 2.23: F-gold binding to platelets.

A variety of granule contents are released to the exterior and several of them are monitored as markers of release reaction in addition to the released ATP monitored in the above-mentioned studies.[32-39]

White and associates, in a series of ultrastructure studies, have demonstrated fibrinogen binding on platelet surface, during cell-cell interactions, cell-surface interactions, and internalization of fibrinogen, using colloidal gold or latex particles coupled to fibrinogen. Since GPIIb/IIIa is the platelet fibrinogen receptor, it is reasonable to assume that fibrinogen is the adhesive protein involved in GPIIb/IIIa mediated platelet interaction with other platelets as well as vessel wall. It is very well known that the von Willebrand factor (vWF), fibronectin, and vitronectin also can bind to GPIIb/IIIa receptor in thrombin-stimulated platelets. The concept that all the adhesive proteins share a common receptor is further supported by the fact that their binding to GPIIb/IIIa receptor is blocked by synthetic peptide containing Arg-Gly-Asp (RGD) sequence.

According to White, GPIIb/IIIa receptors on platelets in suspension and after surface activation bind a variety of specific antibodies and ligands and transport them across the outside of the plasma membrane by a process of clustering, patching, and capping and endocytosis to the platelet interior (Figs. 2.23 and 2.24). They demonstrated that surface-activated platelets have inexhaustible

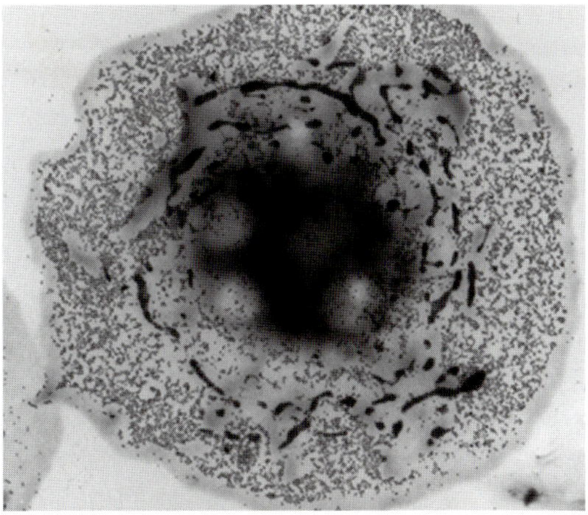

Fig. 2.24: Internalization of fibrinogen.

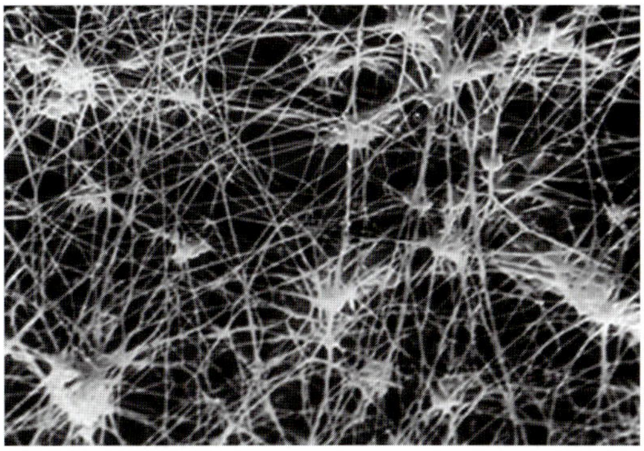

Fig. 2.26: Platelet–fibrin filaments.

population of mobile receptors to participate in the hemostatic process.[38] Figures 2.25A and B show a platelet in the process of spreading on a surface. F-gold particles are seen on the surface, as well as in the OCS.

Figure 2.24 shows a fully spread platelet with F-gold particles on the outer membrane and another platelet approaching for attachment. Figure 2.26 shows platelets interacting with fibrin filaments in a clot. White in his studies to demonstrate the secretory pathways describe his observation as follows: "on exposure to thrombin at concentrations of 1–5 U/mL for 30 seconds or more resulted in intense staining of α granules by osmium. Some granules communicated directly with dilated channels of the OCS, and several were frequently connected to the same canaliculus. The electron-dense substance in swollen granules and channels appeared to be in the process of extrusion through narrow or dilated openings of the OCS onto the platelet surface. Granule-to-granule fusion and formation of sealed vacuoles of fused granule products unstained by tannic acid–osmium were not observed. The findings support the concept that secretion by stimulated human platelets results from development of direct communications between granules and channels of the OCS and subsequent extrusion of products through channel pores to the surrounding medium."[14,20]

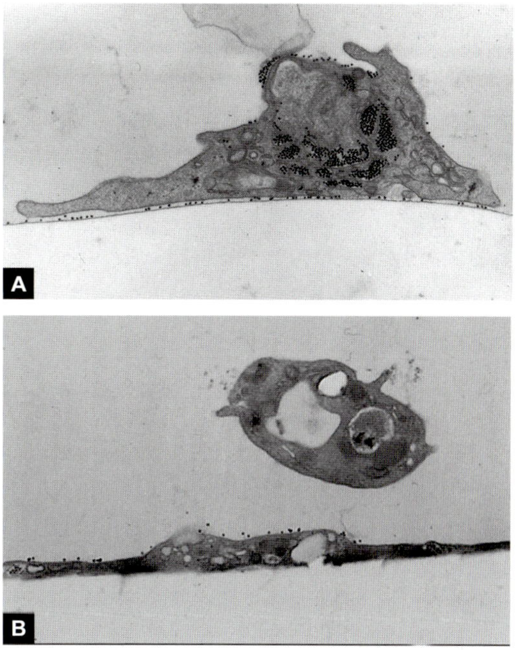

Figs. 2.25A and B: Platelet–surface interactions.

Using similar staining techniques, White and Gerrard provided evidence to suggest that platelet prostaglandin and thromboxane synthesis and an internal calcium store critical to platelet activation are both found in the platelet dense tubular system.[25] Using platelets of patients with afibrinogenemia, Gartner et al. demonstrated that fibrinogen was the receptor for the endogenous lectin of human platelets.[26] Using fibrinogen-coupled gold nanoparticles, they demonstrated the role of fibrinogen in adhesion, aggregation, and vessel wall interactions. Escolar and White using IgG-coupled nanogold particles demonstrated that channels of the surface-connected OCS of human platelets as the common pathway for transport of substances into the cells and as conduits for the discharge of α-granule products secreted during the platelet release reaction.[31] Using PMA, an ingredient of croton oil, White and associates demonstrated that this agent acts primarily on channels and induces activation of platelets without causing shape change.[32,33] White used electron-dense traces (thorium dioxide) extensively to study and demonstrate the activation of platelets and the role of surface membrane receptors, membrane systems, and intermembrane relationship.[28-30]

The platelet release reaction according to White, by and large, involves two primary processes: granule mobilization and contraction to squeeze the granule contents out. Granule mobilization involves fusion of the granule membranes with the surface-connected canalicular system (SCCS) and discharge of the granule contents into the channels. Contraction involves activation of platelet muscle proteins, including thrombosthenin, to produce a forceful expulsion of the granule contents from the SCCS to the exterior,[9,18,21,24,31,34,35] Previous studies from our laboratory have shown that PMA stimulates granule mobilization without shape change, and that the calcium ionophore stimulates platelet contraction. Studies with prostaglandin G_2 (PGG_2) on platelet ultrastructure demonstrated that this agent stimulated contraction and that the effect of PGG_2 was reversible.[37]

PLATELET BIOCHEMISTRY

Collaborating with Bernie Stetland, White demonstrated the calcium uptake by platelet contractile proteins in 1969. They concluded from their studies that "In the presence of ATP, the apparently membrane-free solution inhibited superprecipitation of the platelet contractile protein, thrombosthenin, and the inhibitory activity was abolished by addition of excess calcium ions."[23] These findings were identical to results obtained by others on the behavior of actomyosin in the presence of ATP and relaxing factor from skeletal muscle.[39-45] The relaxing factors extracted from muscle and platelets were thought to be soluble components of the respective cells. In view of the fact that earlier researchers (Bettex-Galland and Luscher) had demonstrated as early as in 1959 the presence of the contractile proteins actin and myosin in platelets; it was assumed that these proteins play a role in platelet contraction, secretion, and clot retraction events.[39-45] White based on his observations, described these contractile proteins as the muscular system of blood platelets.[40] The observation that filopodia of stimulated platelets contain bundles of actin filaments suggested a role for contractile proteins. Further observations by White and associates that a ring of microfilaments surround the granules and facilitate mobilization indicated a role for these contractile proteins in the platelet secretory pathway (Figs. 2.27A and B).

Subsequent studies from our laboratory using calcium-specific fluorophores demonstrated the mobilization of cytosolic calcium during platelet activation.[45-50] In

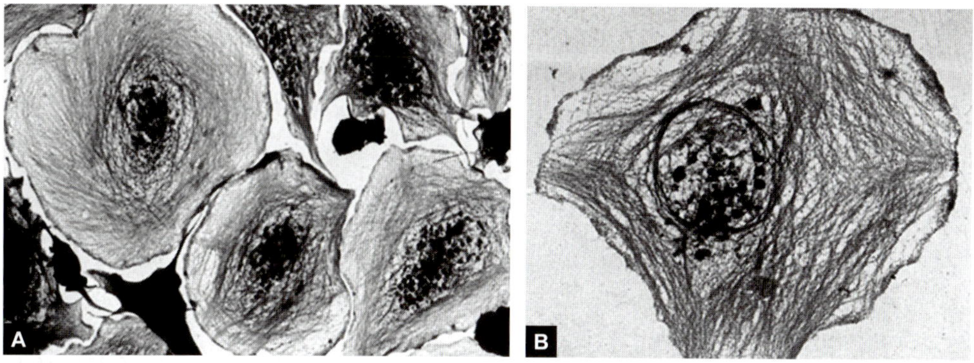

Figs. 2.27A and B: Role of microfilaments on granule mobilization and secretion.

classical muscle contraction process, the release of calcium from sarcoplasmic reticulum increases cytosolic calcium by several folds. This increase in calcium signals muscle contraction via the action of two accessory proteins bound to the actin filaments: tropomyosin and troponin. In nonmuscle cells, contraction seems to be regulated primarily by phosphorylation of one of the light chains of myosin. Using microelectrochemistry and pharmacological approaches, White and associates demonstrated that the F-actin, not the microtubule, regulates platelet dense body secretion.[51]

Intracellular calcium concentration plays a critical role in platelet activation–contraction–secretion coupling.[49] Rao and associates used the calcium-sensitive fluorophores, Quint-2 ester (QAM) its free acid (QFA), and chlortetracycline (CTC) along with ethylenediaminetetraacetic acid (EDTA), an intra- and extracellular calcium-chelating agent to assess the origin and role of calcium in normal platelets, and from patients with storage pool disease. On the basis of the results of their investigation, they concluded that the membranes and membrane systems are the primary source of calcium for platelet activation, with channels of the dense tubular system as the major reservoir. Elevation of cytosolic calcium seems to be essential for contractile events including actin assembly, granule mobilization, contraction, secretion of granule contents, and clot retraction.

White continued to collaborate with experts from all over the world. Since he was a renowned EM expert, people from various disciplines collaborated with him for all their ultrastructural work. He was also involved in the first ever attempt to study the nature of α granules using state-of-the-art proteomic techniques.[21] Using mass spectrometry, they identified 284 nonredundant proteins from intact α granules. New proteins that they discovered in platelet α granules included Scamp2, APLP2, ESAM, and LAMA5.

REFERENCES

1. Pankov R, Yamada KM. Fibronectin at a glance. J Cell Sci. 2002;115:3861-3.
2. Frantz C, Stewart M, Weaver VM. The extracellular matrix at a glance. J Cell Sci. 2010;123:4195-200.
3. Plow EF Hass TA, Zhang L, Loftus J, Smith JW. Ligand binding to integrins. J Biol Chem. 2000;275:21785-8.
4. Beck K, Hunter I, Engel J. Structure and function of laminin: anatomy of a multi-domain glycoprotein. FASEB J. 1990;4(2):148-60.
5. Kehrel B. Platelet-collagen interactions. Semin Thromb Hemost. 1995;21(2):123-9.

6. Rao GH, Fields CG, White JG, Fields GB. Promotion of human platelet adhesion and aggregation by a synthetic, triple-helical "mini-collagen". J Biol Chem. 1994;269(19): 13899-903.
7. Born GVR, Cross MJ. The aggregation of blood platelets. J Physiol. 1963;168:1787-95.
8. Pannicia R, Priora R, Liotta AA, Abbate R. Platelet function tests: a comparative review. Vasc Health Risk Manag. 2015;11:133-48.
9. White JG. Electron microscopic studies of platelet secretion. Prog Hemost Thromb. 1974;2:49-98.
10. White JG. Physicochemical dissection of platelet structural physiology. In: Baldini M, Ebbe S (Eds). Platelets: Production Function, Transfusion and Storage. New York: Grune and Stratton; 1974. pp. 235-52.
11. White JG. Platelet morphology. In: Johnson SA (Ed). The Circulating Platelet. New York: Academic Press; 1971. pp. 45-121.
12. White JG. Shape change. In: Didisheim P, Shimamoto T (Eds). Platelets, Thrombosis and Inhibitors. New York: FK Schatauer-Verlag; 1974. pp. 159-71.
13. White JG. The Ultrastructural cytochemistry and physiology of blood platelets. In: Mostafi FK, Brinkhous KM, (Eds). The Platelet. Baltimore: Williams & Wilkins; 1971. pp. 83-115.
14. White JG, Gerrard JM. Platelet membranes and membrane systems. In: International convention of the American Association of Blood Banks, San Francisco, "Membrane Structure and Function of Human Blood Cells". 1976; 4:61-79.
15. White JG, Gerrard JM. Platelet morphology and the ultrastructure of regulatory mechanisms involved in platelet activation. In: De Gaetano G, Garattini S (Eds). International Symposium on Platelets: A multidisciplinary Approach. New York: Raven Press; 1978. pp. 65-81.
16. White JG, Gerrard JM The ultrastructure of defective platelets. Mol Cell Biochem. 1978;21:109-28.
17. White JG, Gerrard JM Ultrastructural features of abnormal blood platelets. A review. Am J Pathol. 1976;83:589-632.
18. White JG, Rao GH, Gerrard JM. Effects of the ionophore A23187 on blood platelets I: Influence on aggregation and secretion. Am J Pathol. 1974;77(2):135-50.
19. Gerrard JM, White JG, Rao GH. Effects of the ionophore A23187 on the blood platelets 11. Influence on ultrastructure. Am J. Pathol. 1974;77(2):151-66.
20. White JG. Interaction of the membrane systems in blood platelets. Am J Pathol. 1972;66(2):295-312.
21. Maynard DM, Heijnen HFG, Horne MK, White JG, Gahl WA. Proteomic analysis of platelet alpha-granules using mass spectrometry. J Thromb Haemost. 2007;5(9): 1945-55.
22. Walsh PN, Mills D, White JG. Metabolism and function of human platelets washed by albumin density gradient separation. Br J Hematol. 1977;36(2): 281-96.
23. Stetland BE, Heagen BM, White JG. Uptake of calcium by platelet relaxing factor. Nature. 1969;233:521-2.
24. White JG, Krumwiede MD. Further studies of the secretory pathway in thrombin-stimulated human platelets. Blood. 1987;69: 1196-203.
25. Gerrard JM, White JG, Peterson DA. The platelet dense tubular system: Its relationship to prostaglandin synthesis and calcium flux. Thromb Haemost. 1978;40(2):224-31.
26. Gartner TK, Gerrard JM, White JG, Williams DC. Fibrinogen is the receptor for the endogenous lectin of human platelets. Nature. 1981;289:688-90.
27. White JG. Platelet structure. In: Michelson (Ed). Platelets. New York: Elsevier; 2007.
28. White JG, Rao GH. Microtubule coils versus the surface membrane cytoskeleton in maintenance and restoration of platelet discoid shape. Am J Pathol. 1998;152(2):597-609.
29. White JG, Krumwiede MD, Sauk JJ. Microtubule reassembly in surface activated platelets. Blood. 1985;65(6):1494-503.
30. White JG, Rao GH. Effects of a microtubule-stabilizing agent on the response of platelets to vincristine. Blood. 1982;60(2):474-83.
31. Escolar G, White JG. The platelet open canalicular system: a final common pathway. Blood Cells. 1990;17(3):467-95.
32. White JG, Rao GH, Estensen RD. Investigation of the release reaction in platelets exposed

to phorbol myristate acetate. Am J Pathol. 1974;75(2):301-14.
33. Estensen RD, White JG. Ultrastructure features on the platelet response to phorbol myristate acetate. Am J Pathol. 1974;74(3): 441-52.
34. White JG. A search for the platelet secretory pathway using electron dense tracers. Am J Pathol. 1970;58(1):31-49.
35. White JG. The secretory pathway of bovine platelets. Blood. 1986;69(3):878-85.
36. White JG. The transfer of thorium particles from plasma to platelets and platelet granules. Am J Pathol. 1968;53(4):567-75.
37. Gerrard JM, Townsend D, Stoddard S, Witkop CJ, White JG. The influence of prostaglandin G2 on platelet ultrastructure and platelet secretion. Am J Pathol. 1977;86:99-116.
38. White JG. Separate and combined interactions of fibrinogen-gold and latex with surface-activated platelets. Am J Pathol. 1990;137(4):989-98.
39. Bettex-Galland M, Luscher EF. Extraction of an actomyosin-like protein from human thrombocytes. Nature. 1959;184:276-7.
40. Carroll RC, Gerrard JM. Phosphorylation of platelet actin-binding protein during platelet activation. Blood. 1982;59:466-71.
41. Cohen I, Cohen C. A tropomyosin-like protein from human platelets. J Mol Biol. 1972;68: 383-7.
42. Cohen I, Luscher EF. The blood platelet contractile system. Haemostasis. 1975;4:125-43.
43. Cohen I, Kaminski E, De Vries A. Actin-linked regulation of the human platelet contractile system. FEBS Lett. 1973;34:315-7.
44. Cove DH, Crawford N. Platelet contractile proteins: separation and characterization of the actin and myosin-like components. J Mechanochem Cell Motil. 1975;3(2):123-33.
45. White JG. The muscular system of blood platelets. Blood. 1967;30:539.
46. White JG, Gerrard JM. Interaction of microtubules and microfilaments in platelet contractile physiology. Methods Achiev Exp Pathol. 1979;9:1-39.
47. Schollmeyer JV, Rao GH, White JG. An actin-binding protein in human platelets. Am J Pathol. 1978;93:433-46.
48. Rao GH, Peller JD, Semba CP, White JG. Influence of calcium sensitive fluorophores Quin 2 on platelet function. Blood. 1986;67:354-61.
49. Rao GH, Gerrard JM, Witkop CJ, Cohen I, White JG. Origin and role of calcium in platelet activation, contraction-secretion coupling. In: Fiskum G (Ed). Cell Calcium Metabolism. New York: Plenum Publications. 1988. pp. 411-27.
50. Rao GHR, White JG. Aspirin, PGE1, and Quin-2 AM induced platelet dysfunction. Restoration of function by norepinephrine. Prostaglandins Leukot Essent Fatty Acids. 1990;39:141-6.
51. Ge S, White JG, Haynes. Cytoskeletal F-actin, not the circumferential coil of microtubules, regulates platelet dense-body granule secretion. Platelets. 2012;23(4):259-63.

CHAPTER

3

Platelet Morphology and Dysfunction

INTRODUCTION

Platelet production by the bone marrow megakaryocytes is regulated to maintain a constant functional platelet mass in the circulating blood. According to this line of thinking, platelet mass appears to correlate with functional ability than the platelet count alone, since several factors in addition to the platelet count have been shown to modulate the hemostatic function. On the other hand, in clinical situations where there is a need for platelet transfusion, in general, clinicians do not follow this line of approach. They keep transfusing platelet concentrates, till they approach an approved number of platelets in the blood.[1] Thrombopoietin helps maintain the number of circulating platelets by the bone marrow. The liver produces thrombopoietin at a constant rate like many other endogenous modulators and releases into circulation on demand. The circulating platelet count is close to 140,000–400,000/µL. Clinically relevant platelet disorders include abnormal increase in platelet number (thrombocythemia and reactive thrombocytosis), decrease in platelet count (thrombocytopenia), and platelet dysfunctions (hypo- or hyperfunction).

Acquired abnormalities of platelet function are very common and include drug interactions (heparin), pathogen interaction (dengue virus), systemic disorders, and interventional and surgical procedures.[2] Many disorders, such as myeloproliferative, myelodysplastic, uremia, macroglobulinemia, multiple myeloma, cirrhosis can impair platelet function. Hereditary intrinsic platelet disorders are rare and can cause lifelong bleeding tendencies. Diagnosis is confirmed by platelet function tests and ultrastructure studies. Since White and associates have done extensive studies of these rare disorders, we will describe some of them in the following paragraphs. Immune thrombocytopenia (ITP) develops from the interaction of an autoantibody that is directed at a structural platelet antigen. In children, viral antigens may trigger it. ITP worsens during pregnancy and is responsible for maternal morbidity and mortality. Platelet destruction and loss of function can develop as a result of variety of immunological causes (pathogen infections, drugs, connective tissue or lymphoproliferative disorders, and blood transfusions). Thrombocytopenic purpura (TTP), and hemolytic–uremic syndrome (HUS) are characterized by thrombocytopenia and microangiopathic hemolytic anemia.

GLANZMANN THROMBASTHENIA

Ultrastructural studies from various laboratories have demonstrated that membrane defects are common in abnormal cells from patients with inherited hemorrhagic platelet disorders. Thrombasthenia is a classical example of a defect in platelet–platelet interaction (cell–cell interaction). The inability

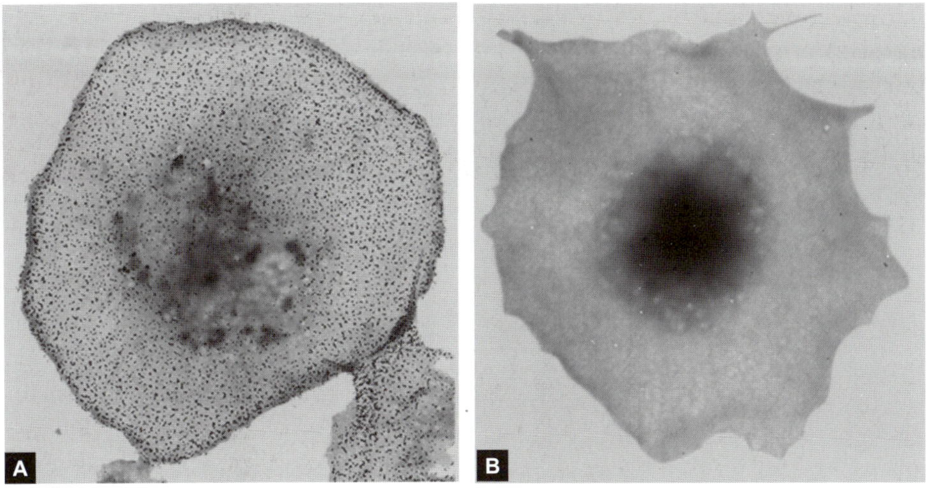

Figs. 3.1A and B: Platelets of Glanzmann thrombasthenia.

of patient's platelets to stick to one another is due to abnormalities of membrane glycoproteins (Figs. 3.1A and B). Glanzmann thrombasthenia (GT) is a rare genetic disorder, which manifests with hemorrhagic conditions. Under the guidance of Professor Mammen Chandy, Christian Medical College (CMC) Vellore, India had highlighted the frequency of GT in South India.[3] GT is a rare autosomal recessive disorder characterized by abnormalities in GPIIβ/IIIα (βII/αIII) receptor proteins. In this context, I would like to mention how bilateral collaboration was established between two great institutions. I was planning our Second International Conference on Thrombosis and Hemostasis at Bengaluru, Karnataka, India and I wanted to invite Dr Barry Coller, Clinical Professor, Mount Sinai School of Medicine, New York. USA. I knew his interest in GT studies and getting patients with this disorder was difficult in United States. I wrote to him that I could facilitate a working relationship with the CMC Vellore group, if he participates in our conference in Bengaluru. He graciously agreed and indeed participated in the SASAT-1996 conference in Bengaluru, which was organized under the leadership of Prof S. S. Iyengar.[4]

As a result of this initiative in 1995, a long-lasting relationship was established between Prof Mammen Chandy of CMC (Currently Director, Tata Memorial Cancer Center, Kolkata) and Prof Barry Coller of New York (Currently at The Rockefeller University, USA). The two groups together were able to work on the molecular diversity of GT in southern India.[5,6] They were able to identify 10 "novel" mutations from 16 unrelated patients, demonstrating the genetic diversity of the disorder in southern India.[5] As an extension of this study, they conducted mRNA splicing and highlighted the role of specific amino acids in structure-function correlations of $\alpha IIb/\beta_3$.[6] Both groups have published their work on prenatal diagnosis of this disease.[7,8] Dr Coller and his staff have continued their studies on the genetic and protein abnormalities responsible for the disease, as well as variants in the genes for the receptor (*ITGA2B* and *ITGB3*). Looking back at the three decades of research progress on this work, it makes me feel happy to note that it has resulted in screening of the *ITGA2B* and *ITGB3* genes in large international cohorts.[9] In this study, researchers were able to sequence the coding of the regions and splice both the genes of 76 affected families and identified 78 genetic variants (55 novel) suspected to cause GT. These seminal studies extend our knowledge of GT and the pathophysiology of an integrin to molecular level.

A variety of molecules are stored within the α and dense granules of the platelet, which upon activation of the platelet, are released into the external environment of the platelet. The storage pool disorders are a result of the deficiency and/or abnormality of either or both types of granules. In these disorders, secretion is hindered, not by the secretory mechanisms, but by the lack of content within the granules. Both granules appear to develop from the homotypic fusion of trans-Golgi vesicles in megakaryocytes as well as from heterotypic fusion of these vesicles with endocytic vesicles from the plasma and plasma membranes.

According to White, the primary congenital release disorders are a heterogeneous group of disorders with a wide variety of underlying defects whose mechanisms are not yet fully elucidated. They can be caused by abnormalities of signal transduction from the membrane (receptor or G-protein defects or mutations), abnormal internal metabolic pathways (mutations or defects of enzymes, i.e. PLC, PKC), abnormal release mechanisms, abnormal structures involved in the release reactions. The common abnormality within this group of defects is the failure to successfully release granule contents upon platelet activation. Release defects are associated with prolonged bleeding time, abnormal in vitro platelet aggregation profile in association with ADP (including an absent secondary wave) and epinephrine and collagen with a blunted or absent secondary wave.

Abnormalities of platelet secretion can be due to deficiency of platelet granules or defects in the signal transduction events that regulate secretion or aggregation. Platelet storage pool disorders can be congenital or acquired and result from a deficiency of granules (α or dense granules, or both) or a defective release of granules at platelet activation. Dense granule storage pool disorders (δ-SPDs) can appear as a singular clinical entity or as part of other hereditary disorders, such as Chediak–Higashi, Hermansky–Pudlak, or Wiskott–Aldrich syndrome (WAS). [14]δ-SPD often shows decreased aggregation response to ADP, epinephrine, and collagen and normal aggregation to arachidonic acid and ristocetin. Ultrastructural abnormalities in these disorders usually show decreased dense granules. Furthermore, α-SPD [gray platelet syndrome (GPS)] has decreased α granules and is usually considered a macrothrombocytopenia. White has described ultrastructural pathology of a variety of rare platelet disorders.[10-39] Additional references can be accessed at the following link at www.labome.org., under James G White, University of Minnesota. (https://www.labome.org/expert/usa/university/white/james-g-white-452177.html).

COMMON PLATELET DISORDERS, BIOCHEMICAL AND CLINICAL FINDINGS

Storage Pool Deficiency

Storage pool deficiencies are a group of disorders caused by problems with platelet granules, which are little sacks containing various proteins, enzymes, and other constituents. There are two types of granules recognized:

α granules and dense granules (dense bodies). Storage pool deficiencies are caused by a lack of granules; by and large, most common ones are caused by a failure of the platelets to empty or release the contents of the granules. Release defects are a diverse group of disorders caused by a problem with the secretory mechanisms. Even though the granules are present within the platelets, their contents are not released upon activation to the circulating blood. Delta storage pool deficiency is caused by a lack of dense granules and the components normally stored within them. This type of bleeding problem can be a feature of other inherited conditions such as Hermansky-Pudlak, Wiskott-Aldrich, and Chediak-Higashi syndrome (CHS). The four major types of congenital platelet storage pool disease identified are dense body deficiency (decreased dense bodies with serotonin and ADP), gray platelet syndrome (decreased α granules and contents), factor V Quebec (protease degradation of α granules), and mixed α-granule/dense body deficiency (decreased α-granules and dense bodies). In δ-SPD, the δ granules (dense bodies) are affected, and in α-SPD, it is the α granules (Table 3.1).

Hermansky–Pudlak Syndrome

Hermansky–Pudlak syndrome (HPS) is a disorder characterized by oculocutaneous albinism, which causes abnormally light coloring of the skin, hair, and eyes. Nine different types

Table 3.1: Platelet disorders, biochemistry and clinical findings.

Platelet disorders	*Biochemistry*	*Clinical findings*
von Willebrand (vWF) (defect in adhesion)	Decreased vWF on platelet membrane	Bleeding mild to severe
Bernard-Soulier (defect in adhesion)	Lacks GpIb/IX, unable to adhere to platelets	Severe bleeding tendencies
Glanzmann thrombasthenia (defect in aggregation)	Lacks GpIIb/IIIa, unable to bind fibrinogen	Varied bleeding possible mucous membranes
Storage pool disease (defect in secretion/release)	Dense granule deficiency, no release	Varied bleeding mild to severe
Hermansky–Pudlak (defect in secretion/release)	Lipid metabolism disorder that causes deficient release of platelet granules	Albinism, mild bleeding
Wiskott–Aldrich (defect in secretion/release)	Structurally abnormal platelets	Severe eczema infections
Chediak–Higashi (defect in secretion/release)	Lack dense bodies and ADP	Albinism, infections hemorrhage
Gray platelet syndrome (defect in secretion/release)	Deficiency of platelet α granules	Mild bleeding
Scott syndrome (defect in coagulation support)	Abnormalities of the platelet surface membrane that fail to promote activation of the blood clotting proteins, which are necessary in the formation of the fibrin clot	

Source: Huebsch LB, Harker LA. Disorders of platelet function. West J Med. 1981;134(2):109-27.

of HPS have been identified (https://ghr.nlm.nih.gov/condition/hermansky-pudlak-syndrome). Several types of HPS have been described in patients from Puerto Rico.[40] Mutations in one of the nine genes (*HPS1, AP3B1, HPS3, HPS4, HPS5, HPS6, DYNBP1, BLOC1S3*, and *PLDN*) are responsible for this disorder. The HPS is a mild bleeding disorder in which the platelets are markedly deficient in the storage pool of adenine nucleotides and serotonin. These products are normal, stored in a specific type of storage organelle, the dense body. HPS platelets appear unable to form these organelles or cannot concentrate the products in them due to an organelle membrane abnormality. Witkop and White shared NIH grants for several years to conduct studies on this rare disorder.[39-44] Majority of patients were from Puerto Rico.

Basically, this is an autosomal recessive disorder causing oculocutaneous albinism and a platelet storage pool deficiency, reflecting defective biosynthesis and/or processing of melanosomes and platelet dense bodies (Figs. 3.2 and 3.3). Four human genes (*HPS1, ADTB3A, HPS3, HPS4*) are associated with four subtypes of HPS. The most common is *HPS1* in which a 16-bp duplication in exon 15 of the HPS gene seems to be the cause of 450 non-Puerto Rican patients.[44-46] Witkop and White studied HPS patients from different parts of the world. I remember fondly the days that I used to visit various hospitals in India to collect hair and platelet samples for their studies. For additional references to their collective work, search Witkop CJ and White JG.

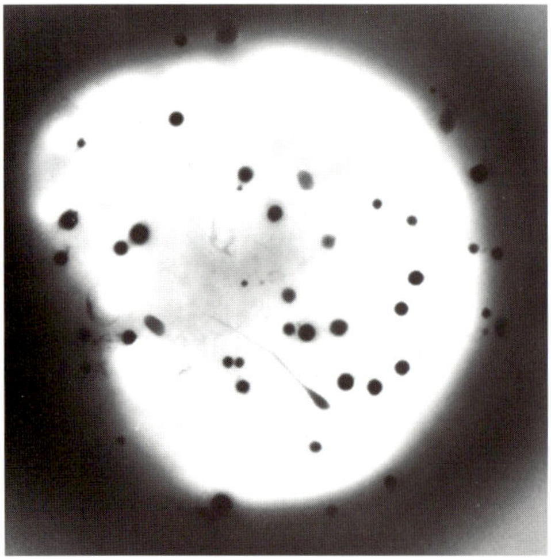

Fig. 3.2: Platelet with dense bodies.

Wiskott–Aldrich Syndrome

Wiskott-Aldrich syndrome (WAS) is characterized by abnormal immune system function and a reduced ability to form blood clots. This condition primarily affects males. Individuals with WAS have microthrombocytopenia, which is a decrease in the number and size of blood cells involved in clotting (platelets). This platelet defect, which is present from birth, can lead to easy bruising or episodes of prolonged bleeding. This syndrome is a rare X-linked primary immunodeficiency condition characterized by repeated infections, hematopoietic malignancies, eczema, and thrombocytopenia. Studies have demonstrated both signaling and cytoskeletal abnormalities in lymphocytes of WAS.[47] The gene responsible for WAS, a disease affecting platelets and lymphocytes, has been cloned and its protein product has been

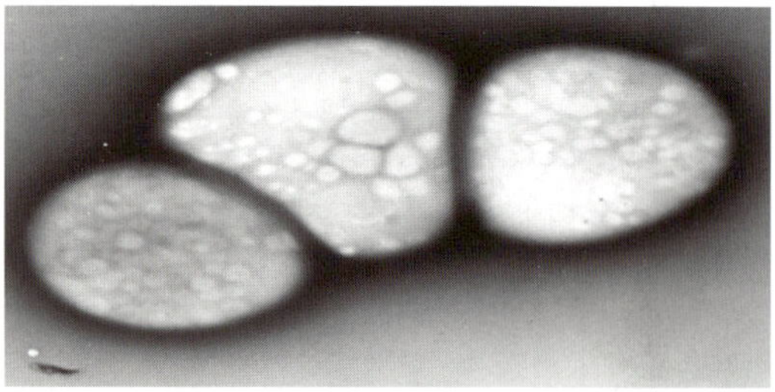

Fig. 3.3: Hermansky–Pudlak syndrome—platelets with no dense bodies.

found to interact with the GTPase Cdo42. WAS protein (WASP) seems to provide a link between Cdc42 and the actin cytoskeleton.[48] This is a complex primary immunodeficiency disorder and its gene product WASP is a key regulator of actin polymerization. Severe manifestation of WAS leads to an early death from infection and bleeding. Currently the only therapy seems to be allogeneic stem cell gene therapy.[49] After successful therapy, the authors concluded that hematopoietic stem cell gene transfer may achieve complete immunological correction without producing the toxic effects implicit in the concept of retrovirus-based stem cell gene transfer.

Chediak–Higashi Syndrome

Giant cytoplasmic granules are the hallmark of the patients with CHS. In addition to the high frequency of giant granules, platelets from most patients with this disorder are deficient in the storage pool of adenine nucleotides and serotonin and the dense bodies in which they are sequestered (Fig. 3.4). CHS is a rare autosomal recessive congenital

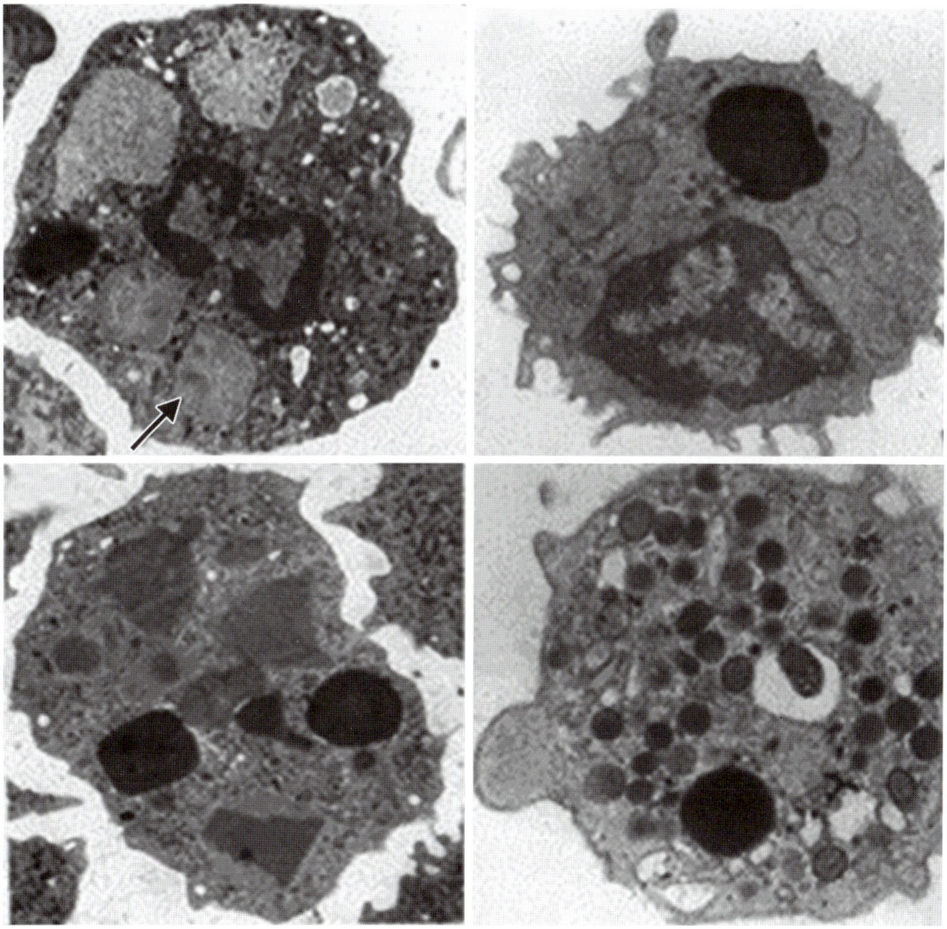

Fig. 3.4: Wiskott–Aldrich syndrome—platelets with giant granule.

immunodeficiency caused my mutations in *CHS1*, a gene encoding a putative lysosomal trafficking protein. Platelets from patients presenting with childhood CHS have been reported to be deficient in dense bodies.[50,51]

Gray Platelet Syndrome

The GPS is another example of an organelle membrane defect. Gray platelets develop normal numbers of dense bodies and lysosomes, but appear selectively unable to form the membranes necessary to enclose α granules. According to White, "by elimination, the only morphologically distinguishable organelle in which gray platelets could be defective is the granule secreting B thromboglobulin, fibrinogen, thrombin-sensitive protein, platelet factor 4 and mitogenic factors". He also explored the possibilities that the large number of vacuoles (Figs. 3.5A and B) seen in gray platelets were meant as storage sites for missing products. Since ultrastructural studies revealed that these platelets have α granules less than 15% of normal, further biochemical studies were initiated to characterize the defects.[52] Platelets from both patients had severe deficiencies of platelet factor 4 and β thromboglobulin. They were also deficient in thrombin-sensitive protein, as well as platelet-derived growth factor.

von Willebrand Factor Disease

The defect in von Willebrand factor (vWF) resides within the vWF, which plays an important role in platelet function. Interactive platelet receptor for this protein is GPIb/IX. Abnormalities of vWF may lead to mucocutaneous bleeding similar to that seen in other platelet function defects. This is inherited as autosomal dominant trait with males and females are equally affected.[53] This disease is classified to three types: type 1 includes partial quantitative deficiency, type 2 includes qualitative defects, and type 3 includes virtually complete deficiency of vWF. According De Jong et al. once the vWF is confirmed by functional tests, subtyping tests can classify the patients as von Willebrand disease (vWD) 1, 2, or 3. The performance of some additional

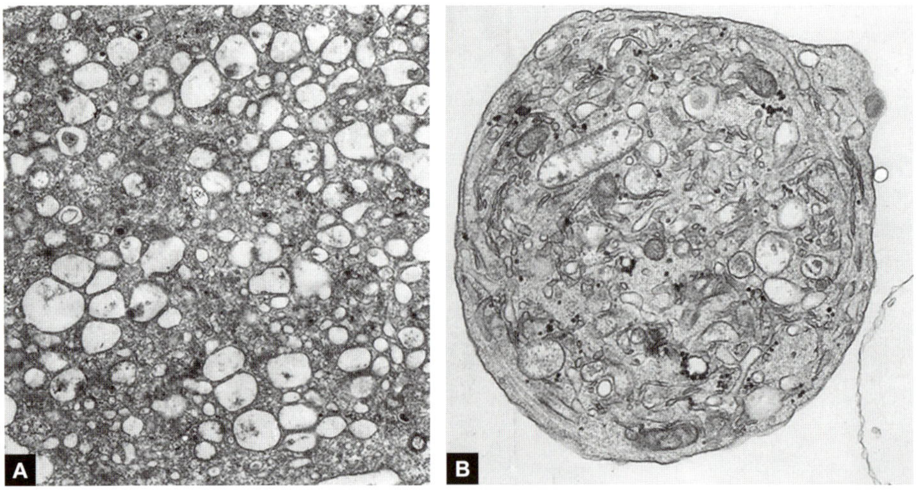

Figs. 3.5A and B: Gray platelets.

assays and analyses, such as vWF propeptide measurements or genetic analyses may help identifying the pathological mechanism behind certain defects or can guide in the choice of treatment.[54]

Bernard–Soulier Syndrome

The abnormal platelets of patients with Bernard-Soulier syndrome (BSS) are capable of adhering to one another, but fail to stick to the site of vessel wall injury. Defective platelet function in this disorder appears related to a marked deficiency or absence of a surface membrane glycoprotein different from the glycoprotein abnormalities of GT. Decreased or absent expression of the GPIb/IX/V receptor due to mutations in the *GP1BA*, *GP1BB*, or *GP9* genes gives rise to BSS (Fig. 3.6).[55]

BSS is characterized by the inability of the platelets to bind to vWF during the initial steps of platelet adhesion because the platelets either lack or have qualitative defect in the platelet membrane glycoprotein GPIb-IX-V complex. Mutations leading to absent expressions or dysfunctions have been uncovered in the gens for GPIbα (CD42b) and GPIX (CD42a). Mutations in GPIbα can lead to platelet-type vWD in which GPIb-1X are expressed normally but bind vWF spontaneously, which leads to platelet aggregation and thrombocytopenia. BSS is nearly always inherited in an autosomal recessive manner, with consanguinity a frequent finding. Just a few representative rare platelet function disorders have been presented in this section. Readers are urged to refer to comprehensive reviews on the molecular basis of these disorders as well as management of such bleeding disorders under clinical conditions.[56-65]

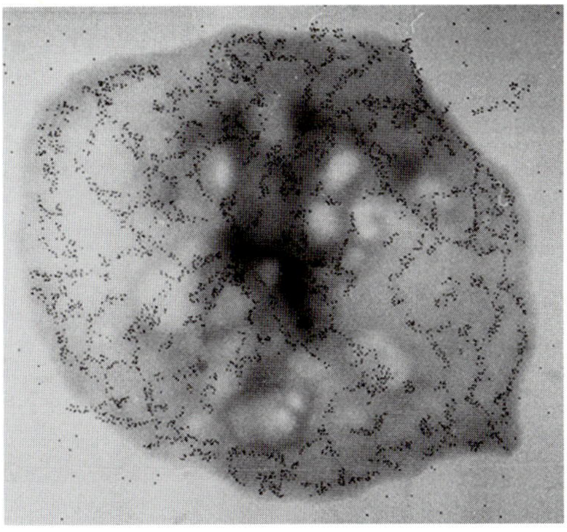

Fig. 3.6: Platelet of BSS patient.

MISCELLANEOUS DYSFUNCTION OF PLATELET FUNCTION

Cyclooxygenase Deficiency

Studies from our laboratory at the University of Minnesota did not reveal "aspirin resistance" in any individuals tested. All the subjects tested responded with aggregation when stimulated with arachidonic acid (AA). However, evaluation of physiology, biochemistry, ultrastructure, and function in a young woman without history of any hemorrhagic problems revealed that her platelets were deficient in cyclooxygenase (COX) activity. Her platelets aggregated in response to thrombin, ADP, and collagen but failed to respond to AA even at as high a concentration as 2 mM. Amounts of ^{14}C-AA released after stirring with thrombin were similar to normal platelets. However, evaluation of prostaglandin synthesis after stirring with radiolabeled AA revealed no evidence of endoperoxides or thromboxane synthesis, although products of lipoxygenase were produced in normal amounts. Preexposure to 5 uM epinephrine, a concentration that gave only a primary wave response to AA resulted in normalization of her platelet response to AA. These observations may explain why patients with platelet COX deficiency have mild absent bleeding symptoms.[66] In a separate study, we demonstrated that a mechanism of membrane modulation, mediated by α-adrenergic receptors cooperatively linked to the endoperoxide and thromboxane receptor can secure irreversible aggregation response in normal and abnormal platelets despite absence of secretion (ADP) and prostaglandin synthesis.

Endoperoxide/Thromboxane Receptor Dysfunction

Extending these studies, we were able to demonstrate existence of such dysfunctions in dog platelets and the ability of the mechanism of membrane modulation to restore the function in these defective platelets.[67,68] Dogs have platelets, which are heterogeneous in regard to their aggregation response to arachidonate. Since prostaglandin metabolism is intact in these platelets, the observed dysfunction appears to be the result of variable sensitivity to endoperoxide and thromboxane A_2. Preincubation of platelet-rich plasma (PRP) with epinephrine uniformly transforms PRP, which does not aggregate with upon exposure to arachidonate alone into arachidonate responsive.[67] Johnson and associates demonstrated that in most of dogs, mongrel or purpose bred, have platelets that generate TXA_2 but fail to aggregate irreversibly or secrete granule contents.[68] These TXA-insensitive platelets do not respond to TXA analogs, U46610, or I-BOP. However, 30% of the mongrel have normal platelets that respond to PG-endoperoxides and TXA. Similar to what we found with COX-deficient human platelets, this genetically inherited receptor abnormality in dogs do not cause any bleeding diathesis. Johnson and associates have done extensive studies on the biology of TXA receptor in platelets as well as the Gx_q and Gx_{11} gene expression in platelets.[68-70]

Platelet Dysfunction in Animal Platelets

Animals are used as experimental models in a variety of studies. In addition, millions of animals are used as domesticated pets. Therefore, it is important to understand the subtle difference in the mechanisms involved in hemostasis and thrombosis. From the point of view of medical device developer for instance, preferred route has been to develop their device in animal models, which are relatively nonresponsive for thrombotic episodes. As an example, much of the work on heart valves, stents, and artificial heart is done using animals, such as goats, cows, or horses. Platelets of these animals are less responsive to the activation stimulus than human platelets. Of course from the point of consumers, this is not the best approach. These tests have to be done in animals that have platelets, which are functionally similar to human platelets (porcine or primates). I have had discussions about this dilemma with funding agencies as well as device development companies. In view of the fact that it is convenient to work with these established animal models, which are less risky, the device companies prefer to use these animal models (goats, sheep, cows, or horses). The funding companies also do not want to take any risk and spend additional funds to develop newer better reliable animal models.

White and associates studied ultrastructure, physiology, and function of blood platelets in a variety of animals, including, dogs, cows, horses, sheep, goat, turkeys, camels, elephants, and Beluga whales. We have already described in the preceding paragraphs about our findings on dog platelets. In the following paragraphs, we will describe briefly about our work on platelet function in other animals. Before I get into the details of platelet dysfunction in animals, I would like to mention, for various reasons, each group preferred to work with blood platelets from a different species. For instance, VA medical Center at Minneapolis, Minnesota, researchers preferred to work with dog platelets. At the Mayo Clinic, Rochester, MN, Dr Bowies' group worked with a "vWF model" with pigs. Canadian researchers at McMaster's University studied rabbit platelets. Chocolate City, Hershey Pennsylvania, used cow platelets for their studies. Utah Heart Institute used horse platelets for their studies. This preference was partly due to the availability and partly due to their earlier experience and publication records.

Bovine Platelets

Human platelets react to surface activation by losing their shape, extending pseudopods, converting to dendritic forms, and finally spreading. Bovine platelets do not spread, rather they unfold (Fig 3.7).[71] Surface activation causes them to transform from disks to irregular flattened shapes resembling dendritic platelets. Bovine platelets lack surface-connected open canalicular system (OCS), which serves as a reservoir of membranes for human platelet spreading.[72]

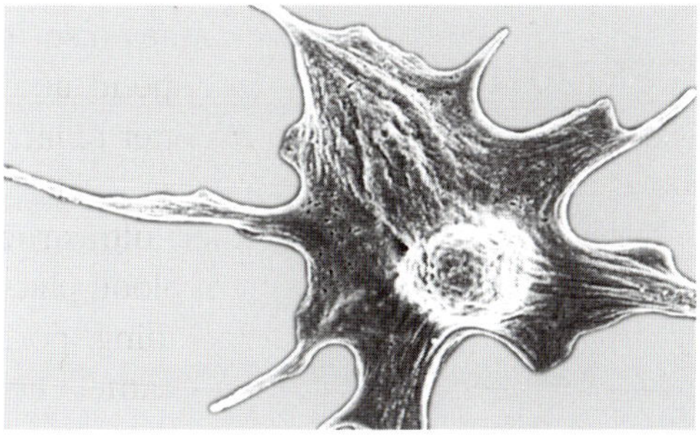

Fig. 3.7: Bovine platelet.

Furthermore, the microtubule coils are more resistant to disassembly in surface-activated bovine platelets. Fibrinogen-gold particles are moved to the interior of human platelets rapidly; bovine platelet receptors hardly internalize F-gold. Human platelets aggregate when mixed with bovine plasma, but bovine platelets do not respond to human plasma. Bovine platelets in citrate buffer poorly react to the subendothelium, whereas suspended in heparinized blood reacted and adhered more readily than human platelets. There seems to be different mechanisms involved in hemostasis in human and bovine species.

Horse Platelets

Collaborating studies were done with the veterinary laboratory at the University of Minnesota on platelet function disorders in racing horses. Platelet function was evaluated in horses with exercise-induced hemorrhage (bleeder) and in control horses (nonbleeder). Platelet aggregation, secretion, and adhesion to rabbit aortic subendothelium were similar for bleeders and nonbleeders. University of Kentucky has maintained a record of all the publications on this topic from 1990 to 2005. See link (http://www2.ca.uky.edu/gluck/images/info%20pages/BibEIPH.pdf). Exercise-induced pulmonary hemorrhage (EPIH) is seen in most race horses and in many other horses used in equine sports. Blood in the tracheobronchial tree is identified in 4–75% of racehorses via endoscopic examination, and hemorrhage is detected by cytological examination of bronchoalveolar lavage in more than 90% of racehorses. Weiss et al. at the University of Minnesota evaluated the platelet function of both bleeder and nonbleeder horses. Platelets readily aggregated in response to ADP, thrombin, collagen, and arachidonic acid. On the basis of their results, they concluded that horses might be predisposed to thrombus formation and subsequent microvascular obstruction.[73] One may also speculate couple of scenarios to explain this phenomenon. When we were trying to do studies on dog platelets, we found that when they are excited, due to the adrenalin rush, platelets would disappear from the circulation (sequestered). However, when the dogs are calm and conditioned to the blood-drawing procedure, we could find normal platelet counts. This fits with the experience of racehorse managers, who observed prior conditioning of thoroughbreds for short periods reduced the incidence of bleeding during the races. On the other hand, adrenaline rush induced by the racing event could produce a thrombotic state in the thoroughbreds, as speculated by Weiss and associates and cause microvascular obstruction. There is a great need for further studies to determine the underlying cause for exercise-induced (adrenalin-induced?) pulmonary hemorrhage.

Turkey Platelets

Turkeys are hypertensive birds compared to mammals of similar size. We studied in vitro synthesis of thrombocyte TXA, 12L-hydorxy-5, 8, 10 heptadecatrienoic acid (HHT), 12L-hydorxy-5, 8, 10, 14 eicosatetraenoic acid (HETE), and aortic prostaglandins (PGs) in 1–10-month-old domestic white turkeys.[74] TXA production was increased and HETE production was markedly reduced in normal thrombocytes. These studies also demonstrated that there was considerable deficiency in PGI_2 production. The vasopressor effect of PGE_1, PGE_2, and PGI_2 was altered in awake turkeys. Both vascular AA metabolism and vasodepressor potencies of PGE_1 and PGI_2 were altered and the activity of lipoxygenase pathway in thrombocytes was limited.

Acquired Platelet Disorders

Several diseases, procedures, and drugs have been associated with acquired platelet function disorders.[2,62,75,76] Hyperglobulinemia associated with multiple myeloma induces a platelet membrane defect resulting in impaired hemostatic function. In uremia associated with any form of renal disease, platelet adhesion and aggregation are decreased. Similarly, chemotherapy may also cause platelet dysfunction. Pathogens, such as dengue virus are known to cause severe loss of circulating platelets.

Numerous drugs can impair platelet function. Drugs reported to block platelet receptor binding or to change platelet membrane charge or permeability include furosemide, penicillin, carbenicillin, lidocaine, phentolamine, and chlorpromazine. Drugs that inhibit transduction of messages received at the platelet surface include caffeine, theophylline, dipyridamole, and papaverine. Drugs that inhibit execution of platelet responses (aggregation, secretion, or thromboxane production) include aspirin, indomethacin, acetaminophen, phenylbutazone, ticlopidine, pentobarbital, and sulfinpyrazone. Heparin-induced thrombocytopenia is well recognized by the clinical community.

REFERENCES

1. Rao GHR, Eastlund T, Jagannathan L. Handbook of Blood Banking and Transfusion Medicine. New Delhi: JP Medical Publishers; 2006.
2. Sharathkumar AA, Shapiro A. Platelet Function Disorders. Canada: World Federation of Hemophilia (WFH); 2008. www.wfh.org
3. Ghosh K. Haematology research in India: past, present, and future. Indian J Hematol Blood Transfus. 2011;27(2):55-64.

4. Rao GHR. Contributions of SASAT and ISAR for our understanding of Cardiometabolic disorders. J Clin Prevent Cardiol. 2016;5(2): 67-72.
5. Nelson EJR, Nair SC, Peretz H, Coller BS, Seligsohn U, Chandy M, et al. Diversity of Glanzmann thrombasthenia in southern India: 10 novel mutations identified among 15 unrelated patients. J Thromb Haemost. 2006;4(8):1730-7.
6. Peretz H, Rosenberg N, Landau M, Usher S, Nelson EJ, Mor-Cohen R, et al. Molecular diversity of Glanzmann thrombasthenia in southern India: new insights into mRNA splicing and structure function correlations of alpha 11b beta 3 integrins (*ITGA2B, ITGB3*). Hum Mutat. 2006;27(4):359-69.
7. Sellighson U, Mibashan RS, Rodeck CH, Nicolaides KH, Millar DS, Coller BS. Prenatal diagnosis of Glanzmann's thrombasthenia. Lancet. 1985;2:1419.
8. Srivastava A, Usher S, Nelson EJ, Jayandharan G, Shaji RV, Chandy M, et al. Prenatal diagnosis of Glanzmann thrombasthenia. Natl Med J India. 2003;16(4):207-8.
9. Nurden AT, Pillois X, Fiore M, Alessi MC, Bonduel M, Dreyfus M, et al. Expanding the mutation spectrum affecting alpha 11 beta3 integrin in Glanzmann thrombasthenia: screening of the *ITGA2B* and *ITGB3* genes in a large international cohort. Hum Mutat. 2015;36(5):548-61.
10. White JG. The Chediak-Higashi syndrome: cytoplasmic sequestration in circulating leukocytes. Blood. 1967;29:435-51.
11. White JG. Ultrastructural defects in congenital disorders of platelet function. Ann N Y Acad Sci. 1972;201:205-33.
12. White JG, Gerrard JM. Ultrastructural features of abnormal blood platelets. A review. Am J Pathol. 1976;83(3):589-632.
13. White JG, Gerrard JM. The ultrastructure of defective human platelets. Mol Cell Biochem. 1978;21(2):109-28.
14. White JG. Ultrastructural studies of the gray platelet syndrome. Am J Pathol. 1979;95(2): 445-62.
15. Gerrard JM, Phillips DR, Rao GHR. Biochemical studies of two patients with gray platelet syndrome. Blood. 1979;66:102-9.
16. White JG. Membrane defects in inherited disorders of platelet function. Am J Pediatr Hematol Oncol. 1982;4(1):83-94.
17. White JG. Platelet granule disorders. Crit RevOncol Hematol. 1986;4(4):337-77.
18. White JG. Inherited abnormalities of the platelet membrane and secretory granules. Hum Pathol. 1987;18(2):123-39.
19. White JG. Platelet spherocytosis: a new bleeding disorder. Am J Hematol. 2002;70:158-66.
20. White JG. Electron dense chains and clusters in human platelets. Platelets. 2002;13: 317-25.
21. White JG, Mattson JC, Nichols WL, Luban NL, Greinacher A. A variant of the Sebastian platelet syndrome with unique neutrophil inclusions. Platelets. 2002;13:121-7.
22. White JG. Giant electron dense chains, clusters, and granules in megakaryocytes and platelets with normal dense bodies: an inherited thrombocytopenic disorder. Platelets. 2003;14:109-21.
23. White JG. Giant electron-dense chains, clusters, and granule sin megakaryocytes and platelets with normal dense bodies: an inherited thrombocytopenic disorder 1. Megakaryocytes. Platelets. 2003;14:53-60.
24. White JG. Giant electron dense chains, clusters and granules in megakaryocytes and platelets in normal dense bodies: an inherited thrombocytopenic disorder 111. Platelet analytical electron microscopy. Platelets. 2003;14:305-12.
25. White JG. The White platelet syndrome: a new autosomal dominant platelet disorder. Platelets. 2004;15:173-84.
26. White JG. Medich giant platelet syndrome: a unique alpha granule deficiency 1. Structure abnormalities. Platelets. 2004;15:345-53.
27. White JG. A "touch" of the White platelet syndrome. Platelets. 2005;16:346-61.
28. White JG. Golgi complexes in hypogranular platelet syndromes. Platelets. 2005;26: 51-60.
29. White JG. Localization of lysosomal enzyme in platelets from patients with the White platelet syndrome. Platelets. 2006;17:231-49.
30. White JG. Some contributions of electron microscopy to knowledge of human platelets. Thromb Haemost. 2007;98:69-72.

31. White JG. Platelet pathology in carriers of the X-linked GATA-1 macrothrombocytopenia. Platelets. 2007;18:620-7.
32. White JG. Platelet pathology in sex-linked GATA-1 dyserythropoietic macrothrombocytopenia 11. Cytochemistry. Platelets. 2007;18:436-50.
33. White JG. Electron microscopy methods for studying platelets structure and function. Methods Mol Biol. 2004;272:47-63.
34. White JG. Platelet storage pool deficiency in Jacobsen syndrome. Platelets. 2007;18:522-7.
35. White JG. Alpha-delta platelet storage pool deficiency in three generations. Platelets. 2007;18:1-10.
36. White JG, Burris SM. Cytoskeletons of X-linked GATA-1, G208S macrothrombocytes are deficient in talin. Platelets. 2008;24:543-50.
37. White JG. The York platelet syndrome: a fourth case with unusual pathologic features. Platelets. 2013;24:44-50.
38. White JG. Rapid ultrastructure detection of success or failure after bone marrow transplantation in Chediak-Higashi syndrome. Platelets. 2013;24:71-4.
39. Witkop CJ, Babcok MN, Rao GHR, Gaudier F, Summers CG, Shanahan F, et al. Albinism and Hermansky-Pudlak syndrome in Puerto Rico. Bol Asoc Med P R. 1990;82:333-9.
40. White JG, Edson JR, Desnick SJ, Witkop CJ. Studies of platelets in a variant of the Hermansky-Pudlak syndrome. Am J Pathol. 1971;63(2):319-32.
41. Witkop CJ, Krumwiede M, Sedano H, White JG. Reliability of absent platelet dense bodies as a diagnostic criterion for Hermansky-Pudlak syndrome. Am J Hematol. 1987;26(4):305-11.
42. White JG, Gerrard JM, Rao GHR, Edson JR, Witkop CJ. Differences in platelet storage pool deficiency (SPD) of Hermansky-Pudlak syndrome and non-albinos. Thromb Diath Haemorrh. 1975;34(1):360-1.
43. Rao GHR, Gerrard JM, Witkop CJ, White JG. Platelet aggregation independent of ADP release or prostaglandin synthesis in patients with Hermansky-Pudlak syndrome. Prostaglandins Med. 1981;6(4):459-72.
44. Hermos CR, Huizing M, Kaiser-Kupfer MI, Gahl WA. Hermansky-Pudlak syndrome type1: gene organization, novel mutations, and clinical and molecular review of non-Puerto Rican case. Hum Mutat. 2002;20(6):482.
45. Shotelersuk V, Dell'Angelica EC, Hartnell L, Bonifacino JS, Gahl WA. A new variant of Hermansky-Pudlak syndrome due to mutation in a gene responsible for vesicle formation. Am J Med. 2000;108:423-7.
46. Oh J, Bailin T, Fukaki K, Feng GH, Ho L, Mao JI, et al. Positional cloning of a gene for Hermansky-Pudlak syndrome, a disorder of cytoplasmic organelles. Nat Genet. 1996;14(3):300-6.
47. Snapper SB, Rosen FS. The Wiskott-Aldrich syndrome protein (WASP): roles in signaling and cytoskeletal organization. Annu Rev Immunol. 1999;17:905-29.
48. Kato M, Miki H, Imai K, Nonoyama S, Suzuki T, Sasakawa C, et al. Wiskott-Aldrich syndrome protein induces actin clustering without direct binding to Cdc42. J Biol Chem. 1999;274(38):27225-30.
49. Boztug K, Schmidt M, Schwarger A, Banerjee PP, Díez IA, Dewey RA, et al. Stem-cell gene therapy for wiskott-aldrich syndrome. N Eng J Med. 2010;363:1918-27.
50. Lozano ML, Rivera J, Sanchez I, Vicente V. Towards the targeted management of Chediak-Higashi syndrome. Orphanet J Rare Dis. 2014;9:132
51. Karim MA, Nagle DL, Kandil HH, Bürger J, Moore KJ, Spritz RA. Mutations in the Chediak-Higashi syndrome gene (CHS1) indicate requirement for the complete 3801 amino acid CHS protein. Hum Mol Genet. 1997;6:1087-9.
52. Gerrard JM, Phillips DR, Rao GHR, Plow EF, Walz DA, Ross R, et al. Biochemical studies of two patients with gray platelet syndrome. J Clin Invest. 1980;66:102-9.
53. Sadler JE, Budde U, Eikenboom J, Favaloro EJ, Hill FG, Holmberg L, et al. Update of the pathophysiology and classification of von Willebrand disease: a report of the subcommittee on von Willebrand factor. J Thromb Haemost. 2006;4(10):2103-14.
54. De Jong A, Eikenboom J. Developments in the diagnostic procedures for von Willebrand disease. J Thromb Haemost. 2016;14(3):449-60.
55. Bolton-Maggs PHB, Chalmers EA, Collins PW, Harrison P, Kitchen S, Liesner RJ, et al. A review of inherited platelet disorders with

guidelines for their management on behalf of the UKHCDO. Br J Haematol. 2006;135:603-33.
56. Simon D, Kunicki T, Nugent D. Platelet function defects. Haemophilia. 2008;14:1240-9.
57. Rao AK. Inherited platelet function disorders: overview and disorders of granules, secretion, and signal transduction. Hematol Oncol Clin North Am. 2013;27(3):585-611.
58. Cox K, Price V, Kahr WH. Inherited platelet disorders: a clinical approach to diagnosis and management. Expert Rev Hematol. 2011;4(4):455-72.
59. Weiss HJ. Congenital disorders of platelet function. Semin Hematol. 1980;17(4):228-41.
60. Weiss HJ. Platelet physiology and abnormalities of platelet function (second of two parts). N Engl J Med. 1975;293(12):580-8.
61. Alamelu H, Liesner RI. Modern management of severe platelet function defects. Br J Haematol. 2010;149:813-23.
62. Konkle BA. Acquired disorders of platelet function. Hematology Am Soc Hematol Educ Program. 2011;2011:391-6.
63. Lassila R. Platelet function tests in bleeding disorders. Semin Thromb Hemost. 2016;42(3); 185-90.
64. Weiss HJ. Platelet physiology and abnormalities of platelet function. N Engl J Med. 1975;293:531-41.
65. Rao AK. Congenital disorders of platelet function: disorders of signal transduction and secretion. AM J Med Sci. 1998;316(2):69-76.
66. Rao GHR, White JG. Epinephrine potentiation of arachidonate-induced aggregation of cyclooxygenase-deficient platelets. Am J Hematol. 1981;11(4):355-66.
67. Johnson GJ, Leis LA, Rao GHR, White JG. Arachidonate-induced platelet aggregation in the dog. Thromb Res. 1979;14:147-54.
68. Johnson GJ, Rao GHR, Leis LA, White JG. Effect of agents that alter cyclic AMP on arachidonate-induced platelet aggregation in the dog. Blood. 1980;55:722-9.
69. Johnson GJ. Platelet thromboxane receptors: biology and function. In: Rao GHR (Ed). Handbook of Platelet Physiology and Pharmacology. Boston: Kluwer Academic Publishers; 1999. pp. 38-79.
70. Johnson GJ, Leis LA, Dunlop PC. Specificity of Gαq and Gα11 gene expression in platelets and erythrocytes: expression of cellular differentiation and species differences. Biochem J. 1996;318:1023-31.
71. Grouse LH, Rao GHR, Weiss DJ, Perman V, White JG. Surface-activated bovine platelets do not spread, they unfold. Am J Pathol. 1990;136:399-408.
72. Rao GHR, Escolar G, White JR, Weiss DJ, Burris S, Ordinas A, et al. Differential response of human and bovine platelets to bovine von Willebrand factor and vascular endothelium. Platelets. 2001;12(3):150-5.
73. Weiss DH, McClay CB, Smith CM, Rao GHR, White JG. Platelet function in the racing thoroughbred: implications for exercise-induced pulmonary hemorrhage. Vet Clin Pathol. 1990;19(2):35-9.
74. Einzig S, Noren GR, Staley NA, White JG, Rao GH. Arachidonic acid metabolism in thrombocytes and vascular tissues of turkeys. Prostaglandins. 1985;30(6):999-1017.
75. Hassan AA, Kroll MH. Acquired disorders of platelet function. Hematology Am Soc Hematol Educ Program. 2005:403-8.
76. Casari C, Bergmeier W. Acquired platelet disorders. Thromb Res. 2016;141(2):S73-5.

CHAPTER 4

Platelet Physiology

Blood platelets have a discoid form in their resting state or inactivated state (Fig. 4.1). A circumferential band of microtubules supports shape. This characteristic shape facilitates their movement in the circulating blood at the periphery of the flow close to the vessel wall. Platelets are only about 20% of the diameter of red blood cells (Fig. 4.2). The normal platelet count is 150,000–350,000/µL of blood.

In view of their size, they make up just a tiny fraction of the blood volume. Platelets are produced from large bone marrow cells called megakaryocytes by a process called fragmentation that releases over 1,000 platelets per megakaryocyte. The hormone that controls development of these parent cells is thrombopoietin. As they lack nucleus, they are not considered as true cells but circulating fragments of cells.

They contain many structures that are essential for the performance of their function, arresting bleeding, and repair of the injured vessel. Their shape, weight, and velocity of circulating blood keep them close to the vessel wall. When platelets are stimulated by cell matrix components of the injured blood vessel, they change their shape, extend pseudopods, and spread on the surface of the injured vessel wall as shown in Figures 4.3 to 4.6. Initially, they become round, extend pseudopods to feel the surface of interaction, and spread on the injured surface. Fully spread platelets are seen in the detergent-extracted preparation (Fig. 4.5) with assembled filamentous actin and adhesion points for cell and surface interactions. This is a dynamic process and involves well-orchestrated biochemical events.

They enter the circulation well packaged with all the required cytoskeletal structures, membrane-associated receptors, biochemical components, signaling, and activation mechanisms.[1-12] They are completely nonsticky in their native state in circulating blood.

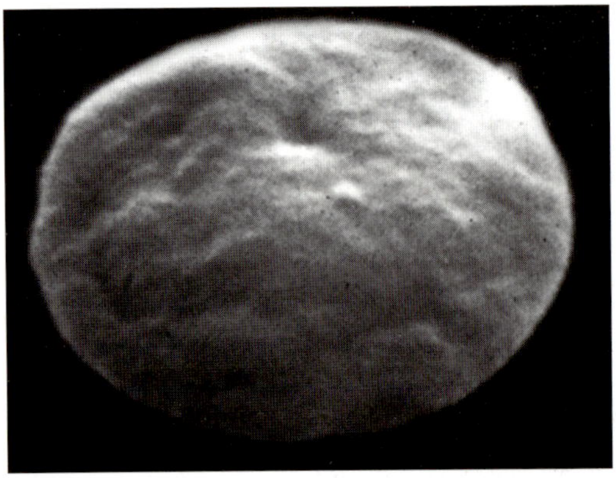

Fig. 4.1: Discoid platelet.

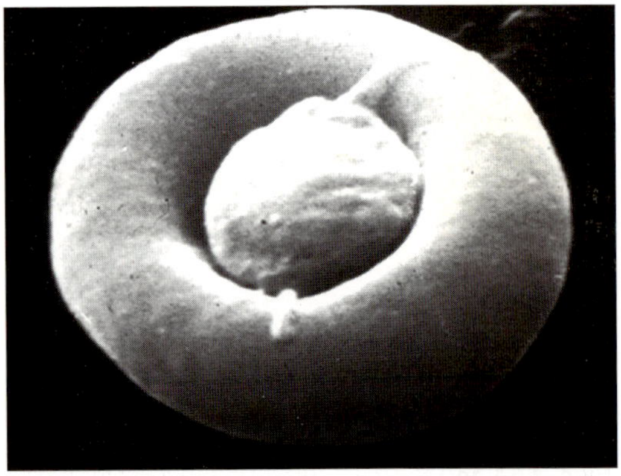

Fig. 4.2: Red blood cell and a platelet.

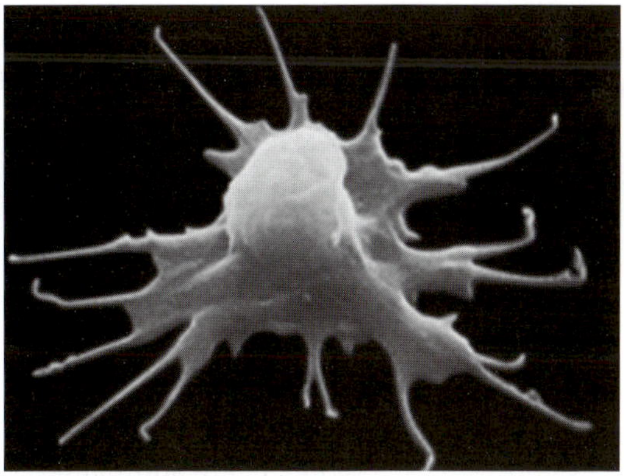

Fig. 4.3: Platelet activation.

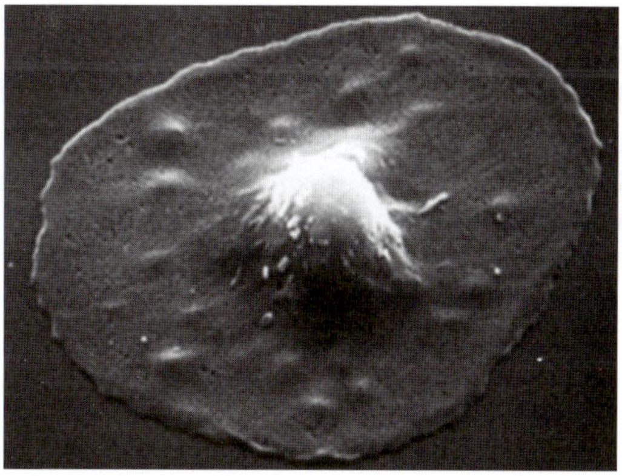

Fig. 4.4: Platelet spreading.

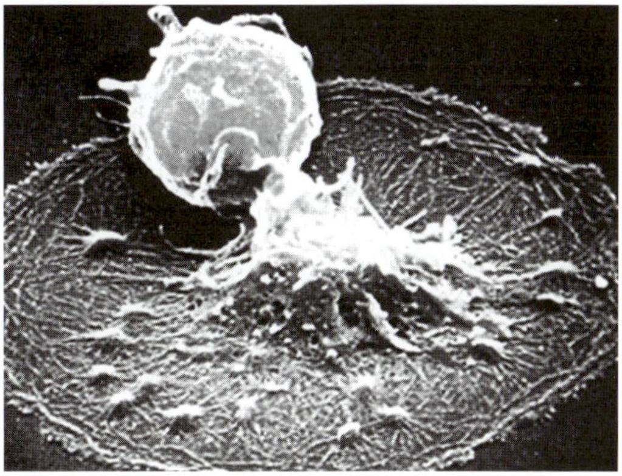

Fig. 4.5: Cell–cell interaction.

They can become sticky with the slightest stimulation. The degree of activation of platelets depends on the strength of the activation stimulus and the information available in the interactive domains of the cell matrix components.[13] The platelet is bestowed with multiple signaling and activation mechanisms.[14,15] Early studies discovered the role of endogenous adenosine diphosphate (ADP) in platelet activation. ADP is stored in high concentrations in dense granules and released from adherent and activated platelets during platelet activation leading to secretion of the granule contents. Serotonin is also stored in platelet granules and is released during

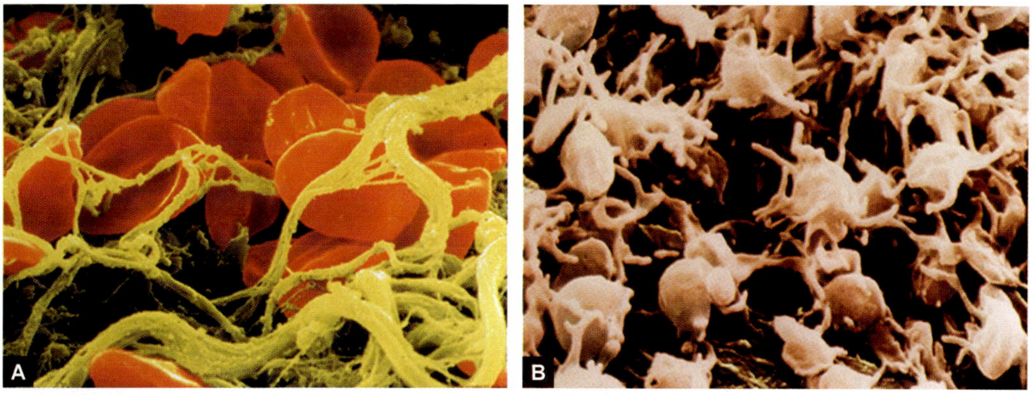

Figs. 4.6A and B: Platelets in circulating blood as well as on injured vessel wall.

platelet activation. Apart from these endogenous agonists, newly formed prostaglandin (PG) endoperoxides (PGG_2, PGH_2) and thromboxanes (TXA_2) also act as potent stimulants. Collagen is a strong thrombogenic substrate. Under high shear force, platelet adhesion is mediated by binding of von Willebrand factor (vWF) immobilized on collagen or on the surface of activated platelets to GPIb. This interaction leads to the activation of GPIIb/IIIa and to stable vWF-mediated aggregates. However, this stimulus seems to be insufficient for stable adhesion. GPVI is the major receptor for collagen, which is necessary for adhesion, aggregation, and degranulation. GPIa acts cooperatively with the major receptor (GPVI) and potentiates the activation process. Thrombin generated endogenously can activate platelets at very low concentrations. It binds the protease-activated receptor (PAR) 1 on the platelet membrane and cleaves a tethered ligand, which binds and activates the receptor. Platelets also express PAR4, which is activated by higher concentration of thrombin.

Ultrastructural as well as biochemical studies have demonstrated ligand binding, receptor activation, and internalization of ligands. Platelet activation promotes accumulation of GPIIb/IIIa at sites in-between activated platelets and between platelets and various surfaces. Ligand binding to integrin and nonintegrin receptors initiates signaling downstream events needed to accomplish various biochemical processes for the generation of second messengers, calcium mobilization, actin assembly, contraction, and secretion of granule contents. These events are in general referred to as "outside-in" signaling. Integrins are composed of extracellular α and β subunits with a cytoplasmic transmembrane tail. The extracellular domain of αIIb subunit consists of a heavy and a light chain. For instance, activation by ADP of $P2Y_{12}$ receptor activates the inactive αIIb β_3 into an active receptor, which can now recognize arginyl-glycyl-aspartate (RGD) tripeptide, the interactive site of fibrinogen. Platelet-membrane glycoprotein (GP) receptors involved in the adhesion and aggregation of platelets include $\alpha_2\beta_1$ (Gpla/IIa) collagen receptor, with recognition amino acid (AA) sequence DGEA; $\alpha_5\beta_1$(GPIc/IIa) fibronectin receptor with recognition AA sequence RGD; $\alpha_6\beta_1$ laminin receptor; $\alpha IIb\beta_3$ (GPIIb/IIIa) Fibrinogen/fibronectin/vWF/vitronectin receptor (RGD); $\alpha v\beta_3$-vitronectn/fibrinogen/fibronectin/vWF (RGD); nonintegrin receptors include GPIb (vWF), and GPIV thrombospondin, collagen (Fig. 4.7).

Integrin $\alpha IIb\beta_3$ is the most abundant of the receptors on platelet membrane. It is also the most thoroughly studied receptor from the point of view of developing antiplatelet therapies. It has a large extracellular domain with a short transmembrane tail. αIIb unit intern has a light chain and a heavy chain with cation-binding sites, which also serve as ligand-binding domains. The β_3 subunit has a cysteine-rich protease-resistant domain, and a ligand-biding domain. For the interaction of integrins with their ligands, to be meaningful for activation, the binding event must be able to regulate signal transduction. Since the integrin-mediated activation is nonenzymatic, signaling is induced by receptor clustering, which increases the avidity of molecular interactions, thereby increasing binding of effector molecules and induction of conformational changes in receptors that create or expose effector-binding sites. It is hard to visualize how a short cytoplasmic tail can convey conformational changes to the large ligand-binding head of the receptor. Extensive studies have been done to monitor the conformational changes and for majority of these studies $\alpha IIb/\beta_3$ has served as the

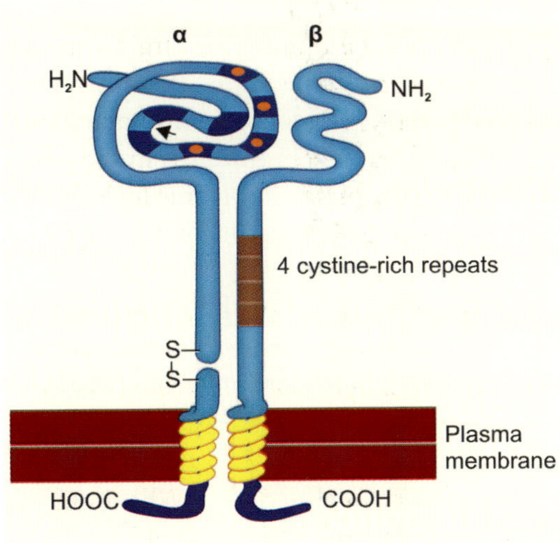

Fig. 4.7: Schematic drawing of a typical integrin dimer.
Source: Lefkovits et al: N Engl J Med. 1995; 332:1553-9.

Collagens	GFOGER	$\alpha_1\beta_1$, $\alpha_2\beta_1$, $\alpha_{10}\beta_1$, $\alpha II\beta_1$
Fibronectin	RGD	$\alpha_5\beta_1$, $\alpha V\beta_3$, $\alpha_8\beta_1$, $\alpha V\beta_1$, $\alpha V\beta_6$, $\alpha IIb\beta_3$
	LDV	$\alpha_4\beta_1$, $\alpha_4\beta_7$
	REDV	$\alpha_4\beta_1$
Laminins	E1′ fragment	$\alpha_1\beta_1$, $\alpha_2\beta_1$, $\alpha_{10}\beta_1$
	E8 fragment	$\alpha_3\beta_1$, $\alpha_6\beta_1$, $\alpha_7\beta_1$, $\alpha_6\beta_4$
Vitronectin	RGD	$\alpha V\beta_3$, $\alpha IIb\beta_3$, $\alpha V\beta_5$, $\alpha V\beta_1$, $\alpha V\beta_8$
Fibrinogen	RGD	$\alpha V\beta_3$
	KQAGDV	$\alpha IIb\beta_3$
von Willebrand factor	RGD	$\alpha IIb\beta_3$, $\alpha V\beta_3$

prototype.[16-19] Although process of integrin activation and ligand binding is understood well at structural level, not much is known about outside-in signaling at the molecular level. Furthermore, studies from our laboratory have demonstrated that the bound fibrinogen to $\alpha IIb/\beta_3$ receptors can be dissociated by lowering cytosolic calcium.[20,21] The process of inactivation, where integrins return to resting state is not known.

The realization that the $\alpha IIb/\beta_3$ integrin mediates the binding of platelets to one another and thus promotes aggregation, thrombus formation and growth, prompted many researchers, to look at this mechanism of platelet activation as a possible area of interest for developing antiplatelet drugs. Researchers from the laboratory of Professor Barry Coller played a major role in the development of monoclonal antibodies for inhibiting $\alpha IIb/\beta_3$-dependent platelet aggregation.[22] Three such $\alpha IIb\beta_3$ antagonists, abciximab, eptifibatide, and tirofiban have received approval of the Food and Drug Administration (FDA) as antiplatelet drugs.[23-27] These $\alpha IIb\beta_3$ antagonists are still widely used for the prevention of periprocedural thrombosis, during percutaneous coronary interventions (PCI). In spite of the success of these antagonists, they cannot be used for secondary prevention of acute coronary events. Aspirin and clopidogrel have been the choice for such prevention strategies. Though these drugs have demonstrated significant clinical benefit, residual morbidity and mortality remain high. In view of these observations, it is felt that antiplatelet therapies that provide more complete inhibition of platelet activation without increases in bleeding risk could considerably decrease residual risk for ischemic events.[28]

Platelet activation by ADP is mediated by two G-protein–coupled receptors, $P2Y_1$ (G_q) and $P2Y_{12}$ (G_{i2}). ADP-mediated activation of $P2Y_1$ receptor leads to the shape change, $P2Y_1$ stimulation leads to the activation of phospholipase C

(PLC) pathway and calcium mobilization, and aggregation of platelets. ADP-mediated activation of $P2Y_{12}$, on the other hand, works through two different mechanisms. α_1 subunit mediates the activation of adenylyl cyclase, protein kinase, and phosphorylation of vasodilator-stimulated phosphoprotein (VASP-P), which leads to the activation of GPIIb/IIIa receptor. On the other hand, the βy subunit by another independent mechanism (via PI3K and Akt1/Akt2) induces dense granule secretion and potentiates aggregation of platelets.[29-31] Jin et al. have demonstrated the presence of two distinct G-protein–coupled receptors on platelets; one coupled to PLC, $P2Y_1$, and the other to inhibition of adenylyl cyclase $P2T_{AC}$.[31] Active metabolite of clopidogrel, an antagonist of ADP-induced aggregation of platelets acts on these receptors. Intraplatelet VASP phosphorylation assay is used for the monitoring of clopidogrel resistance.[32,33]

Thromboxane (TXA) is the final proaggregatory metabolite of substrate arachidonic acid (AA). It is formed via prostaglandin endoperoxide intermediates (PGG_2 and PGH_2) by a specific synthase. Pharmacological studies indicate that TXA receptors in platelets are linked to phospholipase C activation via pertussis toxin–sensitive G proteins. Suggested candidates include, 42 kD G_q and the 60 kD G_e. Thromboxane acts as an amplifying signal for platelet agonist and the response to this eicosanoid is tightly controlled.[34] Offerman et al. have provided evidence to show that G proteins, G_{12} and G_{13} play a functional role in transmembrane signal transduction and suggest that both proteins are involved in pathways leading to platelet activation.[35,36]

Thrombin is the most potent agonist of platelet activation. Thrombin-induced platelet activation involves cleavage of PARs 1 and 4, interaction via GPIbα, with the platelet GPIb/IX/V complex. Glycoprotein Ib belongs to the so-called leucine-rich repeats (LRR) family of proteins. Thrombin is supposed to cleave its receptor's amino-terminal extension to create a new receptor amino terminus, which functions as a tethered ligand and activates the receptor.[37] Thrombin, a protease acts through an unusual proteolytically activated G-protein–coupled receptor.[38] This receptor is designated as PAR3. This receptor mediates thrombin-triggered phosphoinositide hydrolysis needed for formation of second messengers, inositol trisphosphate and diglyceride.

Platelet collagen interaction can be classified into two categories: primary adhesion and secondary reinforcing adhesion. Monomeric and fibrillar collagens support platelet adhesion. Triple-helical structure of collagen and the polymerization of the monomeric collagen are required for collagen-induced platelet aggregation and secretion. GPVI is a platelet membrane protein with a molecular weight of 62 kDa that is identified as a physiological collagen receptor.[39] The GPVI-induced activation mechanism is initiated by tyrosine phosphorylation of the immunoreceptor tyrosine-based activation motif (ITAM) of the FcR-gamma chain and many related proteins transduce the signal. Two prominent receptors, glycoprotein Ia/IIa or integrin $\alpha_2\beta_1$ and glycoprotein VI are associated with intracellular signaling in collagen-mediated platelet activation.[40]

Blood platelets interact with a variety of soluble agonists, such as epinephrine and adenosine diphosphate, many insoluble cell matrix components, including collagen, laminin, and biomaterials used for the construction of invasive medical devices. These interactions stimulate specific receptors and glycoprotein-rich domains (integrins and nonintegrins) on the plasma membrane and lead to the activation of intracellular effector enzymes. The majority of the regulatory events appear to require free calcium. Ionized calcium is the primary bioregulator, and a variety of biochemical mechanisms modulate the level and availability of free cytosolic calcium. Major enzymes that regulate the free calcium levels via second messengers include phospholipase C, phospholipase A_2, and phospholipase D, together with adenylyl and guanylyl cyclases. Activation of phospholipase C results in the hydrolysis of phosphatidyl inositol 4, 5 bisphosphate and formation of second messengers 1, 2 diacylglycerol (DAG) and inositol 1, 4, 5 trisphosphate (IP_3). Diglyceride induces activation of protein kinase C, whereas IP_3 mobilizes calcium from internal membrane stores. Elevation of cytosolic calcium stimulates phospholipase A_2 and liberates arachidonic acid. Free arachidonic acid is transformed to a novel metabolite, thromboxane A_2 by fatty acid synthetase (Cox-1, cyclooxygenase). Thromboxane A_2 is the major metabolite of this pathway and plays a critical role in platelet recruitment, granule mobilization, and secretion. Secretory granules contain a variety of growth factors, mitogens, and inflammatory mediators. Secretion of granules promotes P-selectin expression on the platelet membrane. Furthermore, activation also promotes the expression of acidic lipids on the membrane and tissue factor expression, thus making these cells procoagulant. Fully activated platelets can modulate the function of other circulating blood cells such as leukocytes, monocytes, macrophages, as well as vascular endothelial cells. Agonist-mediated stimulation of platelets promotes the expression of an epitope on glycoprotein IIb/IIIa receptors. Activation of this receptor is essential for the binding of circulating fibrinogen. Fibrinogen forms a bridge between individual platelets and facilitates the thrombus formation. vWF binds platelet GPIbIX complex only at high shear rate unlike fibrinogen, which can bind platelets at low shear. Upregulation in signaling pathways will increase the risk for clinical complications associated with acute coronary events. Downregulation of signal transduction mechanisms may precipitate bleeding diathesis or stroke.

Most soluble agonists, such as ADP, epinephrine, TXA_2, and thrombin-trigger platelet activation through G-protein–coupled receptors (GPCRs). Simulation of these receptors increases cytosolic calcium and activates specific signaling pathways. ADP released from the platelets as well as damaged endothelial cells and erythrocytes activate platelet $P2Y_1$, $P2Y_{12}$, and GPCRs. Thrombin is the most potent agonist and is responsible for converting fibrinogen to fibrin to stabilize hemostatic plugs.

Platelet activation in suspension (circulating blood) or on surfaces is a dynamic process and involves energy consumption, proteolysis, cytoskeletal reorganization, calcium mobilization, contraction, secretion of granule contents, and irreversible aggregation. Some of these events will be discussed in detail in subsequent chapters. Secretion of platelet granule contents and other products generated during activation can be monitored by the analysis of the supernatant plasma or buffers used.[41-46] Binding between platelets and other cell types is primarily mediated by P selectin (CD36), released from α granules to the cell surface. Activated platelets also express CD40L (CD154). Soluble CD40 can induce vascular cells to express E selectin and P selectin and release interleukin (IL) 6. Platelet factor 4 is one of the abundant proteins of the α granules. Majority of platelet activation markers can be assayed with the enzyme-linked immunosorbent assay (ELISA) or Western blot. Flow cytometer also can be used for monitoring platelet activation

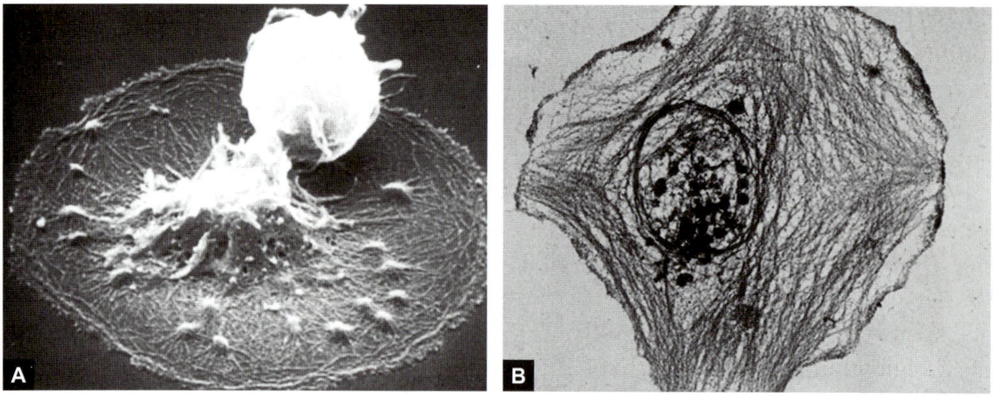

Figs. 4.8A and B: Detergent-insoluble cytoskeleton of spread platelets.

markers on single platelets. Platelets contain at least three types of granules: α-granules, dense granules, and lysosomes. Granule contents include coagulation factors, angiogenic factors, adhesion molecules, cytokines, and chemokines. α-Granules are the most abundant of the storage granules in platelets. They contain adhesive glycoproteins, fibrinolytic inhibitors, immunoglobulins, P selectin, and various chemokines. Dense granules contain catecholamines, such as histamine, serotonin, ADP, adenosine triphosphate (ATP), and calcium.

Various platelet activation pathways as well as biochemical events that support these pathways are intimately coupled with energy metabolism. It has been shown that turnover of cytoplasmic ATP is higher in platelets than in most other cells. According to Holmsen, one-third of the total adenine nucleotides are present in the cytoplasm.[47] Fifty percent of the ADP is bound to the actin and as such is not available for use in metabolic activities. Holmsen and associates monitored energy requirements for various platelet functions. Results of their study showed that various activation responses have different energy requirements, increasing in order: aggregation, < α granule and dense granule secretion < acid hydrolase secretion, phosphatidylinositol breakdown, phosphatidate formation, and arachidonate liberation.[48]

In addition to the energy requirement, platelet activation also requires active participation of actin and actin-binding proteins. Actin represents about fifth of the total platelet proteins. Studies have demonstrated that half of actin in resting platelets is in unpolymerized form stored as 1:1 complex with β_4 thymosin and profilin. Detergent-insoluble cytoskeleton of the resting blood platelet seems to contain 2,000 actin filaments/μm in length (Figs. 4.8A and B).

Activation of platelets by contact with glass (Figs. 4.3 to 4.5) shows within 30 seconds a doubling of polymerized actin content in the cytoskeleton. According to researchers active in this field, the membrane skeleton of the resting platelets is a spectrin-based shell directly attached to the ends of actin filaments and indirectly attached to the same filaments by actin-binding protein molecules connecting GPIb/IX complexes.[49] Various manifestations of platelet activation are achieved by reorganization of components of the contractile system and microtubular systems. Elevated cytosolic calcium triggers the actin–myosin interaction and the developing force. Anchoring of the contractile fibers to membranes is crucial for the platelet contractile manifestations.[50]

So far, we have covered platelet morphology, ultrastructure, membrane systems, glycoprotein-rich transmembrane domains, and their role in platelet physiology and activation. During activation, platelets develop a number of distinguishable structural elements including a delimited plasma membrane; invaginations of the surface membrane that form the open canalicular system (OCS); a closed-channel network of residual endoplasmic reticulum that form the dense tubular system (DTS); a spectrin-based membrane skeleton; an actin-based cytoskeletal network; a peripheral band of microtubules; and numerous organclles including α granules, dense granules, peroxisomes, lysosomes, and mitochondria. Platelet can become sticky and adhere to surfaces or to each other without contracting or secreting granule contents. Similarly, shape change and internal contraction can develop to a limited degree (reversible phase of activation). Despite the wealth of knowledge developed in recent years, considerable confusion exists in our efforts to fit all pieces of the platelet activation puzzle together, to a chain of events to the way platelet responds to all stimuli.

Various agonists, which stimulate platelets to develop shape change and stickiness, also trigger a process of internal reorganization in platelets. Storage organelles are shifted from their random locations to cell centers where they are enclosed within a close-fitting ring of microfilaments and microtubules (Fig. 4.8B). The process of internal transformation in platelets closely resembles contractile events in smooth muscle cells. This original observation by White and associates has led to a variety of ultrastructural and biochemical studies to define the contractile nature of internal transformation of platelets during activation.[49-52] Platelets contain substantial quantities of muscle proteins including actin, myosin, tropomyosin, α actinin, actin-binding proteins, filamin, and troponin.[53-55] Some of these proteins are associated with surface membranes and majority to the interior of the cell. Studies have demonstrated the regulatory roles of energy metabolism and cytosolic calcium in platelet activation. Morphological, cytochemical, and biochemical studies have demonstrated that platelets contain dual membrane systems identical to the sarcoplasmic reticulum of smooth muscle cells. The specific organization of the muscular system in platelets facilitates granule mobilization, the extrusion of secreted products, the contraction of aggregates, and thrombus. Various phases of activation are orchestrated by a variety of cytoskeletal rearrangements and biochemical events. Events leading to receptor-mediated, G-protein–coupled activation, phosphoinositide metabolism, formation of second messengers, activation of phospholipase A_2, cell-surface interaction, biocompatibility, and antiplatelet therapies will be described in subsequent chapters.

REFERENCES

1. Marcus AJ, Zucker MB. The Physiology of Blood Platelets. New York: Crune and Stratton; 1965. p. 162.
2. Caen J. Platelet Aggregation. Paris: Masson and Cie; 1971. p. 228.
3. Brinkhous KM, Sherman RW, Mostof FK. The Platelet. Baltimore: Williams and Wilkinson Co; 1971. p. 420.
4. Johnson SA. The Circulating Platelet. New York: Academic Press; 1971.
5. Weiss HJ. Platelets and their role in hemostasis. Ann N Y Acad Sci. 1972;201:1-450.
6. Ciba Foundation. Biochemistry and Pharmacology of Platelets. New York: Elsevier; 1975. p. 352.

7. Caen JP, Cronberg S, Kubisz P. Platelet Physiology and Pathology. New York: Stratton Intercontinental Medical Book Co. 1977. p. 136.
8. de Gaetano G, Garattini S. Platelets: A Multidisciplinary Approach. New York: Raven Press; 1977. p. 485.
9. Kwan HC, Bowie EJW. Thrombosis. Philadelphia: W.B. Saunders; 1982. p. 331.
10. Rao GHR. Handbook of Platelet Physiology and Pharmacology. Boston: Kluwer Academic Publishers; 1999. p. 553.
11. Phillips DR, Shuman MA. Biochemistry of Platelets. New York: Academic Press; 1986. p. 462.
12. Michelson AD. Platelets. New York: Academic Press; 2012. p. 1353.
13. Nachman RL. Thrombosis and atherogenesis: molecular connections. Blood. 1992;79: 1897-906.
14. Seiss W. Molecular mechanisms of platelet activation. Pharmacol Rev. 1989;69:59-178.
15. Zucker MB, Nachmias VT. Platelet activation. Arteriosclerosis. 1985;5:2-18.
16. Campbell ID, Humphries MJ. Integrin structure, activation and interactions. Cold Spring Harb Perspect Biol. 2011;3:a004994.
17. Plow EF, Haas Ta, Zhang L, Loftus J, Smith JW. Ligand binding to integrins. J Biol Chem. 275: 21785-8.
18. Ruoslahti E. Integrins. J Clin Invest. 1991; 87:1-4.
19. Ruoslahti E, Pierschbacher ND. New perspectives in cell adhesion: RGD and Integrins. Science. 1987;238:491-7.
20. Rao GHR, White JG. Disaggregation and reaggregation of irreversibly aggregated platelets: a method for complete evaluation of antiplatelet drugs. Agents Actions 1985;16:425-34.
21. Cox AC, Caroll RC, White JG, Rao GHR. Recycling of platelet phosphorylation and cytoskeletal assembly. J Cell Biol. 1984;98:8-15.
22. Coller BS, Peerschke EI, Scudder LE, Sullivan CA. A murine monoclonal antibody that completely blocks the binding of fibrinogen to platelets produces a thrombasthenic-like state in the normal platelets and binds to glycoprotiens11b and 111a. J Clin Invest. 1983;72:325-38.
23. Plow EF, Pierschbacher MD, Rusolahti E, Marguerie GA, Ginsberg MH. The effect of Arg-Gly-Asp-containing peptides on fibrinogen and von Willebrand factor binding to platelets. Proc Natl Acad Sci U S A. 1985;82:8057-61.
24. Hynes RO. Integrins: a family of cell surface receptors. Cell. 1987;48:549-54.
25. Hynes RO. Integrins: versatility, modulation, and signaling in cell adhesion. Cell. 1992;69:11-25.
26. Shatill SJ, Kim C, Ginzberg MH. The final steps of integrin activation: the end game. Nat Rev Mol Cell Biol. 2103;11:288-300.
27. Bledzka K, Smyth SS, Plow EF. Integrin αIIbβ3: from discovery to efficacious therapeutic target. Circ Res. 2103;112:1189-1200.
28. Jennings LK. Mechanisms of platelet activation: need for new strategies to protect against platelet-mediated atherothrombosis. Thromb Haemost. 2009;102:248-57.
29. Daniel JL, Dangelmaier C, Jin J, Ashby B, Smith JB, Kunapuli SP. Molecular basis for ADP-induced activation: evidence for three distinct ADP receptors on human platelets. J Biol Chem. 1998;273(4):2024-9.
30. Jin J, Daniel JL, Kunapuli SP. Molecular basis of ADP-induced platelet activation 11. The P2Y1 receptor mediates ADP-induced intracellular calcium mobilization and shape change in platelets. J Biol Chem. 1998;273(4): 2030-4.
31. Jin J, Kunapuli SP. Coactivation of two different G protein-coupled receptors is essential for ADP-induced platelet aggregation. Proc Natl Acad Sci U S A. 1998;95(14):8070-4.
32. Aleil B, Ravanat C, Cazenave JP, Rochoux G, Heitz A, Gachet C. Flow cytometric analysis of Intraplatelet VASP phosphorylation for the detection of clopidogrel resistance in patients with ischemic cardiovascular diseases. J Thromb Haemost. 2005;3(1):85-92.
33. Bidet A, Jais C, Puymirat E, Coste P, Nurden A, Jakubowski J, et al. VerifyNow and VASP phosphorylation assays give similar results for patients receiving clopidogrel, but they do not always correlate with platelet aggregation. Platelets. 2012;21:94-100.
34. FitzGerald GA. Mechanisms of platelet activation: thromboxane A2 as an amplifying signal for other agonists. Am J Cardiol. 1991;68(7):B11-5.
35. Offerman S, Laugwitz K, Spicher K, Schultz G. G protein of the G12 family are activated via thromboxane A2 and thrombin receptors

in human platelets. Proc Natl Acad Sci U S A. 1994;91:504-8.

36. Offerman S. Activation of platelet function through G protein-coupled receptors. Circ Res. 2006;99:1293-304.
37. VU TH, Hung DT, Wheaton VI, Coughlin SR. Molecular cloning of a functional thrombin receptor reveals a novel proteolytic mechanism for receptor activation. Cell. 1991;64(6):1057-68.
38. Ishihara H, Connolly AJ, Zeng D, Kahn ML, Zheng YW, Timmons C, et al Protease-activated receptor 3 is a second thrombin receptor in humans. Nature. 1997;386:502-6.
39. Moroi M, Jung SM. Platelet glycoprotein V1: its structure and function. Thromb Res. 2004;114(4):221-33.
40. Surin WR, Barthwal MK, Dikshit M. Platelet collagen receptors, signaling and antagonism: emerging approaches for the prevention of intravascular thrombosis. Thromb Res. 2008;122(6):786-803.
41. Rao GHR, White JG, Jachimowicz AA, Witkop CJ. Nucleotide profiles of normal and abnormal platelets by high-pressure liquid chromatography. J Lab Clin Med. 1974;84:839-50.
42. Rao GHR, White JG, Jachimowicz AA, Witkop CJ. An improved method for the extraction of endogenous serotonin. J. Lab Clin Med. 1976;87:129-37.
43. Rao GHR, Peller JD, White JG. Rapid separation of platelet nucleotides by reverse-phase isocratic high-pressure liquid chromatography with a rapidly compressed column. J Chromatography. 1981;226:466-70.
44. Flaumenhaft R, Dilks JR, Rozenvayan N, Monahan-Earley RA, Feng D, Dvorak AM.The actin cytoskeleton differentially regulates platelet α-granule and dense-granule secretion. Blood. 2005;105:3879-87.
45. Brass L. Understanding and evaluating platelet functions. Hematology Am Soc Hematol Educ Program. 2010;2010:387-96.
46. Yun S, Sim E, Goh RI, Park JI, Han JY. Platelet activation: the mechanisms and potential biomarkers. Biomed Res Int. 2016;2016:9060143.
47. Holmsen H. Platelet metabolism and activation. Semin Hematol. 1985;22(3):219-40.
48. Holmsen H, Kaplan KL, Dangelmaier CA. Differential energy requirements for platelet response. A simultaneous study of aggregation, three secretory processes, arachidonate liberation, phosphatidylinositol breakdown and phosphatide production. Biochem J. 1982;208(1):9-18.
49. Hartwig JH. Mechanism of actin rearrangements mediating platelet activation. J Cell Biol. 1992;118:1421-42.
50. Cohen I. The contractile system of blood platelets and its function. Methods Avhiev Exp Pathol. 1979;9:40-86.
51. Pollard TD, Fujiwara, Handin R, Weiss G. Contractile proteins in platelet activation and contraction. Ann NY Acad Sci USA. 1996;283:218-36.
52. Stossel TP. Contractile proteins in cell structure and function. Ann Rev Med. 1978;129:427-57.
53. White, JG, Rao GHR, Gerrard JM. Platelet stimulus activation contraction secretion coupling: a frequently fractured chain of events. In: Mann KG, Taylor FB (Eds). The Regulation of Coagulation. North Holland: Elsevier; 1980.
54. Rao GHR. Signal transduction second messengers and platelet function. J Lab Clin Med. 1993;121:18-20.
55. Rao GHR. Signal transduction, second messengers and platelet pharmacology. Pharmacol. 1994;13:39-44.

CHAPTER 5

Platelet Activation Mechanisms

INTRODUCTION

What is platelet activation? Is tethered adherence of platelets to laminin an activation process? Can we consider binding of ligand to the receptor an activation process? Is expression of an epitope on $\alpha IIb\beta_3$ receptor or change in the configuration of the extracellular ligand-binding sites of the receptor an activation? We can go on asking very many questions, as we do not fully understand the chain of events that underlie various stages or phases of activation. For instance, others and we have described early phase of platelet activation as development of stickiness. In reality, they do not become sticky at all. They adhere to surfaces or to other cells via molecules that are meant for eliciting such reactions. Adhesion can be defined as a platelet activation process where insoluble high-molecular-weight proteins with repetitive structures (collagens, fibronectins, laminins, vitronectin) or surfaces normally in contact with the platelets act as agonists and trigger platelet activation. If one looks at platelet interaction on a denuded endothelium, one can see platelets in various stages of activation (Fig. 5.1). Platelets upon activation change shape, extend pseudopods, feel the surface of interaction, adhere, spread, secrete granule contents to promote the formation of hemostatic plug, and express adhesion molecules.

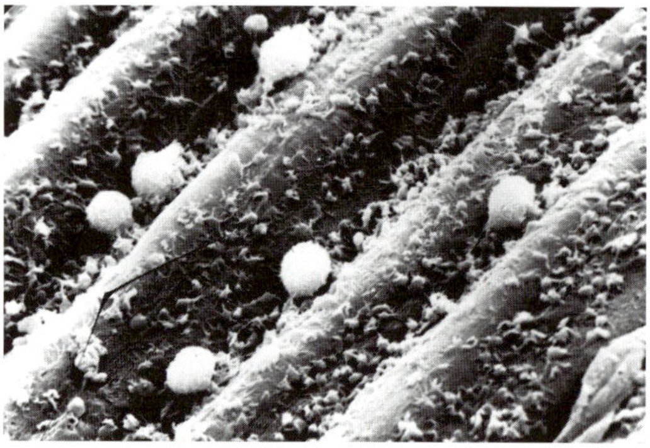

Fig. 5.1: Platelet interaction with injured vessel wall.

In the early days of our research, we used nonphysiological agonists, such as calcium ionophore A23187 and phorbol myristate (PMA) ester to study the mechanism of platelet activation.[1-3] Wte demonstrated that A23187 was able to trigger platelet activation by moving calcium across the membranes and increasing the cytosolic calcium levels. On the other hand, phorbol ester induced selective localization of storage granules resulting in their conversion to distended vacuoles. We also have studied shear-induced platelet activation in flow conditions.[4] What is of great interest to platelet researchers is the fact that no matter how the platelets are activated, the structural changes and biochemical events that follow activation process seem to be common. In view of this observation, in the next few chapters we will discuss common biochemical events that underlie the activation pathways.

SIGNALING PATHWAYS VIA GTP-BINDING PROTEIN–COUPLED RECEPTORS

Soluble agonists, such as thrombin, adenosine diphosphate (ADP), epinephrine, and thromboxane act via G-protein-coupled receptors and initiate the process of activation (Fig. 5.2). GTP-binding proteins (G proteins) act as transducers between seven transmembrane domain receptors and a variety of enzymes and ion channels. In general, G-proteins are made up of three polypeptides: an α subunit of about 39–52 kDa that binds and hydrolyzes GTP, and β and γ subunits of 35–36 kDa and 5–8 kDa, respectively that form a dimeric complex.

According to researchers β and γ subunits are highly conserved while α subunit is different for each G protein. In resting platelets, the α subunit contains a bound GDP and forms an inactive heterodimer with β and γ subunits. When an agonist binds to a G-protein-coupled receptor, it becomes activated and changes its conformation. The subunit

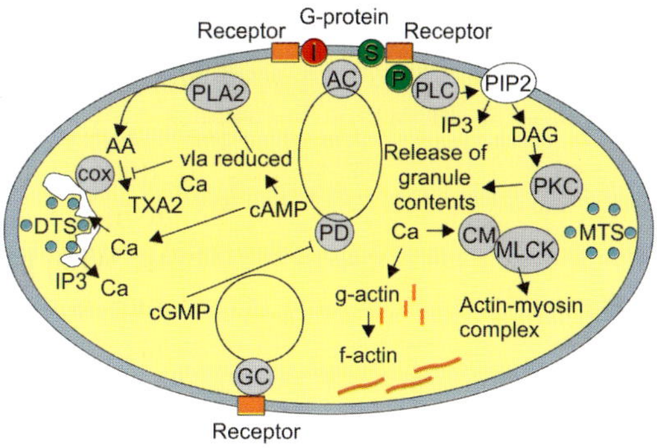

Fig. 5.2: Platelet structure and activation mechanisms.

responds with a conformational change leading to the exchange of its bound GDP for GTP and dissociation of the α-GTP complex from the β-γ complex. The free α-GTP and β-γ subunits each can activate effector enzymes. GTP is hydrolyzed to GDP by the intrinsic GTPase activity of the α subunit.

Over 20 different G-protein α subunits have been identified and divided into four classes based on the amino acid sequences ($G\alpha_s$, $G\alpha_{i3}$, $G\alpha_q$, $G\alpha_{i2}$).[5-8] They are made up of three polypeptides: an α subunit of about 39–52 kDa that binds and hydrolyzes GTP, and β and γ subunits of 35–36 kDa and 5–8 kDa, respectively that form a dimeric complex. Platelet activation via G-protein–coupled receptors involves three major G-protein–mediated signaling pathways that are initiated by the activation of the G proteins, G_q, G_{13}, G_i.[7] According to researchers, the initial interaction of platelets with extracellular matrix (ECM) under high shear and subsequent activation involves the platelet von Willebrand factor (vWF) receptor GPIb/V/IX and the collagen receptor GPVI. This receptor forwards the activation signal via FcRy chain, which induces intracellular signaling process, promoting inside-out activation of integrins such as $\alpha 11b\beta_3$ (GPIIb/IIIa) or $\alpha 2\beta_1$ (GP (Ia/IIa). Interaction of activated integrins with ECM mediates the adhesion of platelets to the injured wall, resulting a monolayer of adherent platelets. The recruitment of additional platelets is mediated by a variety of locally produced or accumulating mediators. These mediators include ADP/ATP, epinephrine, thrombin, and thromboxane. These diffusible mediators act via G-protein–coupled receptors (GPCRs).

Platelet activation by ADP, an endogenous agonist is mediated by three different GPCRs,

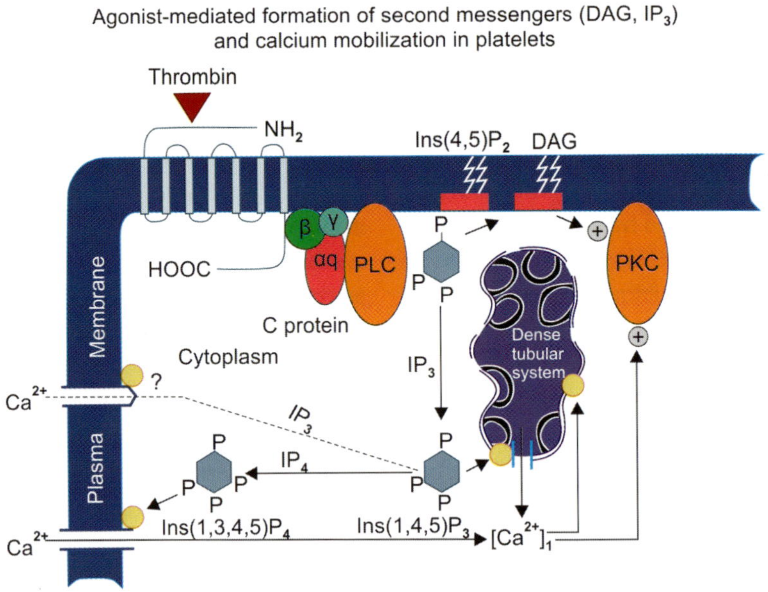

Fig. 5.3: Agonist-mediated activation of G-protein–coupled receptors.

$P2Y_1$ and $P2Y_{12}$. The $P2Y_1$ receptor couples with Gq, $P2Y_{12}$ is coupled with G_i-type of G proteins (G_{i2}). It seems activation of both these receptors are essential to elicit full response of platelets to ADP. Platelet response to low and medium concentrations of thrombin and TXA_2 are reduced in the absence of ADP receptors, suggesting the potentiating action ADP-mediated stimulation. $P2Y_{12}$ receptor is irreversibly inhibited by thienopyridines, such as clopidogrel, a well-known antiplatelet drug. Thrombin formation occurs on cellular surfaces including on the surface of activated platelets. Activation of platelets by this agonist is mediated by protease-activated receptors (PARs), which in turn are coupled to G_q, G_{12}, G_{13}, and G_i family of G-protein receptors. Of the four PARs, PAR1 and PAR4 are present on human platelets. Like ADP, serotonin, epinephrine, TXA_2 functions as a feedback mediator of platelet activation. Thromboxane receptor (TR) is also activated by PG endoperoxides, PGG_2 and PGH_2. TR is coupled to G-protein receptors: G_q, G_{12}, and G_{13}. Epinephrine is known to potentiate the action of other agonists by acting through the α_{2a}-adrenergic receptor. This receptor in platelets is coupled to G_i-type G protein, G_z. Serotonin also serves back as a positive feedback potentiator by activating 5-hydroxytryptamine 2A receptors on platelets, which are G_q coupled. Various chemokines, lysophospholipids, platelet-activating factor also activate platelets via specific receptors. Activation of platelets by chemokines seems to play an important role in the development of atherosclerotic vascular disease.[7]

Agonist-mediated activation of surface membrane G-protein receptors results in the activation of phospholipase (PLCb) through G_q, which induces the formation of inositol trisphosphate and diacylglycerol (DAG) (Fig. 5.3). Inositol trisphosphate (IP_3) mobilizes cytosolic calcium. Activation of protein kinase C (PKC) by DAG and phorbol esters activates $\alpha 11b\beta_3$ receptors.

PHOSPHOINOSITIDE METABOLISM AND PLATELET ACTIVATION

Since the time (1953) Hokin and Hokin recognized the importance of phosphoinositides in cell-signaling events, there is an explosion of studies on the role of phosphoinositols in cell-signaling pathways.[8-14] There are at least 6 well-recognized inositol phospholipids and more than 20 soluble inositol phosphates in cells. Inositol phosphatases are similar to protein phosphatases, in the sense that they inhibit or terminate cellular-signaling reactions. The major phosphatases that were studied in early days of inositol research were those that hydrolyze 1, 4, 5-trisphosphate (ins-1,4,5-P_3) to inositol 1, 4-bisphosphate (ins-1,4-P_2/PIP_2). The classical pathway transforms phosphatidylinositol to phosphatidylinositol bisphosphate (PI-4, 5-P_2/PIP_2) by the action of PI-4 kinases and PI-4-p5 kinases. PIP_2 is the precursor for second messengers, phosphatidylinositol 1, 4, 5-trisphosphate (PIP_3/IP_3) and DAG. Phosphoinositide signaling enzymes are directly associated with membrane receptors. These signaling enzymes include tyrosine kinases, isoforms of PI_3 kinases and phospholipase C.

This family of enzymes (PLC) utilizes PI-4, 5-P_2 (PIP_2) for the generation of second messengers (Fig. 5.4). PIP_2 can also modulate the activity and assembly or disassembly of actin filaments. In addition to the classical G-protein-coupled PLC-mediated inositol-signaling pathway in platelets, some studies have demonstrated the existence of a tyrosine phosphorylation-dependent pathway to activate PLC.[15] In these studies, it was shown that thrombin-induced platelet aggregation as well as secretion of granules could be inhibited by tyrphostin, a specific inhibitor of tyrosine kinase.

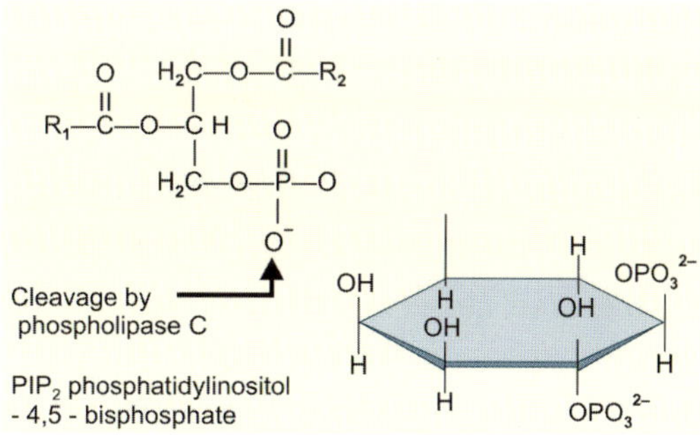

Fig. 5.4: Phospholipase C (PLC) activation and second messenger generation.

LIPID PHOSPHATE PHOSPHATASES AND PLATELET ACTIVATION

Lysophosphatic acid (LPA) and sphingosine 1-phosphate (S1P) are present in biological fluids and activate cells though families of GPCRs.[16-21] These receptors are coupled through $G_{\alpha i}$ that lowers cAMP concentrations, $G_{12/13}$ that stimulates phospholipase D (PLD), and G_q that activates PLC and protein kinases. Enzymes that synthesize or degrade lipid phosphates can modulate many aspects of signaling that are involved in cell division, apoptosis, inflammation, adhesiveness, and migration. Two classes of phosphatidate phosphatases have been studied PAP1 and PAP2. PAP2 is relatively nonspecific for its lipid phosphate substrates since it dephosphorylates LPA, S1P, ceramide-i-phosphate (CIP), and DAG phosphates in addition to phosphatidic acid (PA). The LPPs possess three conserved active site domains and six transmembrane domains. They are expressed on surface membranes as well as internal membranes and control availability of lipid phosphates for signaling events. The phosphatases can control signaling by attenuating the effects of the lipid phosphates and by forming products such as DAG, sphingosine, and ceramide that are also bioactive. Ectophosphatase (e-LPPs) activities of LPPs could thus decrease the activation of PA and S1P receptors and can also promote their uptake into the cell of the dephosphorylated products. Intracellular signaling by DAG, sphingosine, and ceramides can be increased by the e-LPPs. These products can also be rephosphorylated inside the cells to modulate additional signaling events.

PROTEIN PHOSPHORYLATIONS AND PLATELET ACTIVATION

By and large, agonist-mediated stimulation of specific receptors initiate a series of signaling mechanisms leading to the mobilization of cytosolic calcium as well as phosphorylation of certain proteins. In a series of studies, we at the University of Minnesota explored the role of released ADP and thromboxane in platelet activation leading to aggregation. Our studies using platelets from storage pool deficient patients demonstrated that released ADP was not essential for eliciting irreversible aggregation response.[22] Using aspirin-treated platelets as well as platelets from cyclooxygenase-deficient patients, we demonstrated that released ADP as well as PG endoperoxides or thromboxane are not essential for irreversible aggregation of platelets.[23,24] We also demonstrated the need for activation of GPIIb/IIIa receptors and fibrinogen binding in irreversible aggregation. We further demonstrated that irreversibly aggregated platelets could be disaggregated using agents that lower cytosolic calcium and reaggregated by using the dual agonists epinephrine and ADP or thrombin (Fig. 5.5). Association and disassociation of fibrinogen accompanied these cycles of aggregation and disaggregation to the platelets. These cycles of activation and deactivation of platelets were accompanied by phosphorylation and dephosphorylation of selective cytoskeletal proteins.[25] Kabuchi et al. in a series of studies demonstrated that DAGs are directly involved in the transmembrane control of protein phosphorylation through calcium-activated phospholipid-dependent protein kinase.[26] Using diglyceride and calcium ionophore, they demonstrated platelet activation and release of serotonin. Studies from our laboratory at the University of Minnesota had already demonstrated the influence of ionophore on platelet ultrastructure, aggregation, and secretion.

Studies from Nishizuka and associates have demonstrated that agonist-induced hydrolysis of other membrane phospholipids, such as choline phospholipids by PLD and PLA_2, may also take part in cell signaling in addition to the classical inositol phospholipids hydrolyzed by PLC (Fig. 5.6). Prolonged activation of protein kinase C seems to be essential for long-term cellular responses.[27-29]

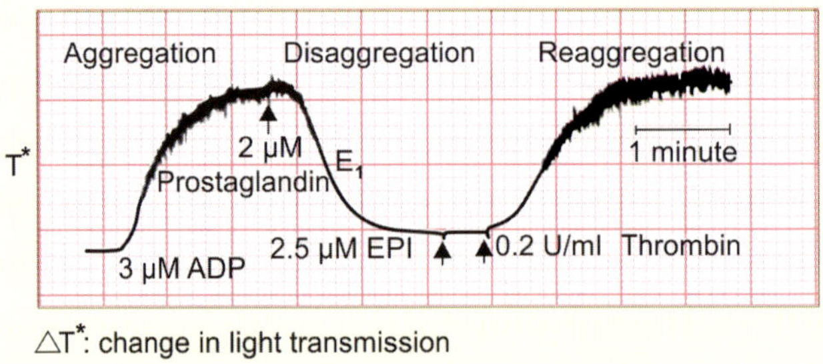

Fig. 5.5: Platelet aggregation, disaggregation, and reaggregation cycles.

Surface membranes of platelets serve as barrier from extracellular environment. However, they also serve as store for a variety of lipids, which upon hydrolysis by phospholipases (PLC, PLD, PLA) rapidly generate structurally diversified intracellular and extracellular lipid-derived mediators of activation.[30] As we have discussed earlier, cell activation is accompanied by calcium mobilization phosphorylation of specific proteins and cytoskeletal reorganization. Lipid mediators, second messengers, eicosanoids, platelet-activating factor (PAF), ceramides, cytokines, leukotrienes, and lipoxins play an essential role in signaling pathways as well as cell–cell communication and cell–surface communication.

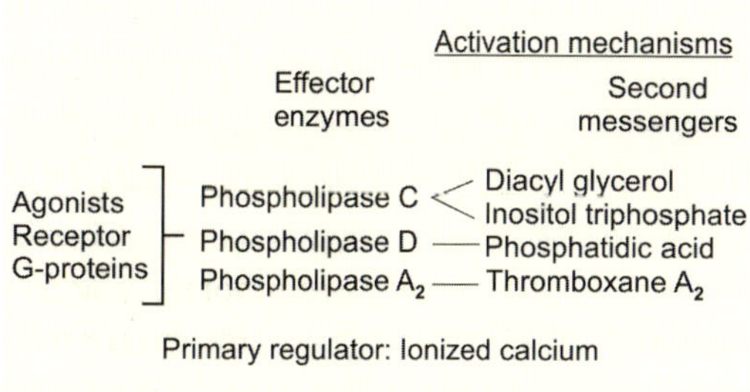

Fig. 5.6: Signal transduction mechanisms by phospholipase C (PLC), PLD, and PLA_2.

GPCRs, also known as seven-transmembrane domain receptors (as they pass through the cell membrane seven times), constitute a large family of receptors that sense molecules outside the cell and activate inside signal transduction pathways and initiate cellular responses.

It is well established that DAG and IP_3 are crucial cellular messengers. DAG can activate the protein kinase C and IP_3 has been shown to mobilize cytosolic calcium from internal membrane stores. Although majority of agonists seem to induce cellular signaling via PLC pathway, there are some agonists that use PLD pathway and generate PA. Others, and we have demonstrated the unique way of signaling initiated by phorbol esters that can use both PLC and PLD pathways (Figs. 5.7 and 5.8). Phorbol ester, which directly activates

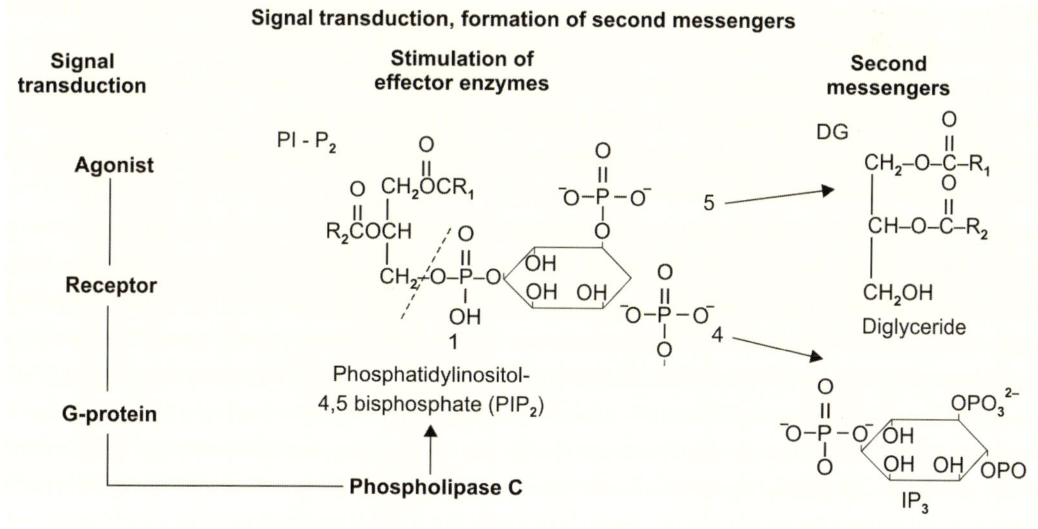

Fig. 5.7: Signaling via phospholipase C pathway.

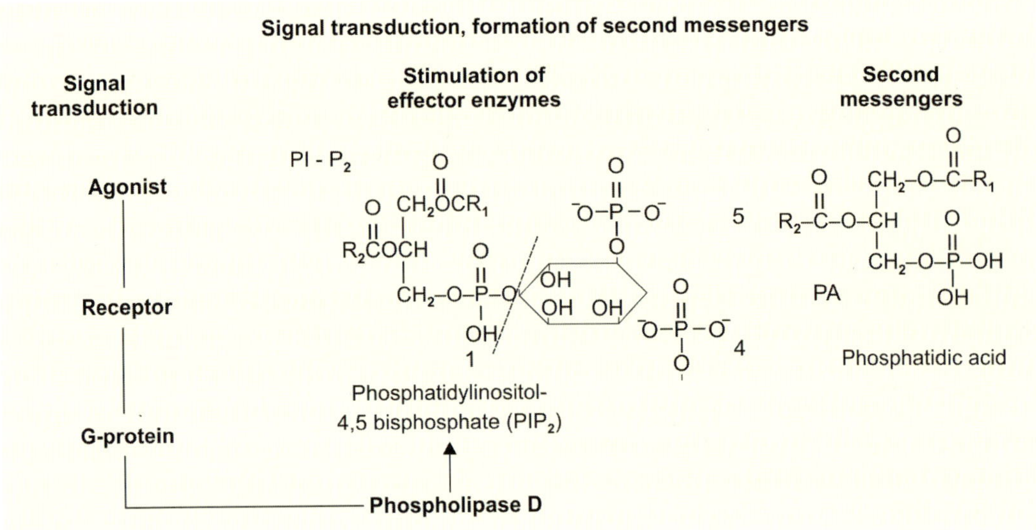

Fig. 5.8: Signaling via phospholipase D pathway.

protein kinase C by substituting for diacylglycerols, stimulates 40 K protein phosphorylation and release reaction without inducing DAG formation.

Huang and associates have provided evidence for direct formation of DAG by both PLC and PLD pathways.[30] Anionic phospholipid phosphatidic acid seems to have moderate biological activity. Some studies suggest that it acts via lyso-PA (LPA) and DAGs. Studies from our laboratory as well as that of Denis English at the Indiana University have demonstrated an independent messenger function for phosphatidic acid in moving calcium across membranes.[31] It is supposed to mediate its action via activation of PA-dependent intracellular kinases. From the time we demonstrated using calcium ionophore A23187 to this day, researchers have been trying to show the pivotal role of cytosolic calcium in platelet activation. Gerrard and associates from our laboratory at the University of Minnesota demonstrated the ability of phosphatidic acid, LPAs to move calcium across membranes in vitro and suggested that LPAs cause aggregation by stimulating the release of calcium intracellularly.[32,33]

REFERENCES

1. White JG, Rao GHR, Estensen RD. Investigation of the release reaction in platelets exposed to phorbol myristate acetate. Am J Pathol. 1974;75(2):301-14.
2. White JG, Rao GHR, Gerrard JM. Effects of the ionophore A23187 on blood platelets 1. Influence on aggregation and secretion. Am J Pathol. 1974;77(2):135-50.
3. Gerrard JM, White JG, Rao GHR. Effects of the ionophore on the blood platelets 11. Influence on ultrastructure. Am J Pathol. 1974;77(2);151-66.
4. Johnson GJ, Sharda AV, Rao GHR, Ereth MH, Laxson DD, Owen WG. Measurement of shear-activated platelet aggregate formation in non-anticoagulated blood: utility in detection of clopidogrel-aspirin-induced platelet dysfunction. Clin Appl Thromb Hemost. 2012;18:140-9.

5. Kaziro Y, Itoh H, Kozasa T, Nakafuku M, Satoh T. Structure and function of signal-transducing GTP-binding proteins. Annu Rev Biochem. 1991;60:349-400.
6. Simon MI, Strathmann MP, Gautam N. Diversity of G proteins in signal transduction. Science. 1991;252:802-8.
7. Offerman S. Activation of platelet function through G protein-coupled receptors. Circ Res. 2006;99(12):1293-1304.
8. Hokin MR, Hokin LE. Enzyme secretion and the incorporation of P32 into phosphoinositides of pancreas slices. J Biol Chem. 1953;203:967-77.
9. Anderson TA, Boronekove IV, Doughman SD, Kunz J, Loijens JC. Phosphatidylinositol phosphate kinases, a multifaceted family of signaling enzymes. J Biol Chem. 1999;274:9907-10.
10. Irvine RF, Schell M. Back in the water: the return of the inositol phosphates. Nat Rev Mol Cell Biol. 2001;2(5):327-38.
11. Majerus PW, Kisseleva MV, Norris FA. The role of phosphates in inositol signaling reactions. J Biol Chem. 1999;274:10669-72.
12. Rameh LE, Cantley LC. The role of phosphoinositide 3-kinase lipid products in cell function. J Biol Chem. 1999;274:8347-50.
13. Shear SB. The versatility of inositol phosphates as cellular signals. Biochim Biophys Acta. 1998;1436:49-67.
14. Min SH, Abrams CS. Regulation of platelet plug formation by phosphoinositide metabolism. Blood. 2013;122:1358-65.
15. Guinebault C, Payrastre B, Sultan C, Mauco G, Breton M, Levy-Toledano S, et al. Tyrosine kinase and phosphoinositide metabolism in thrombin-stimulated human platelets. Biochem J. 1993;292:851-6.
16. Brindley DN. Lipid phosphate phosphatases and related proteins: signaling functions in development, cell division and cancer. J Biol Chem. 2004;92:900-12.
17. Brindley DN, Waggoner DW. Mammalian lipid phosphate phosphohydrolases. J Biol Chem. 1998;273:24281-4.
18. Brindley DN, English D Piquil C, Buri K, Ling ZC. Lipid phosphate phosphatases regulate signal transduction through glycerolipids and sphingolipids. Biochim Biophys Acta. 2002;1582:33-44.
19. English D, Welch Z, Kovala AT, Harvey K, Volpert OV, Brindley DN, et al. Sphingosine 1-phosphate released from platelets during clotting accounts for the potent endothelial cell chemotactic activity of blood serum and provides a novel link between haemostasis and angiogenesis. FASEB J. 2000;14:2255-65.
20. Tigyi G, Parill AL. Molecular mechanisms of lysophosphatidic acid. Prog Lipid Res. 2003;42:498-526.
21. Yatomi Y, Ruan F, Hakamori S, Igarashi Y. Sphingosine-1-phosphate: a platelet activating sphingolipids released from agonist-stimulated human platelets. Blood. 1995;86: 193-202.
22. Rao GHR, Gerrard JM, Witkop CK, White JG. Platelet aggregation independent of ADP release or prostaglandin synthesis in patients with Hermansky-Pudlak syndrome. Prostaglandins Med. 1981;6:459-72.
23. Rao GHR, White JG. Epinephrine potentiation of arachidonate-induced aggregation of cyclooxygenase deficient platelets. Am J Hematol. 1981;11:355-66.
24. Rao GHR, Johnson GJ, White JG. Influence of epinephrine on the aggregation response of aspirin treated platelets. Prostaglandins Med. 1980;5:45-58.
25. Cox AC, Carroll RC, White JG, Rao GHR. Recycling of platelet phosphorylation and cytoskeletal assembly. J Cell Biol. 1984;98:8-15.
26. Kabuchi K, Takai Y, Sawamura M, Hoshijima M, Fujikura T, Nishizuka Y. Synergistic functions of protein phosphorylation and calcium mobilization in platelet activation. J Biol Chem. 1983;258:6701-4.
27. Nishizuka Y. Protein kinase C and lipid signaling for sustained cellular responses. FASEB J. 1995;9(7):484-96.
28. Nishizuka Y. Studies and perspectives of protein kinase C. Science. 1986;233:305-12.
29. Nishizuka Y. Intracellular signaling by hydrolysis of phospholipids and activation of protein kinase C. Science. 1992;258:607-14.
30. Huang C, Cabot MC. Phorbol diesters stimulate accumulation of phosphatidate,

phosphatidylethanol and diacylglycerols in three cell types. Evidence for the indirect formation of phosphatidylcholine-derived diacylglycerols by a phospholipase D pathway and direct formation of diacylglycerols by a phospholipase C pathway. J Biol Chem. 1990; 265:14858-63.

31. English D, Cui Y, Siddiqui RA. Messenger functions of phosphatidic acid. Chem Phys Lipids. 1996;80:(1-2):117-32.
32. Gerrard JM, Buttler AM, Peterson DA, White JG. Phosphatidic acid releases calcium from a platelet membrane fraction in vitro. Prostaglandins Med. 1978;1(5): 387-96.
33. Gerrard JM, Kindom SE, Peterson DA, Peller J, Krantz KE, White JG. Lysophosphatidic acid. Influence on platelet aggregation and intracellular calcium flux. Am J Pathol. 1979;96(2):423-38.

CHAPTER 6

Role of Calcium in Platelet Activation

We have described so far, how soluble and insoluble macromolecules interact with surface membrane receptors or integrins, non-integrin domains, and initiate outside-in signaling pathways. Activation mechanisms including action of enzymes, phosphorylation of proteins, and rearrangement of cytoskeletal proteins seems to depend on the availability of cytosolic ionized calcium. There are several sources of calcium including extracellular, membrane-associated, and intracellular. The widely favored hypothesis suggests that the calcium concentrations increase due to the entry of extracellular (A23187 studies) calcium through the plasma membrane (PM) and the mobilization of stored intracellular calcium from two pools. One is the dense tubular system (DTS) and the other is lysosome-like acidic organelle. DTS releases calcium via signal transduction pathway of inositol-1, 4, 5-trisphosphate and the latter via nicotinic acid adenine dinucleotide phosphate. Membrane-associated channels are responsible for extracellular calcium entry, which is regulated by a Ca^{2+} sensor molecule in intracellular stores and a calcium release-activated calcium modulator. For relaxation or deactivation, two different pumps operate and remove the intracellular free calcium. One is the sarcoplasmic (endoplasmic) reticulum Ca^{2+} ATPase, which pumps back the free calcium to intracellular stores, the other is the plasma membrane Ca^{2+} ATPase, which pumps calcium out of the cells, to maintain normal resting levels (Fig. 6.1).

Although it is presumed that cytosolic calcium mobilization is the final common pathway for platelet activation, the sources and exact molecular mechanisms involved in this process are not clearly understood.[1-11] Chief sources of calcium in the platelet environment include the surrounding plasma, mitochondria, membranes covering the cell surface, lining of the open canalicular system, and the dense tubular system. Studies from our laboratory at the University of Minnesota explored the sources of calcium in platelet aggregation and secretion using three different calcium chelators.

In these studies, we used calcium-sensitive fluorophore Quin-2 ester, its free

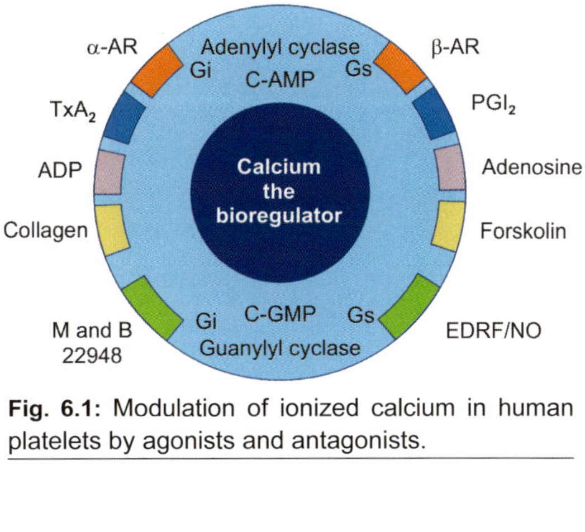

Fig. 6.1: Modulation of ionized calcium in human platelets by agonists and antagonists.

acid (QFA) and chlortetracycline (CTC) along with ethylenediaminetetraacetic acid (EDTA) as intra- and extracellular calcium chelating agents to assess the origin and function of calcium in normal platelets and cells from patients with storage pool deficiency [Hermansky-Pudlak Syndrome (HPS)] and α-granule deficiency [gray platelet syndrome (GPS)]. Rises in cytosolic calcium levels following exposure to thrombin in the presence of EDTA were as great in HPS and GPS as in control platelets indicating that dense bodies and α granules were not the source of cytosolic calcium flux. Treatment of platelets with sodium azide or ethidium bromide to poison mitochondria had no effect on cytosolic calcium levels or the elevation of calcium after exposure to thrombin. In order to complex surface membrane, intracellular and extracellular calcium, respectively, CTC, QAM, and QFA were employed. Chelation at any site was sufficient to block single agonist-induced secretion and irreversible aggregation. However, sensitivity of the refractory cells to agonists could be restored by pretreatment with epinephrine. A combination of any two chelators (CTC + QZM, CTC + QFA, or QZM + QFA) completely blocked secretion, aggregation, and clot retraction. The results of these studies indicate that membranes and membrane systems are the primary stores of calcium for platelet activation, with channels of the dense tubular system as the major reservoir. Elevation of cytoplasmic calcium appears essential for contractile events, including secretion and clot retraction.

Platelets possess various adhesion receptors and agonist-interactive domains on the surface membranes. They respond to a variety of stimuli including shear force. Irrespective of various stimulating agents triggering activation sequence in their own specific ways, they all seem to lead to an increase in intracellular calcium concentration. Calcium is an essential second messenger, regulating a variety of calcium-dependent processes, such as reorganization of actin cytoskeleton necessary for shape change, spreading, inside-out activation of integrin $\alpha IIb\beta_3$ receptor indispensable for fibrinogen binding and aggregation, contraction, and secretion of granule contents. It is well established that agonist-mediated activation of platelets results in the increased levels of cytosolic calcium via inositol phospholipid (IP_3) pathway, and Ca^{2+} entry through the plasma membrane by a process referred to as store-operated calcium entry (SOCE). Recent studies have demonstrated that stromal interaction molecule 1 (STIM1), a Ca^{2+} sensor molecule in intracellular stores, and the four transmembrane proteins, orail, are the key players in platelet SOCE.[2]

The calcium-dependent regulator protein, calmodulin, is a small-molecular-weight polypeptide, which plays an important role in regulating the effect of ionized calcium on contractile proteins. This protein has been reported to stimulate phospholipase A_2 activity in isolated membranes. Trifluoperazine is a potent inhibitor of calmodulin-sensitive enzymes. Walenga and associates have demonstrated that this compound inhibits production of all arachidonic acid metabolites, both cyclooxygenase as well as lipoxygenase, in thrombin-stimulated platelets.[12] When platelets are stimulated, two reactions, which are stimulated, are the hydrolysis of phospholipids by phospholipase A_2 to release arachidonic acid and the cleavage of phosphatidylinositol to diglyceride and 1,2-cyclic inositol phosphate.[13-15] Diglyceride is converted to phosphatidic acid by diglyceride kinase or it may be hydrolyzed to free fatty acids and glycerol by diglyceride lipase. This process seems to be the major source for arachidonic acid in stimulated platelets. Calmodulin also has been shown to have a role in myosin phosphorylation in stimulated platelets. In addition, because of its role as an activator of calcium-modulated enzymes, calmodulin seem to regulate the assembly and disassembly of microtubules. In unstimulated platelets, little myosin light chain (MLC) is in phosphorylated state and remains in solution. Inhibition of calmodulin has been shown to prevent MLC phosphorylation as well as its incorporation into the platelet cytoskeleton.[16] It has been shown that the cytosolic regulatory protein, calmodulin, has an important role in modulation of receptor function. It directly binds to conserved juxtamembrane motifs within the cytoplasmic domains of both GPVI and GPIb-IX-V.

It is well known that morphology and function of platelet depend on the nature and location of intracellular polymeric cytoskeletal structures. The main cytoskeletal structures in platelets are those of microtubules, microfilaments, actin, and myosin. Role of calcium is pivotal in modulating various biochemical events, as actin myosin and various contractile proteins have essential role in all of the events following platelet activation. White described platelets as the muscular system of the blood platelets.[17] In his studies on the interaction of the membrane systems, he concluded, "They appear to be normal constituents of the cells' anatomy, and are unique in the sense that similar organizations of membranous channels have not been observed in other blood cells. In fact, the only other type of cell with an arrangement of channel system resembling complexes in platelet is muscle."[18,19] Takubo and associates of Osaka University, Japan, using fluorescence microscopy have observed the distribution of contractile proteins, myosin, filamentous actin, α actinin, tropomyosin, and vinculin in surface-activated spreading of human platelets.[20,21] It is believed that these contractile proteins are reorganized and reassembled in activated platelets during platelet function.[22-30] Lind and associates demonstrated reversible appearance of high-affinity complexes of profilin and gelsolin with actin in extracts of platelets undergoing activation and actin assembly.[28] The calcium-dependent assembly of actin with gelsolin was reversible and dissociation of gelsolin was correlated with the association of actin with the cytoskeleton. Japanese researchers have demonstrated that when platelets are preactivated with receptor-dependent agonists, ADP or thrombin, the same agonist could not induce cytoskeletal assembly repeatedly. However, according to them, in case of receptor-independent stimulus, cryoactivation, the assembly was induced not only by the receptor-dependent but also by independent stimulus. They concluded that the desensitization lay in the transmission of stimuli from receptors to cytoskeletal proteins.[22]

Ionized calcium plays a pivotal role in agonist interaction with specific binding sites, receptor activation, transmembrane signaling events, cytoskeletal rearrangements, activation of various enzymes, generation of second messengers, calcium mobilization, regulation of contractile proteins, contraction, secretion of granule contents, and contraction of clots. Studies from our laboratory using calcium chelators demonstrated the need for calcium in the surrounding plasma for agonist-receptor interaction as well as for transmembrane calcium flux. Studies with calcium-sensitive ionophore, A23187 demonstrated that just the calcium influx by the ionophore was enough to cause platelet activation and secretion independent of agonist-mediated receptor stimulus. Our studies with chelators of membrane-associated calcium demonstrated the need of calcium at the

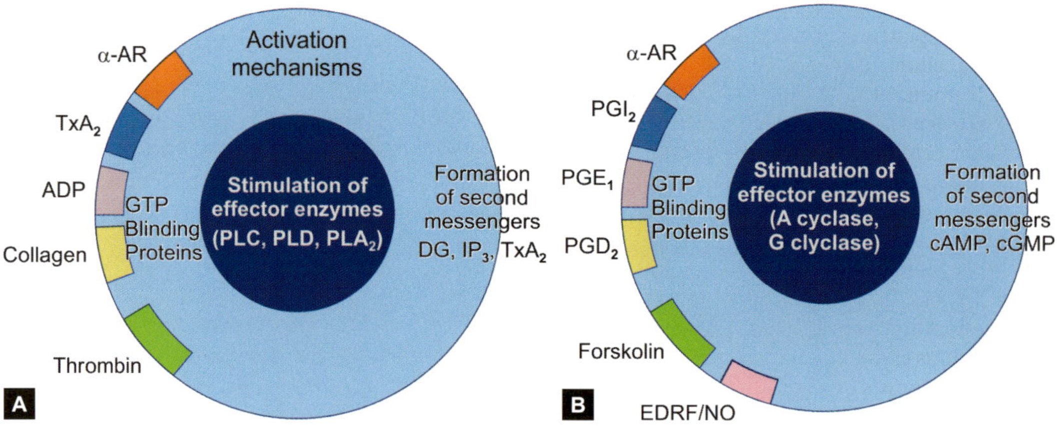

Figs. 6.2A and B: Signal transduction mechanism: Platelet activation and inactivation.

membrane for activation of enzymes, signaling events, and cytoskeletal reorganization. We also showed the specific role of cytosolic calcium by using Quin-2 ester, a cell-permeable calcium chelators. Platelets in which we blocked the increase in cytosolic calcium were able to stick to the surface as well as aggregate in the absence of secretion of granule contents.

A series of studies done in our laboratory demonstrated a common phenomenon of platelet activation (Figs. 6.2A and B). Agonists interacting with specific receptor sites initiated transmembrane signaling events via classical inositol trisphosphate pathway to increase cytosolic calcium levels and generate second messengers IP_3 and diacylglycerol (DAG). Antagonists, on the other hand, lowered the elevated levels of cytosolic calcium via adenylyl cyclase and guanylyl cyclases by generating second messengers, cAMP and cGMP. We were further able to demonstrate that agonist-mediated events like $aIIb\beta_3$ receptor activation, fibrinogen binding, and phosphorylation of proteins could be reversed by exposure to agents that elevated cyclic nucleotides, which lowered cytosolic calcium. We were able to reaggregate the disaggregated platelets again by stimulating them with dual agonists. We believe that these events are strictly modulated by the availability of calcium to promote the signaling events associated with activation and this entire process is reversible including phosphorylation events and cytoskeletal rearrangements, by modulation of calcium levels, via modulation of the levels of cyclic nucleotides.[30,31]

REFERENCES

1. Varga-Szabo D, Braun A, Nieswandt B. Calcium signaling in platelets. J Thromb Hemost. 2009;7:1057-66.
2. Rink TJ, Sage SO. Calcium signaling in human platelets. Annu Rev Physiol. 1990;52:431-49.
3. Chakrabarti R, Chakrabarti R. Calcium signaling in non-excitable cells: Ca2+ release and influx are independent events linked to plasma membrane Ca2+ entry channels. J Cell Biochem. 2006;99(6):1503-16.
4. Sano K, Takai Y, Yamanishi J, Nishizuka Y. A role of calcium-activated phospholipid-dependent protein kinase in human platelet activation. Comparison of thrombin and collagen actions. J Biol Chem. 1983;258:2010-3.
5. Brass L, Shattil SJ. Changes in surface-bound and exchangeable calcium during platelet activation. J Biol Chem. 1982;257(23):14000-5.

6. Charo IF, Feinman RD, Detwiler TC. Inhibition of platelet secretion by an antagonist of intracellular calcium. Biochem Biophys Res Commun. 1976;72:1462-7.
7. Detwiler TL, Charo IF, Feinman RD. Evidence that calcium regulates platelet function. Thromb Haemost. 1978;404:207-11.
8. Feinman RD, Detwiler TC. Platelet secretion induced by cation ionophores. Nature. 1974;249:172-3.
9. Feinstein MD. Release of intracellular membrane-bound calcium precede onset of stimulus-induced exocytosis in platelets. Biochem Biophys Res Commun. 1980;93:593-600.
10. White JG, Rao GHR, Gerrard JM. Effects of the ionophore A23187 on blood platelets 1. Influence on aggregation and secretion. 1974;77(2):135-49.
11. Rao GHR, Gerrard JM, Cohen I et al. Origin and role of calcium in platelet activation—A contraction-secreting coupling, in Cell Calcium Metabolism, Fiskum, G (Ed). Plenum Press: New York, 1989. p. 411-25.
12. Walenga RW, Opas EE, Feinstein MB. Differential effects of calmodulin antagonists on phospholipase A_2 and C in thrombin-stimulated platelets. J Biol Chem. 1981;256:12523-8.
13. Getz TM, Dangelmaier CA, Jin J, Daniel JL, Kunapuli SP. Differential phosphorylation of myosin light chain (Thr) 18 and (Ser) 19 and functional implications in platelets. J Thromb Haemost. 2010;8(10):2283-93.
14. Aburima A, Wraith KS, Rasian Z, Law R, Magwenzi S, Naseem KM. cAMP signaling regulates platelet myosin light chain (MLC) phosphorylation and shape change through targeting the RhoA-Rho kinase-MLC phosphatase signaling pathway. Blood. 2013;122(20):3533-45.
15. Nishikawa M, Hidaka H. Role of calmodulin in platelet aggregation. Structure-activity relationship of calmodulin antagonists. J Clin Invest. 1982;69:1348-55.
16. Fox JE, Phillips DR. Role of phosphorylation in mediating the association of myosin with the cytoskeletal structure of human platelets. J Biol Chem. 1982;257:4120-6.
17. White JG. The muscular system of blood platelets. Blood. 1967;30:359.
18. White JG. The sub membrane filaments of blood platelets. Am J Pathol. 1967;56:267-77.
19. White JG. Interactions of the membrane systems in blood platelets. Am J Pathol. 1972;66:295-312.
20. Cove DH, Crawford N. Platelet contractile proteins: separation and characterization of the actin and myosin-like components. J Mechanochem Cell Motil. 1975;3(2):123-33.
21. Adelstein RS, Pollard TD, Kuehl WM. Isolation and characterization of myosin and two myosin fragments from human platelets. Proc Natl Acad Sci U S A. 1971;68(11):2703-7.
22. Takubo T, Hino M. Suzuki K, Tatsumi N. Relative distribution of myosin, actin and alpha-actinin in surface-activated, spreading platelets. Eur J Haematol. 1998;60(5):307-9.
23. Takubo T Hirso M, Suzuki K, Tatsumi N. Localization of myosin, actin, alpha actinin, tropomyosin and vinculin in surface-activated, spreading human platelets. Biotech Histochem. 1998;73(6):310-5.
24. Fox JE, Phillips DR. Polymerization and organization of actin filaments within platelets. Semin Hematol. 1983;20(4):243-60.
25. Imada T, Saito Y, Shimada H, Kikuchi T, Takagi J, Inada Y. Specific desensitization in the cytoskeletal assembly of platelet by receptor-dependent activations. Thromb Res. 1986;41(1):119-25.
26. Hartwig JH, Chambers KA, Stossel TP. Association of Gelsolin with actin filaments and cell membranes of macrophages and platelets. J Cell Biol. 1989;108:467-79.
27. Berridge MJ. Inositol trisphosphate and diacylglycerols as second messengers. Biochemistry. 1984;220:345-60.
28. Lind SE, Janmey PA, Chaponnier C, Herbert TJ, Stossel TP. Reversible binding of actin to gelsolin and profiling in human platelet extracts. J Cell Biol. 1987;105:833-42.
29. Sun H, Lin K, Yin H. Gelsolin modulates phospholipase C activity in vivo through phospholipid binding. J Cell Biol. 1997;138(4):811-20.
30. Rao GHR, White JG. Disaggregation and reaggregation or irreversibly aggregated platelets: a method for more complete evaluation of antiplatelet drugs. Agents Actions. 1985;16(5):425-34.
31. Cox, AC, Carroll RC, White JG, Rao GHR. Recycling of platelet phosphorylation and cytoskeletal assembly. J Cell Biol. 1984;98:8-15.

Eicosanoid Metabolism and Platelet Function

CHAPTER 7

The eicosanoids include prostaglandins (PGs), thromboxanes (TXs), leukotrienes (LTs), and lipoxins (LXs). The PGs and TXs are collectively identified as prostanoids (Fig. 7.1). The nomenclature of the prostanoids includes a subscript number, which refers to the number of carbon-carbon double bonds that exist in the molecule. The majority of the biologically active PGs and TXs are referred to as series 2 (diene) molecules, due to the presence of two carbon-carbon double bonds. Similarly, molecules of the series 3 (triene) and 4 (tetraene) also have been described. Predominant LTs are series 4 molecules. Earlier studies on prostaglandins originally showed that they were synthesized in the prostate glands. In fact, I remember the days in the 70s, when we used to go to Hormel facility in Austin, Minnesota, to collect freshly harvested sheep seminal vesicle glands for the preparation of prostanoids. By doing extensive comparative studies, we localized the synthesis of prostanoids to the dense tubular system of platelets.[1]

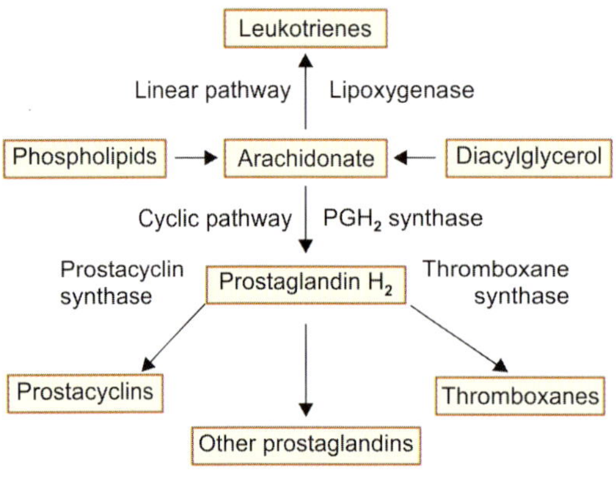

Fig. 7.1: Eicosanoid synthesis.

The principal eicosanoids of biological significance are derived from the substrate arachidonic acid (AA), a 20 carbon fatty acid.[2-10] The major source of AA is through its release from cellular phospholipids associated with membrane stores. Within the platelets, it resides predominantly at the C-2 position of the membrane phospholipids, and is released by the activation of phospholipase A_2 (PLA_2). Common phospholipids of platelets include phosphatidyl choline (PC), phosphatidyl ethanolamine (PE), phosphatidyl serine (PE), and phosphatidyl inositol (PI). More than 15% of the dry weight of the platelets is lipid, of which 80% is phospholipids.[2] Major platelet lipids include cholesterol (30%), phosphatidyl choline (26%), phosphatidyl ethanolamine (8.6%), sphingomyelin (11.6%), and phosphatidyl inositol (2.7%). Phosphatidyl choline contains primarily palmitic acid or stearic acid at carbon 1 and oleic or linoleic acid at carbon 2 positions. Phosphatidyl ethanolamine contains palmitic or stearic acid on carbon 1 and a long-chain unsaturated fatty acid on carbon 2. Phosphatidyl serine contains fatty acid composition similar to PE. Phosphatidyl inositol contains exclusively stearic acid at carbon 1 and arachidonic acid at position 2. Molecules with phosphorylated inositol are called phosphoinositides.

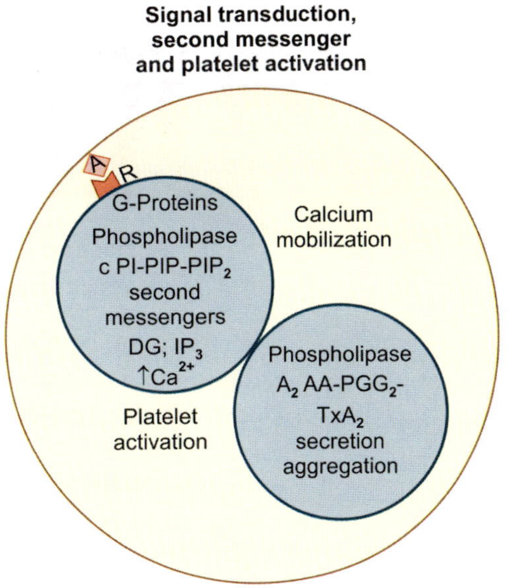

Fig. 7.2: Signal transduction pathways.

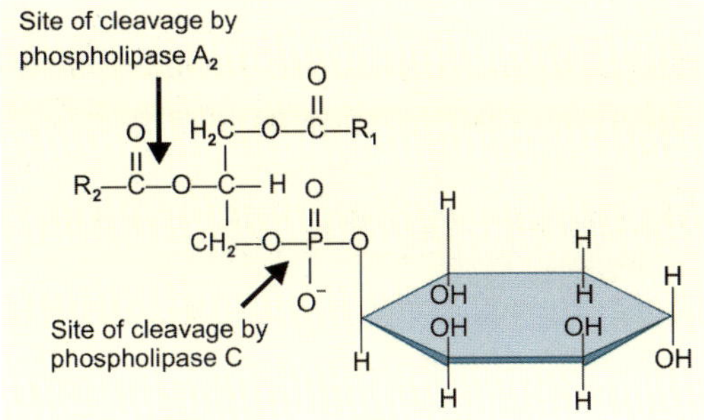

Fig. 7.3: Phosphatidylinositol metabolism.

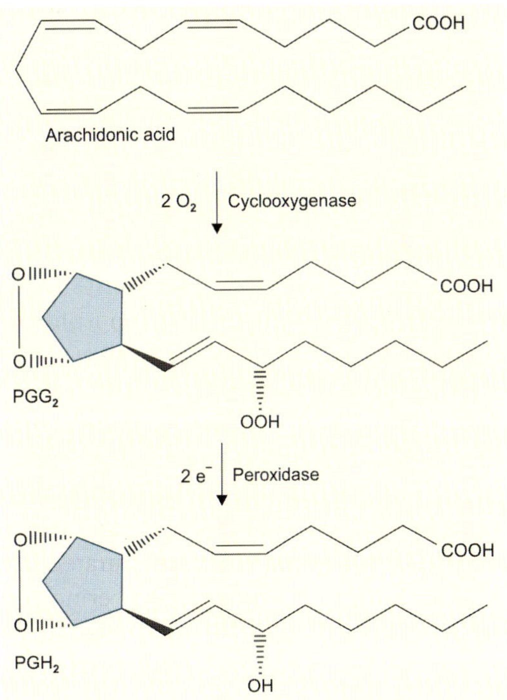

Fig. 7.4: Arachidonic acid metabolism PGG_2 and PGH_2.

We have discussed so far how agonist interaction with specific receptors or integrin domains initiates signaling mechanism via G-protein–coupled transmembrane domains and activate phospholipase C and generate second messenger's diglyceride (DG) and inositol trisphosphate (IP_3). We also have discussed the role of IP_3 in calcium mobilization from internal membrane stores (Fig. 7.2).

Elevation of calcium activates PLA_2 and liberates AA from the phospholipids (PLA_2). Phospholipase is an important enzyme, whose activity is responsible for the release of AA from the C-2 position of the membrane phospholipids (Fig. 7.3). At least 30 enzymes have been identified with phospholipase A activity. PLA_2 enzyme is regulated by phosphorylation. Synthesis of AA, a polyunsaturated fatty acid (PUFA) of 20 carbon atoms with four sites of unsaturation, begins with a CoA-activated form of linoleic acid (linoleoyl-CoA), which is an 18-carbon fatty acid with two sites of unsaturation.

The process of AA synthesis involves both elongation and two separate desaturation steps. The rate-limiting step in the biosynthesis of eicosanoids is the availability of precursor, esterified AA. The release of AA from phospholipids is mediated by the activation of PLA_2 that is coupled to PLC, intracellular Ca^{2+} rise and protein kinase C (PKC), and tyrosine kinase-mediated protein phosphorylations. In addition, as discussed earlier, phosphatidic acid hydrolysis by PA-specific PLA_2 may also contribute significant amounts of AA for eicosanoid synthesis. Despite numerous studies, the amount and source of AA mobilized during platelet activation remain as a subject of controversy. Mahadevappa and Holub, from Canada, have studied degradation of different molecular species of phosphatidylinositol in thrombin-stimulated human platelets and have provided evidence of preferential degradation of 1-acyl-2-arachidonyl species.[3]

Arachidonic acid plays an important role in cellular signaling as a lipid second messenger involved in the regulation of signaling enzymes, such as PLC-γ, PLC-δ, and PKC-α, -β, and -γ isoforms. AA is a key inflammatory intermediate and also can act as a vasodilator.

Numerous stimuli (ADP, epinephrine, and thrombin) interact with G-protein–coupled receptors (GPCRs) (G_q and $G_{i/o}$) with the net effect being increases in cytosolic calcium and activation of PKC. These events activate the endoplasmic reticulum (ER) membrane–associated $cPLA_{2,}$ which hydrolyzes arachidonic acid from cellular membrane phospholipids, especially from PIP_2. Once liberated, AA is converted to transient endoperoxides PPG_2 and PGH_2 by cyclooxygenase (Cox-1, Cox-2: PGG/H synthase) enzymes. These transient metabolites are converted in platelets to thromboxane (TXA_2), a potent agonist and a vasoconstrictor and to prostacyclin (PGI_2) a vasodilator, in endothelial cells (Fig. 7.5). Since we are discussing second messengers, it is worth mentioning that all newly formed biologically active metabolites are called second messengers [DG, IP_3, PG intermediates (PPG_2, PGH_2), TXA, cAMP, and cGMP] (Fig. 7.6).

Each of the eicosanoids function via interaction with cell surface receptors that are members of the GPCR family. There are at least 10 characterized prostaglandin receptors. Receptors that bind the D family of lipids are called DP receptors; those that bind E family prostaglandins are called EP receptors; those that bind F family prostaglandins are called FP receptors; those that bind prostacyclin (PGI_2) are called IP receptors, and those that bind the thromboxane are called the TP receptors.

Yoshimoto and associates were the first to demonstrate that heme is required for enhancing the activity of prostaglandin-synthesizing enzymes.[10] Miyamoto and associates purified the prostaglandin synthetase and showed that either free or protein-bound heme was required for its activity, and only protoheme was active.[11] Ultrastructural studies from our laboratory at the University of Minnesota using an iron-reactive drug diaminobenzidine reported that enzymes involved in endoperoxide synthesis are localized in the dense tubular system of human platelets. Using a cell-free system, we showed that ferrous iron and heme can induce oxidation of polyenoic acids and the extent of oxidation was related to the degree of unsaturation in the fatty acids.[12-26] Heme or iron chelators, as well as several known inhibitors of cyclooxygenase, blocked this reaction.[23] Ferrous iron chelators and heme-complexing agents inhibited prostaglandin synthesis as well as platelet function. In vivo studies using a short-acting drug, ibuprofen and an irreversible inhibitor of cyclooxygenase, aspirin, confirmed our findings that the majority of prostaglandin synthesis inhibitors exert their effect by interfering with heme-AA interaction.[24] On the basis of our studies, we have presented a novel concept of heme-AA interaction.[26] We have extended these ideas further to provide an alternative explanation as to the possible mechanism by which polyenoic acids could compete for this

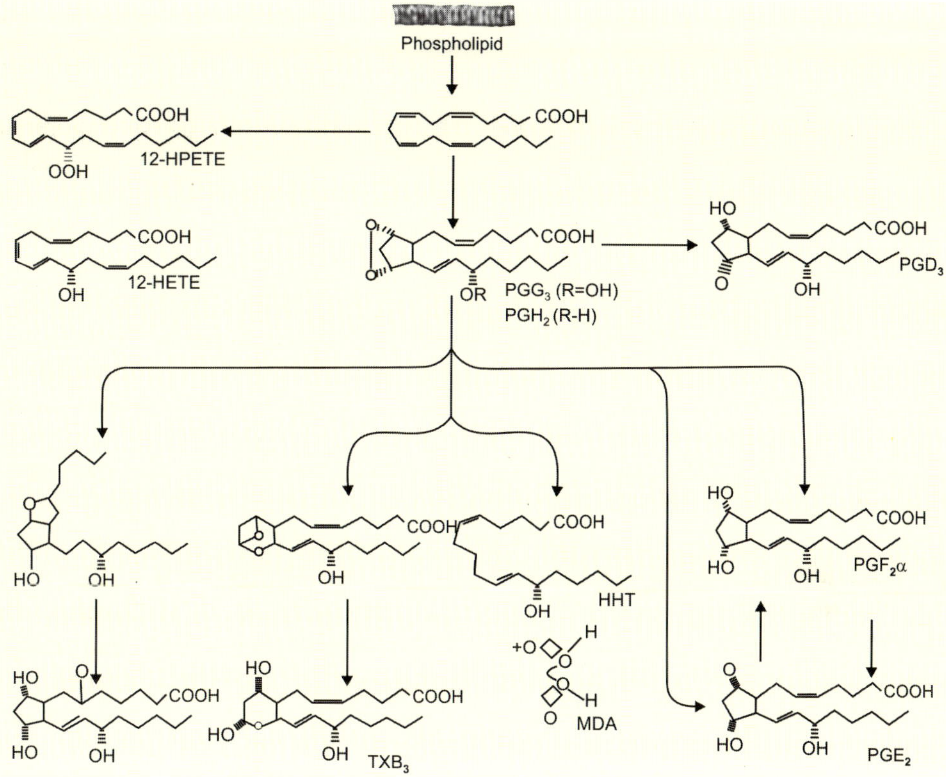

Fig. 7.5: Arachidonic acid metabolism.

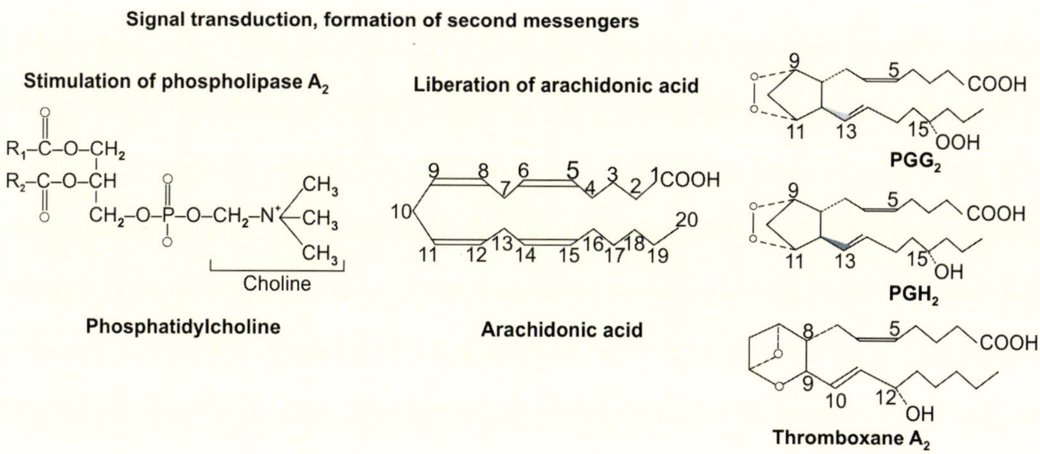

Fig. 7.6: Second messengers of arachidonic acid metabolism.

heme-associated site on the enzyme cyclooxygenase and prevent the conversion of the favored substrate AA.[26]

The prostanoids are part of a family of biologically active lipids derived from the action of cyclooxygenase or prostaglandin synthases, upon the 20-carbon fatty acids. They can be further divided into three main groups, the prostaglandins, prostacyclins, and thromboxanes. The Nobel prize for physiology and medicine in 1982 was given to Professors Samuelsson, John Vane, and Sune Bergstrom for their discoveries in this field. Eicosanoids, including prostanoids, are not stored within cells but are synthesized as required in response to stimuli. Early 70s was the golden age for prostanoids research.[27-37] It was demonstrated by Samuelsson's group at Karolinska Institute, Sweden, that free fatty acids are acted upon by one of two related enzymes, Cox-1 and Cox-2 (alternately termed endoperoxide H synthase-1 and -2: PGHS). Both enzymes catalyze the same two reactions at different sites. Cyclooxygenase reaction in which two molecules of oxygen are added to AA to form bicyclic endoperoxide with further hydroperoxy group in position 15 to form PGG_2. The hydroperoxide is then reduced by a functionally coupled peroxidase to form prostaglandin (PGH_2). The same group from Sweden elucidated the structure of biologically active thromboxane and prostacyclin molecules.[30,32] Willis elucidated the mechanism of action of aspirin on human platelets.[31] He showed that aspirin-like drugs blocked the enzymatic conversion of AA to hitherto undiscovered factor, labile aggregation-stimulating factor.

In spite of the fact that acetyl salicylic acid, aspirin, has been in use for over hundred years, before 1971, little was known about the real mechanism of action of aspirin-like drugs.[31-43] Roth and associates demonstrated that aspirin selectively acetylates the hydroxyl group (Fig. 7.7) of one-serine residue (Ser 530), located 70 amino acids from the C terminus of the enzyme.[41] It was also shown that when the purified enzyme is acetylated, only Cox, not the hydroperoxidase, activity is inhibited. At low concentrations, aspirin selectively acetylates PGHS rapidly. At high concentrations, aspirin will also nonspecifically acetylate a variety of proteins and nucleic acids.[43] Studies from our laboratory have demonstrated the effect of high doses of aspirin on the membrane fluidity of platelets.[44]

Several studies demonstrated the presence of heme iron in the purified Cox enzyme preparations.[40-42] Studies from our laboratory using cell-free systems also demonstrated the heme involvement in PG synthesis and concluded that aspirin-like drugs exert their effect by interfering with heme-AA interactions.[26] Heme or iron chelators as well as several known inhibitors of cyclooxygenase blocked this interaction. Ferrous iron chelators as well as heme-complexing agents inhibited prostaglandin synthesis as well as platelet function.[23]

Pharmacological studies in humans have shown that 65-mg of aspirin given orally

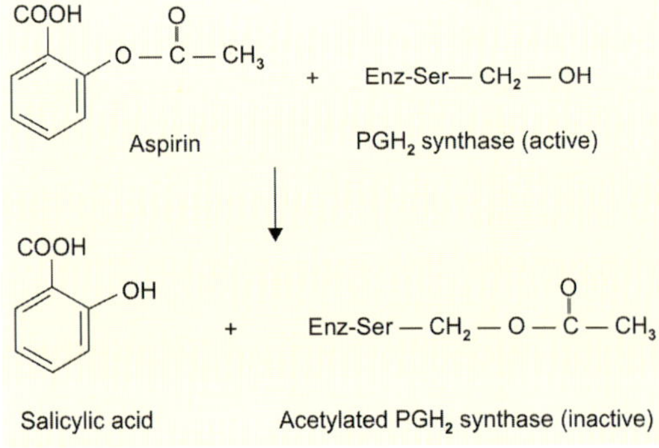

Fig. 7.7: Aspirin-mediated inhibition of Cox enzymes.

will yield plasma aspirin levels of 128 μm at 10 minutes, 56 μm at 25 minutes, and 18 μm at 1 hour. Jafe and Weksler have shown that 6.2 μm aspirin for 1 hour inhibits platelet as well as endothelial cell PG production. They also demonstrated that low-dose aspirin was equally effective in preventing both platelet and endothelial cell Cox enzymes. However, they have shown that endothelial cells can produce PGs once the enzyme is resynthesized.[45] In view of such observations, various researchers recommended a low to medium dose of aspirin for cardiovascular disease (CVD) prophylaxis. Beneficial effects of such doses of aspirin were demonstrated in number of clinical trials of aspirin.[46,47] Studies to achieve this differential production of platelet thromboxane and vascular prostacyclin by administering low-dose aspirin have not been successful.

Dyerberg and Bang in their classic paper described that Eskimos have significantly longer bleeding time.[48,49] Their platelets also contained higher levels of omega-3 fatty acids. It is generally believed that intake of long-chain omega fatty acids also affects bleeding times in human subjects.[50,51] Murthy and associates from Winnipeg, Canada, did a double-blind randomized study in which they gave volunteers 12 g of flax oil containing 55% α-linoleic acid, a precursor of eicosapentaenoic acid (EPA; 20:5) and docosahexaenoic acid (DHA; 20:6) and identical wheat germ oil for 3 months. They did not find any increase in bleeding time in these subjects.[52] They further concluded, on the basis of their studies, that not even one single study has produced the levels of long-chain fatty acids that are comparable to those reported in platelets of Greenland Eskimos. Epidemiological studies suggesting beneficial effects of fish diets in lowering CVDs in Greenland Eskimos and Japanese fisherman have prompted many dietary studies aimed at using long-chain fatty acids in diets for prevention of CVD. Fish fat, fish oil, and various commercial products containing fish lipids are rich in polyenoic acids of the n-3 series: eicosapentaenoic acid and docosahexaenoic acid. Earlier studies suggested that benefits of such a diet were related to the formation of triene or tetraene series of prostacyclin (PGI_3 or PGI_4) and thromboxanes (TXA_3 and TXA_4), which differ in their properties from the diene prostanoids: prostacyclin (PGI_2) and TXA_2.[36,37]

Studies from our laboratory at the University of Minnesota using radiolabeled EPA and DHA have shown that these fatty acids are poorly used by vascular and platelet cyclooxygenases.[53,54] Even sheep vesicular gland converts these fatty acids in very low yield. Oral ingestion of two capsules of EPA (Shaklee Products: EPA 300 mg, DHA 130 mg) per day for 60 days or 15 capsules per day for 3 days had no significant effect on agonist-induced aggregation of platelets[54] We also demonstrated that exogenously added EPA and DHA block the platelet aggregation and the second-wave response of platelets to the action of agonists, such as epinephrine, ADP, and thrombin. DHA also inhibited the conversion of labeled AA to prostaglandins.[25] On the basis of these observations, we speculated that the polyenoic acids, if released in the vicinity of Cox enzymes, may compete for the active site of the enzyme and thereby inhibit the AA conversion to PGs. Results of our studies suggest that polyenoic acid–induced inhibition of platelet function may be related to their ability to compete with substrate arachidonic acid for the active heme-interactive site on the enzyme rather than to the inhibitory metabolites formed via vascular cyclooxygenase or lipoxygenase pathways.[25,26] Although the evidence from randomized clinical studies is lacking, use of long-chain fatty acids,

EPA/DHA as antiplatelet drugs is attractive and worth investigating further. The ratio of long-chain fatty acid that ensures moderate suppression of platelet aggregation without increasing bleeding time may be useful.

As we have discussed in earlier paragraphs, AA metabolism and formation of second messenger PGG_2, PGH_2, and thromboxane, seems to be an integral part of signaling mechanisms in platelet activation sequence (Fig. 7.2). We were a part of this "golden age" of prostanoid research worldwide.[1-54] During this long period of investigation, we found that a fair majority of domesticated mongrel dogs have platelets that do not respond to AA-mediated activation (Fig. 7.8A). However, platelets of these dogs do make prostaglandin endoperoxides and thromboxane like those dogs that respond in a normal fashion.[55,56] These nonresponding dogs do not present with any excessive bleeding episodes. During our studies on eicosanoids, we did come across a young woman whose platelets did not respond to the action of AA.[57] Her platelets responded with reversible aggregation to the action of ADP and thrombin, similar to aspirin-treated platelets. Just at that time, we had discovered a phenomenon that we described as "membrane modulation," which was capable of restoring the response of drug-induced refractory platelets.[55-64] Membrane modulation is mediated by epinephrine and acts via α-adrenergic receptor modulation.[63] Epinephrine was able to restore the response of nonresponding dog platelets as well as that of Cox-deficient platelets to the action of AA. We tested this phenomenon with aspirin-treated platelets. Aspirin-exposed platelets obtained from volunteers did not respond to AA stimulation. However, when exposed to AA in presence of epinephrine, they responded with irreversible aggregation (Fig. 7.8B). We demonstrated similar corrective effect on platelet-vessel interaction using aspirin-treated platelets.[64]

Folts and associates at Wisconsin have developed an in vivo model for initiation of thrombus in a stenosed coronary artery of dogs. In this model, when thrombus growth occurs, it results in cyclic flow reductions. Aspirin prevents formation of thrombus under the same experimental conditions. However, infusion of physiological doses of epinephrine stimulates aspirin-exposed platelets to

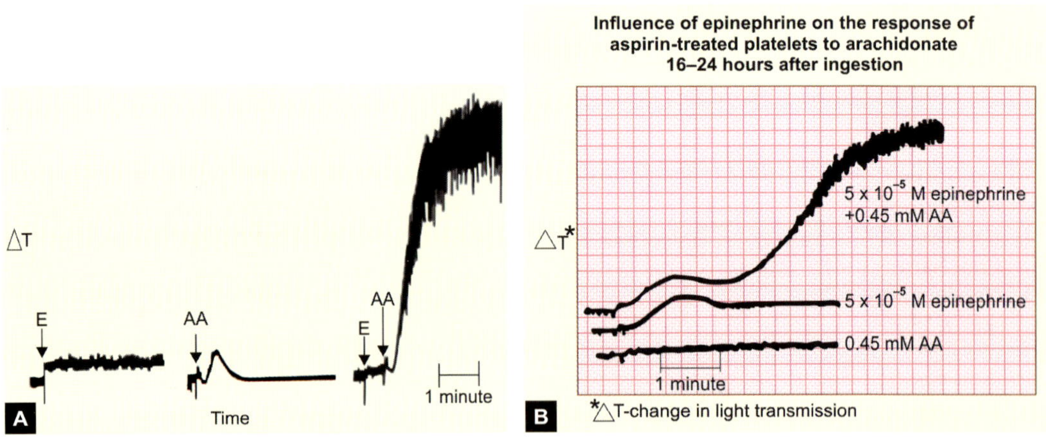

Figs. 7.8A and B: (A) Response of dog platelets to arachidonic acid. (B) Reversal of aspirin effect by epinephrine.

collect within the area of stenosis. Verapamil, which antagonizes epinephrine action, when infused in these dogs, prevents epinephrine-mediated correction of aspirin-exposed platelets.[59] Studies in stenosed canine arteries as well as our studies on platelet–vessel wall interactions have demonstrated that epinephrine can indeed neutralize the protective action of aspirin under flow conditions.

REFERENCES

1. Gerrard JM, White JG, Rao GHR, Townsend D. Localization of platelet prostaglandin production in the platelet dense tubular system. Am J Pathol.1976;83:283-99.
2. Purdon D. Phospholipid metabolism in platelets. Mod Meth Pharmacol. 1987;4:13-23.
3. Mahadevappa VG, Holub BJ. Degradation of different molecular species of phosphatidyl inositol in thrombin-stimulated human platelets. Evidence of preferential degradation of1-acyl-2-arachidonyl species. J Biol Chem. 1983;258:5337-9.
4. Rana RS, Hokin LE. Role of phosphoinositides in transmembrane signaling. Physiol Rev. 1990;70:115-64.
5. Hokin LE. Receptors and phosphoinositide generated second messengers. Annu Rev Biochem. 1986;54:205-35.
6. Nishizuka Y. Turnover of inositol phospholipids and signal transduction. Science. 1984;225:1365-70.
7. Abdel-Latiff AA. Calcium-mobilizing receptors, phosphoinositides, generation of second messengers, and contraction in mammalian smooth muscle: historical perspectives and current status. Life Sci. 1989;48(9):757-86.
8. Berridge MJ, Irvine RF. Inositol phosphate: a novel second messenger in signal transduction. Nature. 1984;312:315-21.
9. Needleman P, Whitaker MO, Wyche K, Watters K, Sprecher H, Raz A. Manipulation of platelet aggregation by prostaglandin and their fatty acid precursors: pharmacological basis for a therapeutic approach. Prostaglandins. 1980;19(1):165-81.
10. Yoshimoto A, Ito H, Tomita K. Cofactor requirement of the enzyme synthesizing prostaglandin in bovine seminal vesicles. J Biochem. 1972;68:487-99.
11. Miyamoto T, Ogino B, Yamamoto S, Hayaishi O. Purification of prostaglandin synthetase form bovine vesicular glands. J Biol Chem. 1976;251:2629-36.
12. Peterson DA, Gerrard JM. A hypothesis for the interactions of heme and arachidonic acid in the synthesis of prostaglandins. Med Hypotheses. 1979;5:683-94.
13. Peterson Da, Gerrard JM, Rao GHR, Krick TP, White JG. Ferrous iron mediated oxidation of arachidonic acid. Studies on nitroblue tetrazolium (NBT). Prostaglandins Med. 1978;1:304-17.
14. Peterson DA, Gerrard JM, Rao GHR, White JG. Inhibition of ferrous iron induced oxidation of arachidonic acid by indomethacin. Prostaglandins Med. 1979;2:97-108.
15. Peterson DA, Gerrard JM, Rao GHR, Mills EL, White JG. Interaction of arachidonic acid and heme iron in synthesis of prostaglandins. Adv Prostaglandin Thromboxane Res. 1980;6: 157-61.
16. Peterson DA, Gerrard JM, Rao GHR, White JG. Epinephrine and other activators of prostaglandin endoperoxide synthetase can reduce Fe+++ heme to Fe++ heme. Prostaglandins Med. 1980;5:357-65.
17. Peterson DA, Gerrard JM, Rao GHR, White JG. Reduction of ferric heme to ferrous by lipid peroxides: possible relevance to peroxide tone in the regulation of prostaglandin synthesis. Prostaglandins Med. 1980;4:73-9.
18. Peterson DA, Gerrard JM, Rao GHR, White JG. Salicylic acid inhibition of the irreversible effect of aspirin on prostaglandin synthetase may be due to competition for the enzyme cationic binding site. Prostaglandins Med. 1981;6:161-4.
19. Rao GHR, Gerrard JM, Eaton JW, White JG. Detection of arachidonic acid (AA) free radical formation, an essential step in platelet prostaglandin synthesis. Blood. 1976; 48:977A.
20. Rao GHR, Gerrard JM, Eaton JW, White JG. Arachidonic acid peroxidation, prostaglandin synthesis and platelet function. Photochem Photobiol. 1978;28:845-50.
21. Rao GHR, Gerrard JM, Eaton JW, White JG. The role of iron in prostaglandin synthesis.

Ferrous iron mediated oxidation of arachidonic acid. Prostaglandins Med. 1978;1:55-70.
22. Rao GHR, Burris SM, Gerrard JM, White JG. Inhibition of prostaglandin (PG) synthesis in sheep vesicular gland microsomes by nitroblue tetrazolium (NBT) and vitamin E. Prostaglandins Med. 1979;2:111-21.
23. Rao GHR, Cox AC, Gerrard JM, White JG. Effect of 2,'2'-dipyridyl and related compounds on platelet prostaglandin synthesis and platelet function. Biochem Biophys Acta. 1980;628:468-79.
24. Rao GHR, Johnson GJ, Reddy KR, White JG. Ibuprofen protects platelet cyclooxygenase from inhibition by aspirin. Arteriosclerosis. 1983;3:383-8.
25. Rao GHR, Radha E, White JG. Effect of docosahexaenoic acid (DHA) on arachidonic acid metabolism and platelet function. Biochem Biophys Res Commun. 1983;117:549-56.
26. Rao GHR, White JG. Heme-polyenoic acid interaction and prostaglandin synthesis. In: Bailey, J. M: (1985) Prostaglandins, leukotrienes, and lipoxins: Plenum Press: New York, ISBN 0-306-41980-7; 1985. p. 357-69.
27. Bergstrom S, Samuelsson B. Prostaglandins. Annu Rev Biochem. 1965;34:101-8.
28. Hamberg H, Svensson J Wakabayashi T, Samuelsson B. Isolation and structure of tow endoperoxides that cause platelet aggregation. Proc Natl Acad Sci U S A. 1974;71: 345-459.
29. Hamberg M, Samuelsson B. Prostaglandin endoperoxides. Novel transformations of arachidonic acid in human platelets. Proc Natl Acad Sci U S A. 1974;71:3400-4.
30. Hamberg M Svensson J, Samuelsson B. Thromboxanes: a new group of biologically active compounds derived from prostaglandin endoperoxides. Proc Natl Acad Sci U S A. 1975;72:2994-8.
31. Willis AL. An enzymatic mechanism for the antithrombotic and antihemostatic actions of aspirin. Science. 1974;183:325-7.
32. Whitaker N, Bunting S, Salmon J, Moncada S, Vane JR, Johnson RA, et al. The chemical structure of prostaglandin X (prostacyclin). Prostaglandins. 1976;12:915-28.
33. Samuelsson B. Role of basic science in the development of new medicines: examples from the eicosanoid field. J Biol Chem. 2012;287:10070-80.
34. Moncada S, Vane JR. The discovery of prostacyclin-a fresh insight into arachidonic acid metabolism. In: Kharasch N, Fried J (Eds). Biochemical Aspects of Prostaglandins and Thromboxanes. New York, Academic Press; 1977. pp. 155-77.
35. Moncada S, Vane JR. Arachidonic acid metabolites and the interactions between platelets and blood vessels. N Engl J Med. 1979;300:1142-7.
36. Needleman P, Minkes M, Raz A. Thromboxanes: selective biosynthesis and distinct biological properties. Science. 1976;193:163-5.
37. Needleman P, Wyche A, Raz A. Platelet and blood vessel arachidonate metabolism and interactions. J Clin Invest. 1979;63:839-49.
38. Vane JR, Bakhle YS, Botting RN. Cyclooxygenases 1 and 2. Annu Revarmacol Toxicol. 1998;38:97-120.
39. Vane JR. Inhibition of prostaglandin synthesis as mechanism of action for aspirin-like drugs. Nat New Biol. 1971;231:232-5.
40. Hemler M, Lands WEM, Smith WL. Purification of the cyclooxygenase that forms prostaglandins: demonstration of two forms of iron in the holoenzymes. J Biol Chem. 1976;251:5575-9.
41. Roth GJ, Majerus PW. The mechanism of the effect of Aspirin on human platelets: 1 Acetylation of a particulate fractions protein. J Clin Invest. 1975;56:624-32.
42. De Witt DL, El-Harith EA, Kraemer SA, Andrews MJ, Yao EF, Armstrong RL, et al. The aspirin and heme-binding sites of ovine and murine prostaglandin synthases. J Biol Chem. 1990;265:5192-8.
43. Vane JR, Botting RM. The mechanism of action of aspirin. Thromb Res. 2003;110(5-6):255-8.
44. Smith CM, Burris SM. Rao GHR, White JG. Epinephrine-induced reversal of aspirin effects on platelet membrane deformability. Thromb Res. 1988;51:35-44.
45. Jafe EA, Weksler BB. Recovery of endothelial prostacyclin production after inhibition by low doses of aspirin. J Clin Invest. 1979;63: 532-5.
46. Rao GHR, Reddy KR, White JG. Low dose aspirin, platelet function and prostaglandin

synthesis: Influence of epinephrine and alpha-adrenergic blockade. Prostaglandins Med. 1981;6:485-94.

47. Antithrombotic Trialists (ATT) Collaboration; Baigent C, Blackwell L, Collins R, Emberson J, Godwin J, Peto R, et al. Aspirin in the primary and secondary prevention of vascular disease: collaborative meta-analysis of individual participant data from randomized trials. Lancet. 2009;373(9678):1849-60.
48. Dyerberg J, Bang HO, Hjorne N. Fatty acid composition of the plasma lipids in Greenland Eskimos. Am J Clin Nutr 1975;28: 958-66.
49. Dyerberg J, Bang HO. Haemostatic function and platelet polyunsaturated fatty acids in Eskimos. Lancet. 1979;314(2):433-5.
50. Goodnight SH. Effects of dietary fish oil and omega-3 fatty acids on platelets and blood vessels. Semin Thromb Hemost. 1988;14: 285-9.
51. Lands WEM, Samuelsson B. Phospholipid precursors of prostaglandins. Biochim Biophys Acta. 1968;164:426-9.
52. Murthy M. Polyenoic acids and platelet function. In: Rao GHR (Ed). Handbook of Platelet Physiology and Pharmacology. Boston: Kluwer Academic Publishers; 1999. pp. 269-93.
53. Rao GHR, Kishore NP, Peller JD, White JG. Influence of polyenoic acids on arachidonic acid metabolism and platelet function. In: Gallo LL (Ed). Cardiovascular Disease. New York: Springer; 1985. pp. 405-505.
54. Rao GHR, Mahadevappa VG, Hill TD, White JG. Arachidonic acid oxidation and platelet function. In: Reddy CC, Hamilton GA, Madyastha KM (Eds). Biological Oxidation Systems. (New York: Academic Press; 1990. pp. 779-90.
55. Johnson GJ, Leis LA, Rao GHR. Arachidonate-induced platelet aggregation in the dog. Thromb Res. 1979;14:147-54.
56. Johnson JW, Rao GHR, Leis L, White JG. Effects of agents, which alter cyclic AMP on arachidonate-induced platelet aggregation in the dog. Blood. 1980;55:722-9.
57. Rao GHR, White JG. Epinephrine potentiation of arachidonate-induced aggregation of cyclooxygenase deficient platelets. Am J Hematol. 1981;11:355-66.
58. Rao GHR, Johnson JG, White JG. Influence of epinephrine on the aggregation response of aspirin-treated platelets. Prostaglandins Med. 1980;6:5-45.
59. Bonebrake FC, Bethra B, Folts HD, Rao GHR. Verapamil combined with aspirin for inhibiting epinephrine stimulated thrombus formation in stenosed canine arteries. Coron Artery Dis. 1991;2:487-92.
60. Rao GHR. Influence of anti-platelet drugs on platelet vessel wall interactions. Prostaglandins Leukot Med. 1987;30:133-45.
61. Rao GHR, White JG. Epinephrine-induced platelet membrane modulation. In: Myers K, Barnes CD (Eds). Platelet Amine Storage Granules. Boca Raton: CRC Press; 1992. pp. 117-95.
62. Rao GHR, Escolar G, Zavoral J, White JG. Influence of adrenergic receptor blockade on aspirin induced inhibition of platelet function. Platelets. 1990;1:145-50.
63. Rao GHR, Johnson GW, Reddy KR, White JG. Ibuprofen protects platelet cyclooxygenase from irreversible inhibition by aspirin. Arteriosclerosis. 1983;117(2):549-55.
64. Rao GHR, Escolar G, White JG. Epinephrine reverses the inhibitory influence of aspirin on platelet-vessel wall interactions. Thromb Res. 1986;44(1):65-74.

CHAPTER 8

Calcium Modulation by Cyclic Nucleotides

Blood platelets play a very important role in the pathogenesis of atherosclerosis, interaction with the vessel wall, thrombus formation, thrombus growth, and coagulation. In other words, development of thrombotic state involves four main factors: alterations in the vessel wall physiology, the interaction of formed elements of blood, activation of coagulation factors, and blood flow dynamics. In the arterial thrombosis, the major part in the initiation and growth of thrombi is played by platelets and fibrinogen. In view of these observations, for the development of drugs that inhibit platelet function, it is helpful to understand the various biochemical mechanisms, which contribute to thrombus formation, so that novel antiplatelet drugs could be developed. In this mini review, we will discuss some of the early discoveries in our laboratory at the University of Minnesota that led us to understand the mechanisms involved in adhesion, shape change, spreading, aggregation, secretion of granule contents, thrombus formation, and thrombus growth. As this is an article that expresses my point of view on the topic, I have taken liberties to summarize our work of over three decades. The results of these studies have been presented in various national and international conferences over the years, as such may not be easily accessible. Moreover, it is hard to understand the overall findings without reading all those published articles. Without that collective knowledge, it would be difficult to design novel antiplatelet therapies, which would be the subject of my next overview to be published in this journal.

In the early 70s, it was believed that agonists activated platelets by as yet unknown mechanism, caused release of granule contents, including serotonin, adenosine diphosphate, and calcium. It was assumed that released components acted as recruiting agents as well as potentiators of platelet activation and aggregation. Studies from our laboratory for the first time demonstrated that calcium ionophore (A23187) by moving calcium across the membranes was able to induce aggregation, contraction, as well as release of the internal contents. I would say that it was a remarkable observation. We were able to show in this study that the antibiotic ionophore was able to move calcium across the membrane, facilitate the release of internal membrane-bound calcium, promote the conversion of soluble actin to filamentous actin, induce contraction, and release of the granule contents. We also demonstrated that the agents that elevate cAMP inhibited this process.[1] Further studies from our laboratory demonstrated the similarity between the ionophore-induced platelet activation and that of changes induced by natural platelet agonists like collagen and thrombin.[2] Now that we knew that elevation of cytosolic calcium was key to contraction and secretion pathways, we had to explore how agonists mobilize intracellular calcium.

Since we were located close to Hormel Meat Packing Plant at Austin, Minnesota, where we had easy access to freshly harvested sheep vesicular glands (SVGs), we were able to obtain these glands and show that one could obtain labile lipid platelet agonists capable of aggregating aspirin-treated platelets.[3] Studies from our laboratory for the first time demonstrated the localization of the prostaglandin synthetase in the platelet dense tubular system.[4] My associate, Jonathan Gerrard, using arachidonic acid, endoperoxides, and ionophore as agonists demonstrated calcium mobilization and phosphorylation of platelet proteins.[5] We were also able to demonstrate agonist-mediated calcium mobilization using calcium-specific fluorophores.[6-10] During the same period, Prof Nelson D Goldberg of the University of Minnesota published an article to explain a phenomenon of "Yin/Yang hypothesis" to describe a concept of biological regulation, in which two cellular components, cyclic adenosine monophosphate (cAMP) and cyclic guanosine monophosphate (cGMP), are envisioned to provide the facilitatory or supportive role in modulating a variety of biological events.[8] In Chinese philosophy, Yin and Yang describes how opposite or contrary forces are actually complementary, interconnected, and interdependent to each other as they interrelate to one another. We were quite impressed by the work of Prof Goldberg and were very much interested in demonstrating such an effect in platelet activation and deactivation. Therefore, we collaborated with his group and published an abstract in the Journal of Clinical Investigation in 1973. (I was not able to get this abstract by internet search). This is the way I have summarized our observations in an abstract on my Research gate site: "In those days when cGMP ruled, most cellular events or that is what the experts in Nelson Goldberg's laboratory believed, these studies were done to demonstrate that there was a role for cGMP in modulation of platelet physiology and function. However, later studies demonstrated that elevation of cGMP by "nitroso" compounds, as well as nitric oxide inhibited platelet activation." One exception for this observation is cGMP elevation by ascorbic acid. The ascorbic acid–induced increase in cGMP does not lead to aggregation; the exact role for this observation begs explanation.

On the basis of our studies at the University of Minnesota, platelet activation story goes something like this (Fig. 8.1). One or more agonists interact with the platelet lipid membrane–associated, glycoprotein-rich receptors. The agonist's interaction with specific receptors results in transmembrane signaling via transmembrane proteins, such as GTP-binding proteins. Receptor-mediated signaling results in the hydrolysis of GTP to GDP and activation of phospholipase C (PLC). This enzyme acts on membrane-associated phospholipids (inositol phosphates) and generates second messengers like inositol 1-4'-5' trisphosphate (IP_3) and diacylglycerol (2-DAG). Inositol trisphosphate mobilizes cytosolic calcium from membrane stores and elevates free cytosolic calcium. This elevation in cytosolic-free calcium activates phospholipase A_2 (PlA_2) and releases arachidonic acid (AA). This fatty acid is further converted by cyclooxygenase (Cox) enzymes to prostaglandin endoperoxides (PGH_2, PGG_2) and thromboxanes (TXA_2), proaggregatory, vasoconstrictory metabolites. These active metabolites of AA are released to the exterior of the cells and they in turn activate specific receptors on platelet membranes. This is one of the common pathways to activate GPIIb/IIIa receptors on platelets. Once these receptors are activated, they can recognize the active

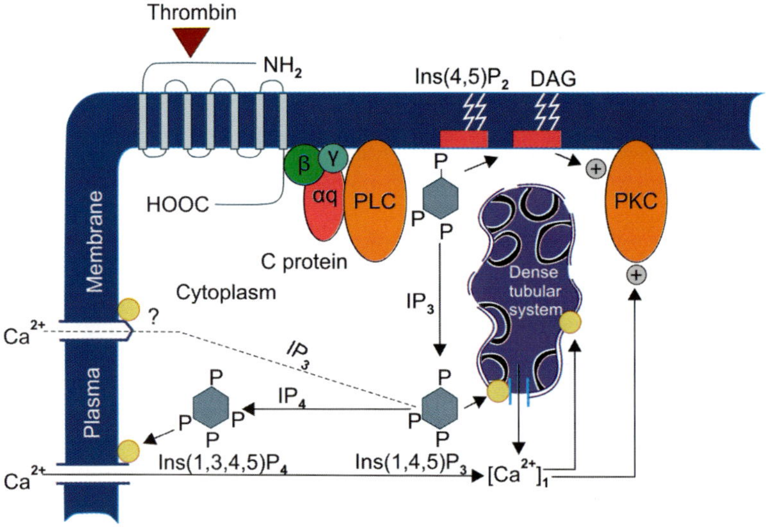

Fig. 8.1: Agonist-mediated formation of second messengers (DAG, IP_3) and calcium mobilization in platelets.

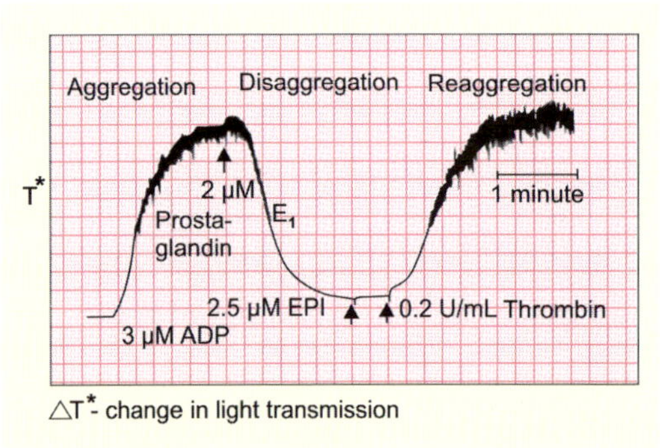

Fig. 8.2: Platelet aggregation, disaggregation and reaggregation.

binding site on fibrinogen that contains the peptide; Arg-Gly-Asp (RGD) containing the following sequence of amino acids and brings platelets together (aggregation or thrombus formation). As far as the morphology and cytoskeletal changes are concerned, platelets when activated, change shape, extend pseudopods, spread on the surface, assemble filamentous actin, contract and secrete granule contents. Series of studies from our laboratory demonstrated that platelet deactivation was achieved by lowering the elevated levels of cytosolic free calcium by the second messengers, cAMP and cGMP.

By this time, studies from our laboratory as well as that of others had demonstrated that platelet aggregation was dependent on GPIIb/IIIa activation and fibrinogen binding. In a series of elegant studies, we were able to demonstrate that one could dissociate bound fibrinogen from aggregated platelets by lowering cytosolic calcium (Fig. 8.2).[5,11-13] These studies further demonstrated that fibrinogen binding, which paralleled irreversible aggregation was accompanied by phosphorylation of specific proteins and the disaggregation and reaggregation cycles were accompanied by disassociation and reassociation of fibrinogen and protein phosphorylation cycles.[5,14]

Having explained basic mechanisms involved in receptor-mediated activation of PLC, calcium mobilization, stimulation of PLA_2, release of AA, generation of second messengers, PGG_2, PGH_2, TXA_2, cAMP, cGMP, and modulation of cytosolic calcium, we turned our attention to define the mechanisms involved in adhesion, spreading irreversible aggregation, and platelet vessel wall interactions.[14-29] Using platelets of patients with Hermansky-Pudlak syndrome, which are devoid of granules, we demonstrated irreversible aggregation independent of release of granule contents.[11,16]

Using cyclooxygenase-deficient platelets, we demonstrated irreversible aggregation independent of prostaglandins.[11,18] Deploying Quin-2 AM a calcium fluorophores and a chelating agent, we demonstrated adhesion and irreversible aggregation of platelets independent of cytosolic calcium. Using denuded rabbit aorta, we demonstrated that commonly used antiplatelet drugs did not prevent platelet–vessel wall interactions.[17,26]

Summarizing the work of four decades in our laboratory at the University of Minnesota in a short overview is a herculean task. However, it is important to understand the salient findings, so that we can figure out why some of the drugs failed and some were successful. For instance, collective knowledge from our group as well as that of others regarding the activation of GPIIb/IIIa receptor as a prerequisite for fibrinogen, and the sequence of amino acids that are recognized by the activated receptor (RGD) played an important role in the development of RGD mimics, as well as the monoclonal antibody abciximab (ReoPro).[30,31] Platelets do not recognize this RGD sequence in soluble fibrinogen circulating in the blood; once the GPIIb/IIIa receptor is activated, then they can find this binding site. Whereas, once the fibrinogen is bound on a surface, this binding site is exposed and activation of the receptor is not essential for platelets to interact with the surface-bound fibrinogen. Contrary to this phenomenon, platelet GPIb receptor does not need any activation to bind von Willebrand factor protein. However, this globular protein can interact with platelets only at very high shear force (arterial circulation). Our studies very clearly demonstrated that drug-induced refractoriness of platelets could be overcome by the action of multiple agonists or by epinephrine-induced mechanism of membrane modulation.[29-34] Since platelet interactions with the vessel wall was mediated by extracellular matrix components, commonly used antiplatelet drugs failed to inhibit these interactions.[12,25,26]

From the very first report from our laboratory in 70s, in which we had demonstrated a raise in cGMP in parallel with irreversible aggregation and release of granule contents, there had been considerable conflicting reports on the role of cyclic nucleotides in platelet function.[8,35,36] Noble laureate Louis Ignarro, in his chapter on the regulation of polymorphonuclear leukocyte, macrophage, and platelet function, writes, "Recent advances in the fields of cyclic nucleotide and biological regulation have made it clear, however, that a second cyclic nucleotide cGMP serves as important, and perhaps obligatory, function in the bioregulation of cellular processes (Refers to our 1973 abstract). Much of the work involving cGMP suggests that it may function to mediate or signal cellular processes that are ultimately antagonistic or opposite in direction to those mediated by cAMP."[37] Studies from our laboratory as well as that of others have demonstrated the inhibitory role of agents that elevate cAMP as well as cGMP.[20-22] According to recent studies, the activation of human platelets seems to be inhibited by two intracellular pathways, regulated by either cAMP- or cGMP-elevating agents.[38] These studies have demonstrated that inhibitory effect of these antagonists to be mediated by the phosphorylation of vasodilator-stimulated phosphoprotein (VASP). Our results on the inhibitory role of cGMP on platelet function, similar to that of cAMP, have been confirmed by studies from many other laboratories including the Welcome Laboratories under the leadership of Salvador Moncada.[39,40]

In conclusion, studies from our laboratory at the University of Minnesota as well as that of others have demonstrated that agonist-mediated receptor stimulation leads to the activation of PLC and formation of second messengers, DAG and inositol trisphosphate and mobilization of cytosolic-free calcium. Elevation in intracellular calcium activates PLA_2 and facilitates the release of AA. This fatty acid is further converted to active metabolites, PGH_2, PGG_2, and TXA_2. Thromboxanes promote fibrinogen binding, irreversible aggregation, and the release of granule contents, including serotonin and ADP. Agents that promote irreversible aggregation facilitate fibrinogen binding and those drugs that dissociate this process do so by lowering the cytosolic calcium levels. Endogenous antagonists, such as PGE_1, PGI_2, and NO exert their inhibitory effect on platelet function by the action of cyclic nucleotides, cAMP and cGMP. Epinephrine-induced modulation of α-adrenergic receptor restores the action of agonists in drug-induced refractory platelets. As far as the role of cyclic nucleotides is considered, the observations are consistent with the concept that cyclic nucleotides' participation in the biological regulation may be modulated by cytoplasmic cations and that a change in intracellular cyclic nucleotides and appropriate cations serve to promote the participation of both regulatory effectors.[41] Antiplatelet drugs such as aspirin, indomethacin, and PGE_1 do not inhibit platelet interactions with the vessel wall. On the basis of this collective knowledge, novel antiplatelet drugs should be developed for the prevention of acute vascular events.

REFERENCES

1. White, JG, Rao GHR, Gerrard JM. Effects of ionophore A23187 on blood platelets 1. Influences on aggregation and secretion. Am J Pathol. 1974;77:135-50.
2. Gerrard JM, White JG, Rao GHR. Effects of the ionophore A23187 on blood platelets 11. Influence on ultrastructure. Am J Pathol. 1974;77:151-66.
3. Gerrard JM, White JG Rao GHR, Krivit W, Witkop CJ. Labile aggregation stimulating substance (LASS): the factor from storage pool deficient platelets correcting defective aggregation and release of aspirin treated normal platelets. Br J Hematol. 1975;29(4):657-65.
4. Gerrard JM, White JG, Rao GHR, Townsend D. Localization of prostaglandin production in the platelet dense tubular system. Am J Pathol. 1976;83:283-98.
5. Gerrard JM, Buttler AM, Graff G, Stoddard SF, White JG. Prostaglandin endoperoxides promote calcium release from platelet membrane fraction in vitro. Prostaglandins Med. 1978;1(5):373-85.
6. Gerrard JM, Carroll, RC. Stimulation of platelet protein phosphorylation by arachidonic acid and endoperoxides analogues. Prostaglandins. 1981;22:82-94.
7. Rao GHR, Peller JD, White JG. Measurement of ionized calcium with a new generation calcium indicator. Biochem Biophys Res Commun. 1985;132:652-7.
8. White JG, Goldberg ND, Estensen RD, Haddox MK, Rao GHR. Rapid increase in platelet cyclic 3',5'-guanosine monophosphate (cGMP) levels in association with irreversible aggregation, degranulation and secretion. J Clin Invest. 1973;52:89a.
9. Rao GHR, Peller JD, Semba CP, White JG. Influence of the calcium-sensitive fluorophore, Quin-2 AM on platelet function. Blood. 1986;67:354-61.
10. Rao GHR, White JG. Aspirin, PGE1 and Quin-2 AM-induced platelet dysfunction: restoration of function by noradrenalin. Prostaglandins Leukot Essent Fatty Acids. 1990;39:141-6.
11. Rao GHR, Gerrard JM, Witkop CJ, White JG. Platelet aggregation independent of ADP release or prostaglandin synthesis in patients

with Hermansky-Pudlak syndrome. Prostaglandins Med. 1981;6:459-62.
12. Rao GHR, Escolar G, White JG. Epinephrine reverses the inhibitory influence of aspirin on platelet-vessel wall interactions. Thromb Res. 1986;1;44:65-74.
13. Rao GHR. Influence of anti-platelet drugs on platelet-vessel wall interactions. Prostaglandins Leukot Med. 1987;30:133-45.
14. Rao GHR, White JG. Disaggregation and reaggregation of "irreversibly" aggregated platelets: a method for more complete evaluation of antiplatelet drugs. Agents Actions. 1978;16:425-34.
15. Cox AC, Caroll RG, White JG, Rao GHR. Recycling of platelet phosphorylation and cytoskeletal assembly. J Cell Biol. 1978;16:425-34.
16. Graber SE, Hawiger J. Evidence that changes in platelet cyclic AMP levels regulate the fibrinogen receptor on human platelets. J Biol Chem. 1982;257:14606-9.
17. Rao GHR, Gerrard JM, Witkop CJ, White JG. Platelet aggregation independent of ADP release or prostaglandin synthesis in patients with the Hermansky-Pudlak syndrome. Prostaglandins Med. 1981;6:459-72.
18. Rao GHR, White JG. Epinephrine potentiation of arachidonate-induced aggregation of cyclooxygenase deficient platelets. Am J Hematol. 1981;11:355-66.
19. Folts JD, Rowe CG, Rao GHR. Problem with aspirin as anti-thrombotic agent in coronary artery disease. Lancet. 1988;1:937-8.
20. Krsihnamurthi S, Wheeler-Jones CPD, Patel Y, Sadowska K, Kakkar VV, Rao GHR. Nitroprusside inhibits platelet function primarily by inhibiting calcium mobilization. Biochem Soc Trans. 1990;18:468-70.
21. Rao GHR, Krishnamurhti S, Raij L, White JG. Influence of nitric oxide on agonist-mediated calcium mobilization in platelets. Biochem Med Metab Biol. 1990;43:271-5.
22. Rao GHR, Raij L, Lester B, White JG. Inhibition of agonist-induced human platelet activation by nitric oxide. In: Moncada S, Higgs EA (Eds). Proceedings Roy Society Symposium. New York: Elsevier Publishing Company; 1990. pp. 355-67.
23. Rao GHR, Fareed J, White JG. Influence of heparins on inositol 1, 4, 5-trisphosphate induced calcium mobilization in permeabilized human platelets. Biochem Med Metab Biol. 1991;45: 171-80.
24. Rao GHR, Wilson RF, White CW, White JG. Influence of thrombolytic agents on human platelet function Thromb Res. 1991;62: 319-34.
25. Bonebrake FL, Bertha B, Folts JD, Rao GHR. Verapamil combined with aspirin for inhibiting epinephrine-stimulated platelet thrombus formation in stenosed canine coronary arteries. Coron Artery Dis. 1991;2:487-92.
26. Rao GHR, Smith CM, White JG. Influence of calcium antagonists on thrombin-induced calcium mobilization and platelet vesselwall interactions. Biochem Med Metab Biol. 1992;47:226-31.
27. Rao GHR, Smith CM, Doni MG, White JG. Intracellular calcium imaging in adherent human platelets. Arteriosclerosis Thromb. 1994;5:95-105.
28. Padoni E, Alexander A, Carvalline L, Rao GHR, Doni MG. Human platelet activation is inhibited by the occupancy of glycoprotein 11b/111a receptor. Arch Biochem Biophys. 1996;333:407-13.
29. Nagarajan SR, Devadas B, Malecha JW, Lu HF, Ruminski PG, Rico JG, et al. R-isomers of Arg-Gly-Asp (RGD) mimics as potent a_v/B_3 inhibitors. Biorg Med Chem. 2007;15:3783-800.
30. Coller BS, Folts JD, Scudder LE, Smith SR. Antithrombotic effect of a monoclonal antibody to the platelet glycoprotein 11b/11a receptor in an experimental animal model. Blood. 1986;68(3):783-6.
31. Coller BS Peerschke, Scudder LE, Sullivan CA. Studies with a murine monoclonal antibody that abolishes ristocetin-induced binding of von Willebrand factor to platelets: additional evidence in support of GP1B as a platelet receptor for von Willebrand factor. Blood. 1983;61(1):99-110.
32. Rao GHR, Schmid HHO, Reddy KR, White JG. Human platelet activation by an alkyl acetyl analogue of phosphatidylcholine. Biochem Biophys Acta. 1982;715:205-14.
33. Rao GHR, White JG. Platelet activating factor causes human platelet aggregation through the mechanism of membrane modulation. Prostaglandins Leukot Med. 1982;9:459-72.
34. Rao GHR, White JG. Epinephrine-induced platelet membrane modulation. In: Myers K (Ed). Platelet Amine Storage Granules. Academic Press: New York, 1989.

35. Claesson H, Malmsten C. On the interrelationship of prostaglandin endoperoxides G2 and cyclic nucleotides in platelet function. Eur J Biochem. 1977;76:277-84.
36. Weiss A, Baenziner NL, Atkinson JP. Platelet release reaction and intracellular cGMP. Blood. 1978;52:524-31.
37. Ignarro LJ. Regulation of polymorphonuclear leukocyte, macrophage, and platelet function. In: Hadden JW, Coffey RG, Spreafico F (Eds). Immunopharmacology, Vol. 3. Plenum Publishing: New York, 1977. p. 61.
38. Walter U, Eigenthaler M, Geiger J, Reinhard M. Role of cyclic nucleotide-dependent protein kinase and their common substrate VASP in the regulation of human platelets. Adv Exp Med Biol. 1993;344:237-49.
39. Loscaizo L. N-acetyl cysteine potentiates inhibition of platelet aggregation by nitroglycerine. J Clin Invest. 1985;76:703-8.
40. Moncada S, Higgs A. The L-arginine-nitric oxide pathway. N Engl J Med. 1993;329:2002-12.
41. Goldberg ND, Haddox MK, Zelig CE, Nicol SE, Acott TS, Glass DB. Cyclic GMP, cyclic AMP and the Yin Yang hypothesis of biological regulation. J Clin Invest. 1976;67:641-5.

Reproduced with permission from: Wolter Kluwer Permissions Team Jan 28, 2017. Article published in Journal of Clinical and Preventive Cardiology: 5(3):99-103, 2016. DOI:10.4103/2250-3528.191101

CHAPTER 9

Pharmacology of Antiplatelet Drugs

By and large, the choices of drugs for antiplatelet prophylaxis, worldwide currently, are aspirin, clopidogrel, or a combination of the two with appropriate combinations.[1-6] Health data compiled from more than 190 countries by the American Heart Association show heart disease as the number one global cause of death with 17.3 million deaths each year, according to "Heart Disease and Stroke Statistics—2015 Update: A Report from the American Association." That number is expected to rise to more than 23.6 million by 2030. A World Health Organization report says that people with cardiovascular disease, who are at high risk due to the presence of one or more risk factors, such as hypertension, diabetes, and hyperlipidemia need early detection and management of the identified risks, counseling, and medicines as appropriate. Noncommunicable Disease (NCD) Risk Factor Task Collaboration in their seminal article in *Lancet* (April 2016) concluded that if the post 2000 trends continue in the incidence and rise in diabetes, the probability of meeting the global target of halting the rise in the prevalence of diabetes by 2025 level worldwide would be lower than 1%. According to the Institute of Health Matric and Evaluation (IHME), today 2.1 billion people—nearly 30% of the global population are either obese or overweight—a new, first-of-a-kind analysis of trend data from 180 countries.[7] Since 1980, obesity has increased worldwide by twofold and type 2 diabetes by fourfold. Patients with diabetes have a two- to threefold higher risk for developing cardiovascular disease (CVD) and cerebrovascular disease (CBD). India currently has over 65 million type 2 diabetics and equal number of prediabetics. According to published literature, a large percentage of these individuals develop CVD or CBD. Major complication leading to death is, by and large, due to vessel thrombosis, ischemia, resulting in heart attacks, or stroke.

The role of blood platelets in the pathogenesis of atherosclerosis, thrombosis, thromboembolism, and stroke is well established.[8-23] In view of this recognized role played by platelets in the complications associated with coronary artery disease and cerebral artery disease, there is considerable interest in the pharmacology of platelet activation inhibitory drugs.[15] Earlier studies on platelet biochemistry, physiology, and function suggests that the release of granule contents is essential for recruitment of cells, irreversible aggregation, and formation of thrombi.[24] The most prominent structural features of a platelet are three types of granules: dense bodies (dense core, dense granules), α, and lysosomal granules. Early literature suggests that released ADP as well as newly synthesized endoperoxides and thromboxane play a role in the activation of other cells and recruitment of them for thrombus growth. There are a host of cytokines, chemokines, and growth factors released by platelets upon activation.

Studies from our laboratory demonstrated that circulating levels of catecholamines could induce stickiness in blood platelets. If the levels are not high enough, the minimally activated platelets could reverse back into their normal inactivated state. This intrinsic mechanism of catecholamine-induced membrane modulation is capable of restoring the sensitivity of drug-induced refractory platelets to the action of agonists. The restoration of sensitivity to various agonists is not dependent on the potentiation of various activating and signaling mechanism, such as phosphatide inositol metabolism, formation of second messengers: diglyceride and inositol trisphosphate, elevation of cytosolic calcium, activation of phospholipases, release of arachidonic acid (AA), formation of endoperoxides, thromboxanes, assembly of cytosolic actin, contraction of cytoskeletal proteins, or release of granule contents.[25-33] The mechanism of membrane modulation is mediated by α-adrenergic receptor stimulation, and is dependent on the availability of membrane-associated calcium.

In an article published in 2009, Rendu and associates write, "Dense granules contain small nonprotein molecules that are secreted to recruit other platelets. F-granules contain large adhesion and healing proteins. Lysosomes contain hydrolases that are able to eliminate the circulating platelet aggregates. The extrusion of storage granules' contents to the platelet's environment occurs according to regulated secretion events: movements of granules, apposition and fusion of granule, and plasma membranes. Typical platelet disorders resulting from a storage granule abnormality are referred to as storage pool defect and are characterized by prolonged bleeding time.[34] In spite of the fact that our earlier studies have demonstrated the existence of an intrinsic mechanism of membrane modulation that is capable of restoring the function of platelets independent of release reaction, we find references to this mechanism and its key role in platelet function."

Biochemical pathways associated with agonist-mediated platelet activation are initiated with ligand binding to the specific platelet membrane receptors or glycoprotein-rich integrin, nonintegrin domains. Ligand receptor interaction leads to transmembrane signal transduction via GTP-binding proteins and activation of phospholipase C, leading to the hydrolysis of phosphatidyl inositol 4,5-bisphosphate (PIP_2) and formation of second messengers 1,2-diacylglycerol (DAG) and inositol 1,4,5-trisphosphate (IP_3). Diglyceride stimulates protein kinase C and IP_3 mobilizes cytosolic calcium. Elevation of cytosolic calcium activates phospholipase A_2 and liberates AA from the membrane phospholipids. Free AA is converted by cyclooxygenases to prostaglandin endoperoxides (PGG_2/PGH_2) and by thromboxane synthase to thromboxane A_2 (TXA_2). Thromboxane is the major metabolite and facilitates platelet recruitment and secretion of granule contents. Promising antiplatelet drugs can be screened to prevent all of the above activation mechanisms or just prevent some discrete responses. On the basis of the information available on the specific mechanisms involved in platelet activation, antiplatelet or antithrombotic drugs were developed to prevent or disrupt discrete steps in the activation signaling pathways.

Some of the antiplatelet or antithrombotic drugs include cyclooxygenase inhibitors, thromboxane synthetase inhibitors (receptor antagonists), stimulators of adenylyl and guanylyl cyclases, phosphodiesterase inhibitors, serine protease inhibitors, and calcium antagonists (Fig. 9.1).

AGENTS MODULATING PLATELET FUNCTION

Antagonist/ inhibitors	Platelet adhesion
von Willebrand factor	Glycoprotein GPIb receptor antibody
	Antibody to von Willebrand factor
	Inactive von Willebrand factor fragments
Platelet aggregation and signaling pathways:	
Cyclooxygenase	Aspirin, ibuprofen, indomethacin
Thromboxane synthetase	Dazoxiben
Thromboxane synthase and receptor	Thromboxane A_2 receptor blocker
ADP	Ticlopidine, clopidogrel
Thrombin	Hirudin, hirulag, argatroban
Serotonin	Ketanserin
Platelet-activating factor (PAF)	PAF antagonists
Phosphodiesterase (PDE)	Dipyridamole, caffeine
Glycoprotein GPIIb/a receptor	RGD mimetics (intravenous and oral)

From Mousa S: Drug Discovery Today. 2000; 4(12): 552-6.

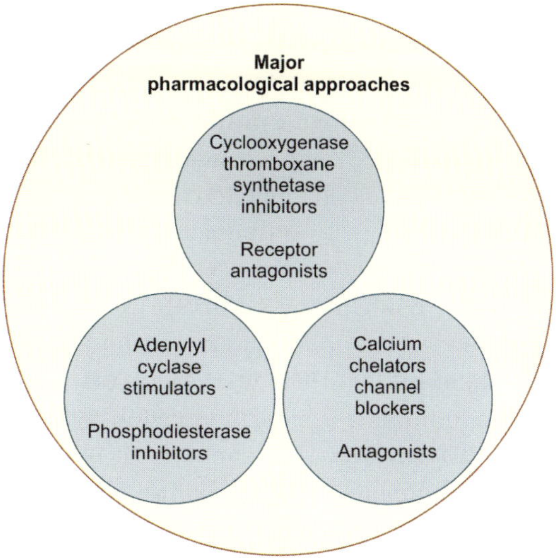

Fig. 9.1: Antiplatelet drugs.

Major pharmacological approaches therefore revolved around prevention of the release of arachidonic acid, blocking conversion of the fatty acid substrate by prostaglandin synthase or to interfere with the availability of ionized calcium. In this chapter, we will describe our studies on arachidonic acid metabolism, role of ferrous iron, and epinephrine in some of these reactions. We will also discuss a unique, "laboratory to clinic" development effort of a successful antiplatelet drug, and brief description of antithrombotic therapies.

Yoshimoto and associates were the first to demonstrate that heme is required for enhancing the activity of prostaglandin synthase enzymes.[35] Ogino et al. found very little iron in purified endoperoxide synthetase but found that the enzyme required metalloporphyrins for its activity.[36] Ultrastructural studies from our laboratory using an iron-reactive drug, diaminobenzidine, reported that enzymes involved in endoperoxide generation are localized in the dense tubular system in human platelets.[37] The fact that heme iron acts as a catalyst for the isolated enzymes and that heme-complexing compounds react with these enzymes in the platelet, dense tubular system (DTS) prompted us to evaluate the role of iron and heme in AA oxidation.[38]

Using a cell-free system, we showed that ferrous iron and heme could induce oxidation of polyenoic acids.[39] We found oxidation of AA by ferrous sulfate a useful model to study the role of iron in lipid oxidation reactions. We employed nitroblue tetrazolium (NBT) for our investigations. Reduction of NBT was accompanied by oxidation of ferrous iron to ferric, suggesting the transfer of four electrons from the ferrous to NBT to reduce the dye. AA was found to be unchanged when extracted indicating that the complex is transient and dissociates easily. NBT reduction was not inhibited by agents, which hydrolyzed superoxide, by catalase, or by agents, which trap hydroxyl radicals. We therefore proposed a model in which NBT traps a radical generated on the AA molecule (Fig. 9.2).

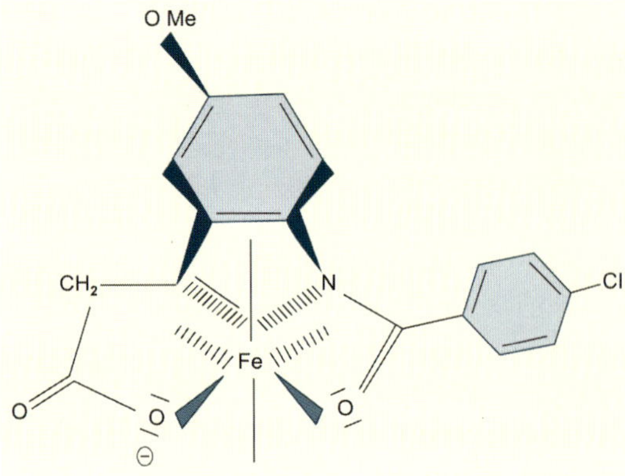

Fig. 9.2: A postulated model for the interaction of ferrous iron and indomethacin, a cyclooxygenase inhibitor. The carboxylate and amide groups of indomethacin are shown interacting with the valences of iron to form this complex. From Peterson et al., 1979, with permission.

AA is the major substrate for production of platelet endoperoxides, thromboxanes, as well as vessel wall-generated prostacyclins.[16] Iron or heme is an essential cofactor for the peroxidase, lipoxygenase, and cyclooxygenase enzyme activities.[40] We explored the interaction of AA with ferrous iron to identify the transient free radical that is formed during such reactions. High-pressure liquid chromatography, chemical ionization and electron-impact mass spectrometry, and nuclear magnetic resonance spectroscopy suggested that the major product was hydroperoxide of AA. Conversion of AA to hydroperoxide was inhibited by the antioxidant 2, 3 tert-butyl-4-hydroxyanisole, the radical scavenger NBT and iron-chelating agents, including ethylenediaminetetraacetic acid (EDTA), imida-zole, and dihydroxybenzoic acid. Iron-induced oxidation of AA was not affected by superoxide dismutase, catalase, or aspirin.

One of the drugs that have been shown to inhibit prostaglandin synthesis is indomethacin.[41] The molecular mechanisms by which indomethacin exerts its inhibitory effects on the prostaglandin endoperoxide synthetase enzyme is unknown. In the late 70s, we explored the possibilities that indomethacin might interact with ferrous iron or heme in the enzyme to exert its inhibitory effect.[42] On the basis of our in vitro studies, Peterson, a close associate of ours, postulated a model for the interaction of ferrous iron and indomethacin as shown in Figure 9.2.

The carboxylase and amide groups of indomethacin are shown interacting with the valence of iron to form this complex. Ibuprofen and tolmetin, two other prostaglandin inhibitors, also inhibit the interaction of ferrous iron with AA suggesting that this might be a general mechanism of action for this type of drugs.[43,44] We also demonstrated that epinephrine and other activators of prostaglandin synthetase could reduce ferric heme to ferrous heme, suggesting that reduction of ferric heme to ferrous heme as an essential step in catalyzing these reactions.[45] We further demonstrated that the lipid peroxides generated in the prostaglandin synthetic pathway via lipoxygenase might also reduce ferric heme to ferrous suggesting a possible relevance for peroxide tone in the regulation of prostaglandin synthesis.[46] Using salicylic acid, a metabolite of acetyl salicylic acid (aspirin), we demonstrated competitive inhibition of aspirin effect by salicylic acid.[47] In view of this observation, we tested the effect of short-acting prostaglandin inhibitor, ibuprofen, on the irreversible inhibitory action of aspirin. We demonstrated that ingestion of ibuprofen before ingesting aspirin effectively prevented the action of aspirin on platelet cyclooxygenase enzymes.[48] We also showed that bidentate compounds like 2, 2-dipyridil, similar to heme-complexing compounds, inhibited platelet prostaglandin synthesis and irreversible aggregation of platelets.[49] Studies from our laboratory in the late 70s, starting from simple in vitro methods to clinical evaluation, demonstrated the mechanism by which aspirin-like compounds exert their effect on platelet and sheep vesicular gland cyclooxygenase enzymes.[50-69]

By this time, studies from our laboratory as well as several other laboratories had demonstrated that activation of platelet IIb/IIIa receptors and fibrinogen binding underlie the mechanism for platelet–platelet attachment, thrombus formation, and growth.[70-79] In addition to these findings, studies with patients who lack these receptors, by Dr Barry Coller and associates at the Rockefeller University, established that the platelet “IIb-IIIa receptor” was an important target for antithrombotic therapy. Several other laboratories also were developing antibodies for the epitope responsible for the activation of IIb/IIIa receptors. Through site-directed mutagenesis, molecular dynamics, electron microscopy, and X-ray crystallography, his laboratory did extensive studies on integrin structure and activation. His laboratory identified a single compound out or more than 33,000 tested that inhibits ligand binding to platelet aIIb-IIIa. Structure-guided modification of this led to a compound (RUC-2) that is approximately 110 times more potent and has a novel mechanism of actions as pure agonist. This compound was modified to improve solubility, and is being developed for prehospital therapy for myocardial infarction.

It is well established that the function of the activated GPIIb/IIIa receptor is to bind fibrinogen during the cascade of thrombosis. Therefore, blockade of the GPIIb/IIIa receptors will prevent aggregation, thrombus formation, and thrombus growth. In 1985, Prof Barry Coller and his associates developed a murine monoclonal antibody, c7E3 Fab, directed against the GPIIb/IIIa receptor. This monoclonal antibody inhibits the binding of fibrinogen to the GPIIb/IIIa receptor, therefore inhibits platelet aggregation (Fig. 9.3). A fragment of this antibody was then used to make a nonimmunogenic compound known as abciximab (ReoPro; Eli Lilly Co, Indianapolis, IN). Abciximab has been studied extensively in clinical trials to assess its efficacy and safety, in platelet-induced clinical complications, such as myocardial infarction and stroke. In the cardiology applications,

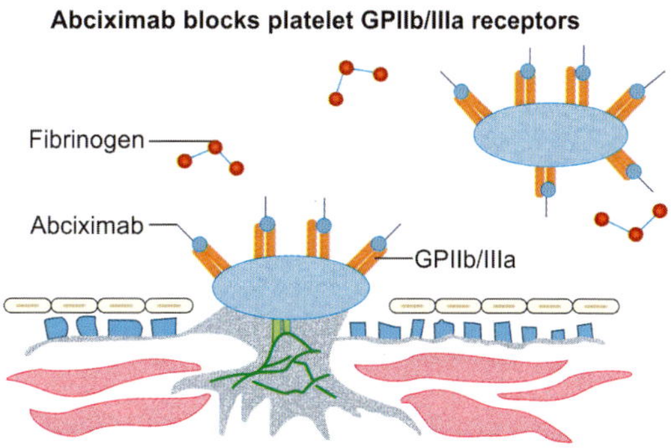

Fig. 9.3: A model for heme-indomethacin interaction. *Courtesy:* Daniel Ericson, SUBc, Inc, Rochester, Minnesota.

abciximab has been found to significantly decrease primary end point of death and reinfarction in multiple clinical trials. The use of abciximab with coronary stenting and angioplasty has been well studied, which implies that abciximab may have similar benefit during carotid and vertebrobasilar angioplasty and stenting.

Abciximab (ReoPro) is a noncompetitive irreversible inhibitor of GPIIb/IIIa. It is the humanized chimeric Fab fragment of the monoclonal mouse antibody 7E3. Eptifibatide and tirofiban are low-molecular-weight competitive and reversible GPIIb/IIIa antagonists, which act specifically on the α-11 subunits of GPIIb/IIIa. Eptifibatide is a cyclic heptapeptide whereas tirofiban is a nonpeptide (peptidomimetic) antagonist. Tirofiban contains the RGD sequence, whereas in eptifibatide the arginine residue is replaced by lysine. Unlike abciximab, which crossreacts with other integrins on the surface of various cell types, eptifibatide and tirofiban specifically act on GPIIb/IIIa receptors. Furthermore, eptifibatide and tirofiban unlike abciximab cannot induce immune response because of their small molecular weights and low affinities to GPIIb/IIIa receptors. On the other hand, owing to their short plasma half-lives, continuous infusion is needed to sustain platelet inhibition.[79,80] The clinical utility of abciximab is based on several trials involving coronary artery intervention procedures: EPIC (high-risk abrupt closure), EPILOG (broad entry criteria), CAPTURE (refractory unstable angina), EPISTENT (stent eligible), and RAPPORT).[81-86]

The fact that the reactive domains of adhesive proteins contain the tripeptide arginine-glycine-aspartic acid (RGD) sequence prompted the researchers to develop peptides as antiplatelet drugs.[87] It was also noticed that enhancing the potency of critical peptides by novel modifications was possible. Prof Kini and associates at the University of Singapore, incorporated proline residues on either sides of the interaction site of an antiplatelet peptide (IARGDMNA) and determined the inhibitory potency of the peptide in whole blood aggregation. Inclusion of one proline residue on either amino or carboxy terminal side of the interaction site enhanced the antiplatelet activity to approximately same extent (1.5–2.5 fold).

Incorporation of proline residues on both sides enhanced the activity 7–13 fold. They concluded that incorporation of proline brackets provides a novel approach to the design and development of more potent peptide drugs and ligands.[88] Currently, three generic platelet glycoprotein inhibitors (GPI) with different antithrombotic properties are in use for intravenous administration: abciximab, eptifibatide, and tirofiban. The development of oral GPIs has been abandoned.

In spite of the fact that there is intense research in the area of drug discovery and development of antiplatelet drugs, we still do not have too much choice when it comes to primary or secondary prevention of clinical complication related to the development of acute vascular events. As mentioned before, the choice of drugs is limited to aspirin and clopidogrel. From the novel drug discovery and development of GPIIb/IIIa antagonists, we learn that there is a great window of opportunity to develop novel drugs to antagonize the activity of this receptor. We are initiating some work at Dayananda Sagar Institutions (DSI), Bengaluru, some basic studies for designing synthetic molecules that can interfere with this critical interaction between GPIIb/IIIa receptor and the RGD sequence of fibrinogen molecule.

Normally, blood flows through arteries and veins smoothly and efficiently, but if there is narrowing of the vessels, hardening of the vessel walls, or if there is a clot, or thrombus, which blocks or alters the flow of the blood, then various clinical complications can occur, including thrombosis.[89] For a long time, just Coumadin and unfractionated heparins were the choice drugs for the prophylaxis of venous thromboembolism. We now have an array of drugs that can be used to prevent or treat thrombosis. A medical student, at the Johns Hopkins University in 1916, first discovered heparin. In 1939, dicumarol was extracted from a mold by a biochemist in University of Wisconsin. These anticoagulants have been used effectively to prevent clots from 1940. Warfarin is taken orally as a tablet and hence its anticoagulant effect is relatively slow. In India, Dr PVN Raju and associates of Gland Pharma (Hyderabad) were the pioneers in producing heparin for clinical use.

In the 70s, three different groups of researchers in Stockholm, London, and Hamilton Ontario, initiated work on the development of low-molecular-weight heparin (LMWH). LMWH is produced by chemically splitting the native heparin into one-third of its original size. It has fewer side effects than heparin [heparin-induced thrombocytopenia (HIT)], and produces a more predictable response. Because the LMWH is injected subcutaneously in a fixed dose without need for anticoagulant monitoring, patients can now be treated at home. Structural chemists began to fabricate or synthesize small molecules that can mimic the action of LMWH. During the development, clinical testing, and approval of the first synthetic heparin by the Food and Drug Administration (FDA), I was an active participant with a group of researchers who were experts in this field (Prof Sam Goldharber, Harvard University, Prof Jawed Fareed, Loyola University, Chicago). The first successful synthetic anticoagulants were fondaparinux and bivalirudin. Newer designer drugs that target single clotting factors that can be taken orally are being developed.

The US FDA decision to approve a synthetic generic heparin derivative without clinical safety or efficacy data raises the possibility that trials might not always be required for the approval of follow-on biologics.[90] The product (enoxaparin) codeveloped by Momenta Pharmaceuticals and Sandoz was approved under generics and was designate to as a substitute for Lovenox, manufactured by Sanofi-Aventis. Enoxaparin is not the first generic approved in the United States. Six other generic biologics have been approved under Abbreviated New Drug Applications (ANDAs). The elucidation of the structure of the antithrombin-binding sequence in heparin has given a large impulse to the design of heparin-like molecules.[91-95] Fondaparinux and idraparinux are examples of such compounds. The new molecule EP426785 exerts antithrombin-mediated antifactor Xa activity together with direct thrombin-inhibiting capacity. EP217609 exerts the same pharmacological profile as EP42675 and it can be neutralized instantaneously by injection of avidin.[94] Discussion of antithrombotic and thrombolytic therapy is beyond the scope of this monograph and readers are urged to seek further information on this topic by reading expert reviews and comprehensive monographs on this topic.[89]

REFERENCES

1. Markus HS, Droste DW, Kaps M, Larrue V, Lees KR, Siebler M, et al. Dual antiplatelet therapy with clopidogrel and aspirin in symptomatic carotid stenosis evaluated using Doppler embolic signal detection. The clopidogrel and aspirin for reduction of emboli in symptomatic carotid stenosis. CARESS trial. Circulation. 2005;111:2233-40.

2. Antithrombotic Trialists' Collaboration. Collaborative meta-analysis of randomised trials of antiplatelet therapy for prevention of death, myocardial infarction, and stroke in high risk patients. BMJ. 2001;324:71-86.
3. CAPRIE Steering Committee. A randomized, blinded trial of Clopidogrel versus aspirin in patients at risk of ischemic events (CAPRIE). Lancet. 1996;348:1329-39.
4. Yusuf S, Zhao F, Mehta SR, Chrolavicius S, Tognoni G, Fox KK; Clopidogrel in Unstable Angina to Prevent Recurrence Events Trial Investigators. Effects of clopidogrel in addition to aspirin in patients with acute coronary syndromes without ST-segment elevation. N Engl J Med. 2001;345:494-502.
5. Payne DA, Jones Cl, Hayes PD, Thompson MM, London NJ, Bell PR, et al. Beneficial effects of clopidogrel combine with Aspirin in reducing cerebral emboli in patients undergoing carotid endarterectomy. Circulation. 2004;109:1476-81.
6. Cadroy Y, Bossaya JP, Thalamas C, Sagnard L, Sakariassen K, Boneu B. Early potent antithrombotic effect with combined aspirin and a loading dose of clopidogrel one experimental arterial thrombosis in humans. Circulation. 2000;101:2823-8.
7. Ng M, Fleming T, Robinson M, Thomson B, Graetz N, Margono C, et al. Global, regional, and national prevalence of overweight and obesity in children and adults during 1980-2013: a systematic analysis of the global burden of disease study 2013. Lancet. 2014;384:766-81.
8. Weiss HJ. Platelets and their role in hemostasis. Ann N Y Acad Sci. 1972;201:1-450.
9. Ciba Foundation. Biochemistry and Pharmacology of Platelets. New York: Elsevier; 1975. p. 352.
10. Weiss HJ. Platelets, Pathophysiology and Antiplatelet Drug Therapy. New York: Alan R. Leiss, Inc.; 1982. p. 165.
11. Mehta JL. Thrombosis and Platelets in Myocardial Ischemia. Philadelphia: FA Davis Co.; 1987. p. 294.
12. Seiss W. Molecular mechanisms of platelet activation. Physiol Rev. 1989;69:58-178.
13. Dusting CJ, MacDonald PS. Prostacyclins and vascular function: implications for hypertension and atherosclerosis. Pharmacol Ther. 1990;48:323-44.
14. Rao GHR. Physiology of blood platelet activation. Ind J Physiol Pharmacol. 1993;37:263-75.
15. Rao GHR, Rao AT. Pharmacology of platelet activation inhibitory drugs. Ind J Physiol Pharmacol. 1994;38:69-84.
16. Marcus AJ. The role of prostaglandins in platelet function. Prog Hematol 1979;11:147-71.
17. Lands WEM. The biosynthesis and metabolism of prostaglandins. Ann Rev Physiol. 1979;41:633-52.
18. Srivastava KC. Prostaglandins and platelet function. S Afr J Sci. 1978;74:290-4.
19. Marcus AJ. The role of lipids in platelet function: with particular reference to the arachidonic acid pathway. J Lipid Res. 1978;19:793-826.
20. Mustard JM, Kinlough-Rathbone RL. Prostaglandins and platelets. Ann Rev Med. 1980;31:86-96.
21. Hammstrom S. Biosynthesis and biological actions of prostaglandins and thromboxanes. Arch Biochem Biophys. 1982;214:431-45.
22. Moncada S. Clinical use of prostacyclins. Adv Med. 1986;22:323-32.
23. Needleman P, Raz A Minkes MS, Ferrendelli JA, Sprecher H. Triene prostaglandins: prostacyclin and thromboxane biosynthesis and unique biological properties. Proc Natl Acad Sci U S A. 1979;76:944-8.
24. Holmsen H, Philos D, Day HJ. The blood platelet release reaction. Eur J Haematol. 1969;6:3-26.
25. White JG, Rao GHR, Gerrard JM. Effects of the ionophore, A23187, on blood platelets 1. Influence on aggregation and secretion. Am J Pathol. 1974;77:135-49.
26. Rao GHR, Reddy KR, White JG. The influence of epinephrine on prostacyclin induced dissociation of ADP aggregated platelets. Prostaglandins Med. 1980;4:385-97.
27. Rao GHR, Johnson GJ, White JG. Influence of epinephrine on the aggregation response of aspirin-treated platelets. Prostaglandins Med. 1980;5:45-58.
28. Rao GHR, Gerrard JM, Witkop CJ, White JG. Platelet aggregation independent of ADP release or prostaglandin synthesis in patients with the Hermansky-Pudlak syndrome. Prostaglandins Med. 1981;6:459-72.
29. Rao GHR, White JG. Epinephrine potentiation of arachidonate-induced aggregation of cyclooxygenase deficient platelets. Am J Pathol. 1981;11:355-66.

30. Cox AC, Carroll RC, White JG, Rao GHR. Recycling of platelet phosphorylation and cytoskeletal assembly. J Cell Biol. 1984;98:8-15.
31. Rao GHR, White JG. Role of arachidonic acid metabolism in human platelet activation and irreversible aggregation. Am J Hematol. 1985;19:339-47.
32. Rao GHR, White JG. Disaggregation of irreversibly aggregated platelets: a method for more complete evaluation of antiplatelet drugs. Agents Actions. 1985;16:425-34.
33. Rao GHR, White JG. Epinephrine-induced membrane modulation. In: Myers K, Barnes CD (Eds). Platelet Amine Storage Granules. New Orleans: CRC Press; 1992. pp. 117-49.
34. Rendu F, Brohard-Bohn B. The platelet release reaction: granule's constituents, secretion and functions. Platelets. 2001;12(5):261-73.
35. Yoshimoto A, Ito H, Tomita K. Cofactor requirement of the enzyme synthesizing prostaglandin in bovine seminal vesicles. J Biochem. 1970;68:487-99.
36. Ogino N, Ohki S, Yamamato S, Hayaishi O. Prostaglandin endoperoxide synthetase from bovine vesicular gland microsomes. Inactivation and activation by heme and other metalloporphyrins. J Biol Chem. 1978;253:5061-8.
37. Gerrard JM, White JG, Rao GHR, Townsend D. Localization of platelet prostaglandin production in the platelet dense tubular system. Am J Pathol. 1976;83:283-99.
38. Rao GHR, White JG. Heme-polyenoic acid interaction and prostaglandin synthesis. In: Bailey, JM: (1985) Plenum Press, New York, 1985. pp. 357-69.
39. Peterson DA, Gerrard JM, Rao GHR, Krick TP, White JG. Ferrous iron mediated oxidation of arachidonic acid: employing nitroblue tetrazolium (NBT). Prostaglandins Med. 1978;1:304-17.
40. Rao GHR, Gerrard JM, Eaton JW, White JG. The role of iron in prostaglandin synthesis: Ferrous iron mediated oxidation of arachidonic acid. Prostaglandins Med. 1978;1:55-70.
41. Vane JR. Inhibition of prostaglandin synthesis as a mechanism of action of aspirin-like drugs. Nat New Biol. 1971;231:232-5.
42. Peterson DA, Gerrard JM, Rao GHR, White JG. Inhibition of ferrous iron induced oxidation of arachidonic acid by indomethacin. Prostaglandins Med. 1979;2:97-108.
43. Peterson DA, Gerrard JM. A hypothesis for the interaction of heme and arachidonic acid in the synthesis of prostaglandins. Med Hypotheses. 1979;5:683-94.
44. Peterson DA, Gerrard JM, Rao GHR, Mills EL, White JG. Interaction of arachidonic acid and heme iron in the synthesis of prostaglandins. Adv Prostaglandin Thromboxane Res. 1980;6:157-61.
45. Peterson, DA, Gerrard JM, Rao GHR, White JG. Epinephrine and other activators of prostaglandin endoperoxide synthetase can reduce ferrous heme to ferric heme. Prostaglandins Med. 1980;4:357-65.
46. Peterson DA, Gerrard JM, Rao GHR, White JG. Reduction of ferric heme to ferrous heme by lipid peroxides: possible relevance to the role of peroxide tone in the regulation of prostaglandin synthesis. Prostaglandins Med. 1980;4:73-9.
47. Peterson DA, Gerrard JM, Rao GHR, White JG. Salicylic acid inhibition of the irreversible effect of aspirin on prostaglandin synthesis may be due to competition for the enzyme cationic site. Prostaglandins Med. 1981;6:161-4.
48. Rao GHR, Reddy KR, White JG. Ibuprofen protects platelet cyclooxygenase from irreversible inhibition by aspirin. Arteriosclerosis. 1983;3:384-8.
49. Rao GHR, Cox AC, Gerrard JM, White JG. Effects of 2,2`-dipyridil and related compounds on platelet prostaglandin synthesis and platelet function. Biochim Biophys Acta. 1980;628:468-79.
50. Rao GHR, Burris SM, Gerrard JM, White JG. Inhibition of prostaglandin (PG) synthesis in sheep vesicular gland microsomes (SVGM) by nitro blue tetrazolium (NBT) and vitamin E. Prostaglandins Med. 1979;2:203-16.
51. Peterson DA, Gerrad JM, Peller J, Rao GHR, White JG. Interaction of zinc with arachidonic acid. Prostaglandins Med. 1981;6:75-90.
52. Peterson DA, Gerrard JM, Rao GHR, White JG. Reduction of heme by lipid peroxides and its potential relevance to understanding the control of cyclooxygenase activity. Prog Lipid Res. 1981;20:299-301.

53. Peterson DA, Gerrard JM Glover SM, Rao GHR, White JG. Epinephrine reduction of heme: implication for understanding the transmission of agonist signal. Science. 1982;215:71-3.
54. Rao GHR. Radha E, White JG. Effect of docosahexaenoic acid (DHA) on arachidonic acid metabolism and platelet function. Biochem Biophys Res Commun. 1983;117:549-56.
55. Rao GHR, White JG. Comparative pharmacology of cyclooxygenase inhibitors. Prostaglandins Leukot Med. 1985;18:119-31.
56. Rao GHR, Hill TD, John V, Vennerstrom JL, White JG, Holmes TJ Jr. Inhibition of platelet aggregation by novel triphenylethylene analogs. Thromb Res. 1986;44:527-38.
57. Rao GHR, Escolar G, White JG. Epinephrine reverses the inhibitory effect of aspirin on platelet-vessel wall interactions. Thromb Res. 1986;44:65-74.
58. Rao GHR, Kishore M, Peller JD, White JG. Influence of polyenoic acids on arachidonic acid metabolism and platelet function. Cardiovasc Dis. 1987:495-505.
59. Rao GHR. Polyenoic acids and platelet function. Adv Essent Fatty Acid Res. 1987:36-49.
60. Folts JD, Rowe CG, Rao GHR. Problem with aspirin as antithrombotic agent in coronary artery disease. Lancet. 1988;1:937.
61. Hill TD, White JG, Rao GHR. Platelet hypersensitivity induced by 1-chloro-2, 4-dinitrobenzene, hydroperoxides and inhibition of lipoxygenase. Thromb Res. 1989;53:447-57.
62. Hill TD, White JG, Rao GHR. Role of glutathione and glutathione peroxidase in human platelet arachidonic acid metabolism. Prostaglandins. 1989;38:21-32.
63. Rao GHR, Mahadevappa VG, Hill TD et al: Arachidonic acid oxidation and platelet function. In: Reddy CC, Hamilton GA, Madyasta KM (Eds). Biological Oxidation Systems. Amsterdam: Academic Press; 1990. pp. 770-90.
64. Sugihara T, Rao GHR, Hebbel RP. Diphenylamine: an unusual antioxidant. Free Rad J. 1993;14;381-7.
65. Rao GHR, Gerrard JM, Murthy M, White JG. Possible mechanisms of epinephrine actions in human platelets that are refractory to arachidonic acid. Biochem Med Metab Biol. 1993;50:322-37.
66. Rao GHR, Parthasarathy S. Antioxidants, atherosclerosis and thrombosis. Prostaglandins Leukot Essent Fatty Acids. 1996;54:155-66.
67. Rao GHR, White JG. Epinephrine and platelet function. J Lab Clin Med. 1997;130:238-39.
68. Rao GHR. Handbook of Platelet Physiology and Pharmacology. Boston: Kluwer Academic Publishers; 1999.
69. Rao GHR. Management of type-2 diabetes by antiplatelet therapies: with special reference to aspirin. Front Biosci. (Scholar Ed) 2011;3:1-15.
70. Rao GHR. Aspirin resistance: clinical significance. J Clin Prevent Cardiol. 2012;479:1980.
71. Rao GHR, Fareed J. Aspirin prophylaxis for the prevention of thrombosis: Expectations and Limitations. Thrombosis. 2012. doi:10.1155/2012/104707.
72. Pardoni E, Alexandre A, Cavalline L, Rao GHR, Doni MG. Human platelet activation is inhibited by the occupancy of glycoprotein IIb/IIIa receptor. Arch Biochem Biophys. 1996;333:407-13.
73. Jackson AP, Yuan Y, Schoenwaelder SM. Role of the platelet integrin glycoprotein IIb/IIIa in intracellular signalling. Thromb Res. 1993;71:159-68.
74. Smyth SS, Parise LV. Regulation of ligand binding to glycoprotein IIb-IIIa (integrin alpha11b beta 3) in isolated platelet membranes. Biochem J. 1993;292:749-58.
75. Smyth SS, Hillery, Parise LV. Fibrinogen binding to purified platelet glycoprotein IIb-IIIa (integrin alpha11b beta 3) is modulated by lipids. J Biol Chem. 1992;5:15568-77.
76. Tomiyama Y, Tsubakio T, Piotrowicz RS, Kurata Y, Loftus JC, Kunicki TJ. The Arg-Gly-Asp (RGD) recognition site of platelet glycoprotein IIb-IIIa on non-activated platelet is accessible to high-affinity macromolecules. Blood. 1992;79:2303-12.
77. Khaspekova SG, Vlasik TN, Byzova TV, Vinogradov DV, Berndt MC, Mazurov AV. Detection of an epitope specific for the dissociated form of glycoprotein IIIa of platelet membrane glycoprotein IIb-IIIa complex and its expression on the surface of adherent platelets. Br J Haematol. 1993;85:332-40.

78. Savage B, Shattil SJ, Ruggeri ZM. Modulation of platelet function through adhesion receptors. A dual role for glycoprotein IIb-IIIa (integrin alpha11 beta 3) mediated by fibrinogen and glycoprotein Ib-von Willebrand factor. J Biol Chem. 1992;267:11300-3006.
79. Kunicki TJ. Platelet membrane glycoproteins and their function: an overview. Blut. 1989;59:30-4.
80. Kalantzi KI, Tsoumani ME, Goudevenos A, Tselepis AD. Pharmacodynamics properties of anti-platelet agents: current knowledge and future perspectives. Expert Rev Clin Pharmacol. 2012;5(3):319-36.
81. Califf RM, Lincoff AM, Tcheng JE, Topol EJ. An overview of the results of EPIC trial. Eur Heart J. 1995;16:43-9.
82. Cho L, Topol EJ, Balog C, Foody JM, Booth JE, Cabot C, et al. Clinical benefits of glycoprotein IIb/IIIa blockade with Abciximab is independent of gender: pooled analysis from EPIC, EPIOLG and EPISTENT trials. J Am Coll Cardiol. 2000;36:381-6.
83. EPIC Investigators. Use of a monoclonal antibody directed against the platelet glycoprotein IIb/IIIa receptor in high-risk coronary angioplasty. N Engl J Med. 1997;336:1689-96.
84. EPILOG Investigators. Platelet glycoprotein IIb/IIIa receptor blockade and low dose heparin during percutaneous coronary revascularization. N Engl J Med. 1997;336:1689-96.
85. EPISTENT Investigators. Enhancement of the safety of coronary stenting with the use of abciximab, a platelet glycoprotein IIb/IIIa inhibitor. Lancet. 1998;352:87-92.
86. Brener SJ, Ellis SG, Sapp SK, Betriu A, Granger CB, Burchenal JE, et al. Predictor of death and reinfarction at 30 days after primary angioplasty: The GUSTO and RAPPORT trials. Am Heart J. 2000;139:476-81.
87. Grant GA. Synthetic Peptides: A User's Guide (Advances in Molecular Biology) 2nd edition. Gregory Grant. New York: Oxford University Press; 2002. p. 390.
88. Kini RM, Evans HJ. A novel approach to the design of potent bioactive peptides by incorporation of proline brackets: antiplatelet effects of Arg-Gly-Asp peptides. FEBS Lett. 1995;375:15-7.
89. Rao GHR. Clinical Handbook of Management of Antithrombotic and Thrombolytic Therapy. New Delhi: Kontentworx; 2014. p. 505.
90. The identity problem. Nat Biotechnol. 2010;28:877.
91. Roy S, Hadri AE, Richard S, Denis F, Holte K, Duffner J, et al. Synthesis and biological evaluation of a unique heparin mimetic hexasaccharide for structure-activity relationship studies. J. Med Chem. 2014;57(11): 4511-20.
92. Lin F, Lian G, Zhou Y. Synthesis of fondaparinux: modular synthesis investigation for heparin synthesis. Carbohydr Res. 2013; 371:32-9.
93. Petitou M, Herault JP, Bernart A, Driguez PA, Duchaussoy P, Lormeau JC, et al: Synthesis of thrombi-inhibiting heparin mimetics without side effects. Nature. 1999;398:417-22.
94. Petitou M, Nancy-Portebois V, Dubreucq G, Motte V, Meuleman D, de Kort M, et al. From heparin to EP217609: the long way to a new pentasaccharide-based neutralisable anticoagulant with an unprecedented pharmacological profile. Thromb Heamost. 2009;102(5):804-10.
95. Petitou M. From heparin to synthetic antithrombotic oilgosacchardies. (Article in French). Bull Acad Natl Med. 2003;187:47-56.

CHAPTER 10

Antiplatelet Therapies

INTRODUCTION

The role of blood components including platelets in initiating inflammation, endothelial dysfunction, atherosclerosis, thrombus formation, thrombus growth, and acute vascular ischemic events, is well established. In view of this recognized role played by platelets, there is considerable interest in understanding the physiology and function of platelets, as well as in the development of novel platelet function inhibitory drugs. The generation of second messengers, calcium mobilization, shape change, adhesion, aggregation, contraction, release of granule contents, thrombus development, thrombus growth, and formation of hemostatic plug at the injured vessel surfaces, in brief, constitutes platelet activation. Some of the known compounds that inhibit platelet activation include inhibitors of arachidonic metabolism (Cox-1 inhibitors; aspirin, ibuprofen, etc.), adenosine diphosphate (ADP) receptor antagonists ($P2Y_{12}$ inhibitors), adenylyl and guanylyl cyclase stimulators, calcium antagonists, and glycoprotein (GP)IIb/IIIa receptor antagonists. Since platelets have multiple mechanisms of achieving in vivo activation, it is difficult to design a novel drug that offers total protection for developing acute ischemic vascular events, without compromising coagulation mechanisms. In view of this complexity, any aggressive antiplatelet therapy results in increased bleeding episodes. Having said that, we feel that there is a great window of opportunity for developing novel antiplatelet therapies. There is also scope for the development of fixed-dose combinations for the primary and secondary management of chronic diseases, such as hypertension, heart disease, and type 2 diabetes.

Atherosclerosis is a chronic, complex, inflammatory disease of the blood vessels, which leads to the narrowing and hardening of the arteries.[1] Thrombosis is another associated multifactorial disease that causes reduction and blockage of the flow of blood to the tissues causing ischemia and tissue injury. Together, these vascular diseases leading to heart attacks and stroke are the leading causes of morbidity and mortality worldwide.[2,3] A variety of risk factors contribute to the pathogenesis of these diseases. Some of the well-known risk factors include smoking, inflammation, endothelial dysfunction, hypertension, diabetes, repeated injury of the vascular tissues, elevated levels of low-density lipoproteins (LDL), low levels of high-density lipoproteins (HDL), visceral adiposity, and sedentary lifestyle. Some of the newer emerging risk factors include increased levels of fibrinogen, elevation of circulating activating factor, circulating endothelial cells, increased stress, depression, decreased levels of vitamin B_{12}, vitamin D, elevated blood phosphorus, C-reactive protein, platelet microparticles, platelet hyperfunction and hypercoagulability. Since the time Framingham trials listed predictors of risk (www.framinghamheartstudy.org/risk) [age, diabetes, smoking, systolic blood pressure, total cholesterol, HDL cholesterol, and body mass index (BMI)] for acute vascular events, there has been great interest in reducing modifiable risks with appropriate intervention. In spite of decades of research in this field, role of platelets in initiation of inflammation, vascular dysfunction, atherosclerosis, ischemic heart disease, and stoke is not very well defined. In this overview, an attempt is made to provide some evidence to support the hypothesis that platelets play a very significant role in the promotion of events leading to acute coronary and cerebrovascular events.[1-18] Unlike other reviews on the subject, no attempt will be made to catalog the results of all the clinical studies. On the other hand, we will try to explain why we have not reaped the benefits of antiplatelet therapy and shed some lights on some novel approaches.[8]

PLATELET PHYSIOLOGY

Blood platelets interact with a variety of soluble agonists such as epinephrine and ADP, many insoluble cell matrix components, including collagen, laminin, and biomaterials used for the construction of invasive medical devices.[1] These interactions stimulate specific receptors and glycoprotein-rich domains (integrins and nonintegrins) on the plasma membrane and lead to the activation of intracellular effector enzymes. The majority of the regulatory events appear to require free cytosolic calcium. Ionized calcium is the primary bioregulator, and a variety of biochemical mechanisms modulate the level and availability of free cytosolic calcium.[13-15] Major enzymes that regulate the free calcium levels via second messengers include phospholipase C, phospholipase A_2, and phospholipase D, together with adenylyl and guanylyl cyclases. Activation of phospholipase C results in the hydrolysis of phosphatidyl inositol 4,5 bisphosphate (PIP_2) and formation of second messengers 1,2-diacylglycerol and inositol 1,4,5 trisphosphate (IP_3) (Fig. 10.1).

Diglyceride induces activation of protein kinase C, which plays a crucial role in signal transduction for a variety of biologically active substances (Nishizuka Y. Nature. 2016;308:693-8.). Inositol trisphosphate mobilizes cytosolic calcium from internal membrane stores (Fig. 10.2). Elevation of cytosolic calcium stimulates phospholipase A_2 and liberates arachidonic acid. Free arachidonic acid is transformed to a novel

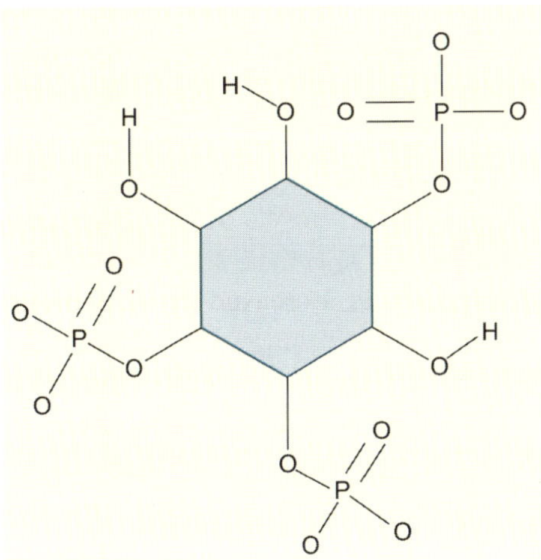

Fig. 10.1: Phosphatidyl inositol 1, 4, 5 trisphosphate.

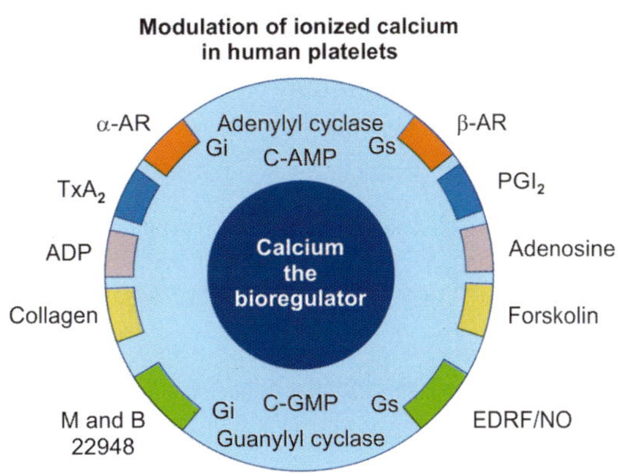

Fig. 10.2: Cellular calcium homeostasis.

metabolite, thromboxane A_2 by fatty acid synthetase (Cox-1, cyclooxygenase). Thromboxane A_2 is the major metabolite of this pathway and plays a critical role in platelet recruitment, granule mobilization, and secretion.[13,14]

Secretory granules contain a variety of growth factors, mitogens and inflammatory mediators. Secretion of granules promotes P-selectin expression on the platelet membrane. Furthermore, activation also promotes the expression of acidic lipids on the membrane and tissue factor expression, thus making these cells procoagulant. Fully activated platelets can modulate the function of other circulating blood cells such as leukocytes, monocytes, macrophages, as well as vascular endothelial cells. Agonist-mediated stimulation of platelets promotes the expression of an epitope on glycoprotein IIb/IIIa receptors. Activation of this receptor is essential for the binding of circulating fibrinogen. Fibrinogen forms a bridge between individual platelets and facilitates the thrombus formation. von Willebrand factor (vWF) binds platelet GPIbIX complex only at high shear rate unlike fibrinogen, which can bind platelets at low shear. Upregulation in signaling pathways will increase the risk for clinical complications associated with acute coronary events. Downregulation of signaling pathways may precipitate bleeding diathesis or hemorrhagic stroke. Based on this knowledge about various activation mechanisms current antiplatelet drugs are being developed for therapeutic applications.[14,16] Having said this, I would like to mention here that aspirin is one of the most researched drugs in the world, and was used for prevention of cardiovascular and cerebrovascular diseases, long before its mechanism of action was researched and the results published by Professor John Vane in 1971. According to Clinical Pharmacist (September, 2014), an estimated 700–1,000 trials are conducted each year. As far as its use as an antiplatelet drug, Antithrombotic Trialists' (ATT) collaboration has done meta-analysis of all clinical trials of aspirin and summarized their findings. The results of these studies will be discussed along with the other newer antiplatelet therapies.

CLINICAL CONDITIONS NEEDING ANTIPLATELET THERAPY

Cardiovascular disease (CVD) is the leading cause of death, accounting for 17.5 million deaths per year, that is expected to exceed 24 million by 2030. Worldwide prevalence of stroke was 33 million in 2010, with some 17 million people with first stroke. Stroke is the second leading cause of death with 12 million deaths worldwide. In view of these statistics from the American Heart and Stroke Association data, it is clear that antiplatelet therapies play an important role in the management of these diseases. Having said that, we should give credit to the significant role primary prevention has played in the reduction of morbidity and mortality. Nearly half of the decline in coronary artery disease (CAD) deaths has been attributed to population-wide risk reduction and another half due to intervention with medical therapies specific to risk factors. Antiplatelet therapies play a significant role in the risk reduction strategies.[19,20]

PHARMACOLOGICAL APPROACHES FOR DEVELOPMENT OF ANTIPLATELET DRUGS

Major pharmacological approaches for prevention of platelet activation include the use of compounds that inhibit release of arachidonic acid (vitamin E), development of receptor antagonists for potent agonists (thromboxane receptor antagonists), cyclooxygenase inhibitors (aspirin, indomethacin, triflusal), stimulators of adenylyl cyclases (adenosine, PGE_1, PGI_2) and guanylyl cyclases (nitric oxide), calcium chelators, calcium antagonists, and calcium channel blockers (Fig. 10.3).

Before discussing studies related to major antiplatelet therapies, for the sake of providing readers some knowledge of the type of antiplatelet studies that have been explored before, we will list a few examples for each class of platelet function inhibitory drugs.[14-16] Cyclooxygenase inhibitors include aspirin, phenylbutazone, ibuprofen, fenoprofen, flurbiprofen, naproxen, BHA, BHT, DPA. Thromboxane synthetase inhibitors include benzydamine, imidazole congeners, 9,11-azo-13 oxa-15 hydroxypropanoic acid, 9,11-azoprosta-5-13 dienoic acid (U-51605). Thromboxane receptor antagonists include vapiprost (SN309), 13 azaprostanoic acid, isoprostane (8epi-PGF_2 α), (3-pyridyl) alkanoic acids. Stimulators of cyclases include adenylyl cyclases; PGE_1, PGI_2, adenosine, forskolin, coleonol, guanylyl cyclases; nitric oxide, nitroglycerine, nitroprusside, Sin-1, nitrosoglutathione, free radicals. Cyclic AMP phosphodiesterase inhibitors include dipyridamole and related compounds RA233, RA433, VK744, VK774, methylxanthines, theophylline, caffeine, papaverine, aminophylline. Serine protease inhibitors include heparin, hirudin, low-molecular-weight heparins, and synthetic biosimilars. Calcium antagonists include cAMP, cGMP, verapamil, nifedipine, diltiazem, Quin-2AM, BAPTA-AM, mepacrine, and trifluoperazine. Studies from our laboratory as well as that of others have demonstrated that none of these agents are capable of effectively blocking platelet interactions with vessel wall or with cell matrix components.[11] In addition, we have to remember that in vivo platelet activation is accomplished by a variety of small molecules, enzymes, peptides, proteins, and cell matrix components. Just blocking one receptor or one pathway will not be able inhibit platelet activation in acute clinical conditions.[14-16]

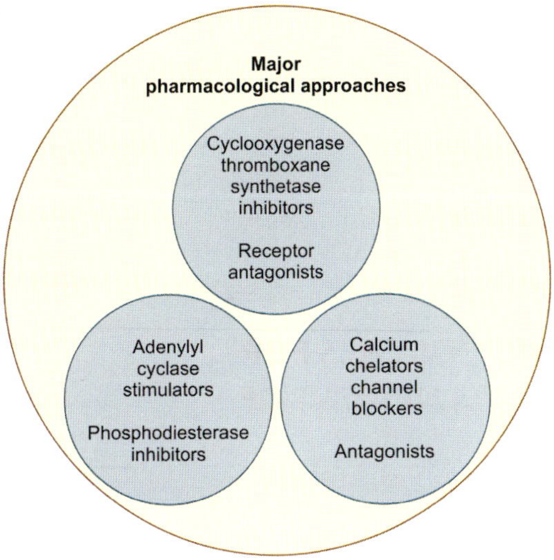

Fig. 10.3: Pharmacology of antiplatelet drugs.

CLINICAL COMPLICATIONS NEEDING ANTIPLATELET THERAPIES

Clinical applications of antiplatelet drugs include conditions such as coronary artery disease (acute myocardial infarction, unstable angina, re-occlusive restenosis), cerebrovascular disease (transient ischemic attack, complete stroke, carotid endarterectomy), peripheral vascular disease (peripheral arterial disease, peripheral venous disease), small vessel disease, and situations where thrombus formation need to be prevented on medical implants, artificial surfaces, preoperational conditions, before and during cardiac and cerebrovascular interventional procedures.[18-27]

One of the great success stories of modern-day discovery of a drug on evidence-based science is the development of GPIIb/IIIa antagonists. Professor Barry S Coller and his associates did extensive work in the development of a monoclonal antibody (10E5) that blocked fibrinogen binding to platelets. Experiments that led to this discovery and the clinical studies that helped them to develop a potent antiplatelet therapy make a superb story in the modern-day drug discovery initiatives. We were fortunate to have Prof Coller as our chief guest at the SASAT-1996 conference in Bengaluru. The GPIIb/IIIa receptor complex numbers between 60,000 and 80,000 copies per platelet and plays a critical role in fibrinogen binding and aggregation of platelets. The clinical data supporting the use of these classes of inhibitors were first established with abciximab [Evaluation of c7E3 in Preventing Ischemic Complications (EPIC) and Evaluation of PTCA to Improve Long-term Outcome by c7E3 GPII B/IIIA Receptor Blockade (EPILOG) trials] and eptifibatide (Integrilin to Minimize Platelet Aggregation and Coronary Thrombosis, IMPACT II and Enhanced Suppression of the Platelet IIb/IIIa Receptor with Integrilin Therapy, ESPRIT). Both were found to achieve significant improvements in reducing the mortality in patients undergoing percutaneous coronary interventions (PCIs).[21-26] Glycoprotein IIb/IIIa inhibitors are antiplatelet drugs that are commonly used in treating patients who have unstable angina, certain types of heart attacks, and in combination with angioplasty with or without stent placement. These drugs are given in combination with heparin or aspirin to prevent clotting before and during invasive cardiac and cerebrovascular procedures. Specific inhibitors of this class of drugs in use include abciximab (ReoPro), eptifibatide (Integrilin), and tirofiban (Aggrastat). These drugs are usually administered as intravenous (IV) injections or IV infusion during hospitalization.

What are some of the concerns related to the use of this class of drugs in antiplatelet therapies? Currently, use of these types of drugs is limited because of the need to administer them by constant intravenous infusion. Since it is not easy to reverse their effect, there are chances of increased bleeding if the dosage is not well within the required limit. There is also some concern about immunogenicity. The second-generation drugs of this class are the group of synthetics that target a GPIIb/IIIa recognition site for an Arg-Gly-Asp sequence found in fibrinogen. When these classes of drugs occupy the receptor site, GPIIb/IIIa is no longer functional as the aggregation receptor. There is continued effort to develop orally active RGD mimics for therapeutic applications. There is a window of opportunity for synthetic chemists to develop novel organic molecules, which can compete for this active site on the platelet membrane and provide an alternative for ReoPro-like molecules, which can be used only by IV route and as such have limited clinical application.

Another class of drugs that were developed on the basis of available scientific evidence is ADP receptor antagonists. Since the time studies by Hellem et al. observed that small molecules from red cells caused platelets to adhere to the glass and aggregate, there is considerable interest in the development of ADP receptor antagonists.[27-35] Clopidogrel versus Aspirin in Patients at Risk of Ischemic Events (CAPRIE) was a randomized, blinded, international trial designed to assess the relative efficacy of clopidogrel (75 mg once daily) and aspirin (325 mg once daily) in reducing the risk of acute vascular events. CAPRIE steering committee concluded that long-term administration of clopidogrel to patients with atherosclerotic vascular disease is more effective than aspirin in reducing the combined risk of ischemic stroke, myocardial infarction, or vascular death. The overall safety profile of clopidogrel is at least as good as that of medium-dose aspirin.[29,34]

CLINICAL TRIALS OF ANTIPLATELET DRUGS

Many clinical trials have evaluated the benefit of long-term use of antiplatelet drugs in reducing clinical vascular complications. Data for aspirin as a drug of choice for the primary prevention strategies comes from ATT, which evaluated 95,456 patients in six clinical trials.[4] Current ACC/AHA guidelines recommend the use of low-dose aspirin for primary prevention.[21] Both aspirin and clopidogrel, the drugs of choice, have been quite effective.[29-35] The ATT was set up to provide updated information about the benefits and hazards, among particular types of patients, of antithrombotic therapy. In the 2002 analyses, 200,000 high-risk individuals in 287 studies were compared. Aspirin was the most widely studied antiplatelet drug. Indirect and direct comparisons suggested that doses of 75–100 mg daily were at least as effective as higher daily doses. In the 2009 analyses, 95,000 low-risk individuals in six primary prevention trials were compared. In the primary prevention trials, the absolute risk of a serious event was an order of magnitude less than in the secondary prevention trials. In secondary prevention trials, aspirin is of substantial benefit. It reduces nonfatal events by much more than it would increase major extracranial bleeds. (BMJ. 2002:234:71-86; Lancet. 2009;373:1849-60). In an earlier article, Sudlow and Baigent (Rao GHR. Handbook of Platelet Physiology and Pharmacology; 1999, Kluwer Publication) reviewed all of the available randomized trial evidence for the effects of antiplatelet therapy in the treatment and prevention of major vascular outcomes as summarized by the ATT collaboration in 1994. The 2002 ATT analyses showed that aspirin or some other antiplatelet regimen was of clear net benefit for those who have occlusive vascular disease. For primary prevention, however, the balance between risks and benefits was less clear.[30-33] Recent studies (meta-analysis) have shown that aspirin prophylaxis for peripheral vascular disease or peripheral arterial disease (PVD/PAD) is not very effective.

In view of the fact that ATT collaboration does not discuss the controversial area of aspirin and clopidogrel resistance, I have briefly discussed this phenomenon. In recent years, several studies have reported the existence of a strange phenomenon of resistance to these drugs.[17,18] However, if one looks at these studies, one can see the flaw in these studies. Aspirin, for instance, is an irreversible inhibitor of cyclooxygenase, an enzyme, which converts substrate arachidonic acid to active metabolites, prostaglandin endoperoxides. The bioactive molecules are further converted to thromboxanes, which are the real agonists that induce platelet activation. In our experience of four decades, we have never found any one whose platelet cyclooxygenases are resistant to the action of aspirin.[17] However, we have demonstrated that if platelets are first exposed to short-acting ibuprofen, then those platelets are resistant to the action of aspirin. Majority of studies, describing aspirin resistance, have based their conclusion on results obtained by functional studies using various platelet agonists other than arachidonic acid. Similarly, clopidogrel studies also should be done, using the specific agonist

ADP, to titrate platelet aggregation response, post-clopidogrel treatment. Having said that, we would like to bring the attention of the readers to the observations in several clinical studies, in which those individuals, who have increased urinary metabolites of thromboxane, in spite of aspirin prophylaxis, are at risk for developing acute CVD events. In view of these reports, it is important to customize the antiplatelet prophylaxis with functional studies as well as by monitoring urinary metabolites.

A new meta-analysis of clopidogrel clinical trials has shown that patients with either one or two loss-of-function CYP2C19 alleles, undergoing PCI on normal doses of clopidogrel, have an increased risk of cardiovascular events, compared with noncarriers. In these studies, the researchers explain that the CYP2C19 enzyme plays a key role in clopidogrel metabolism, and carriers of reduced-function variants in the CYP2C19 gene have lower active clopidogrel metabolite levels and diminished platelet inhibition. The findings of this collaborative meta-analysis demonstrate that common genetic variants in the CYP2C19 gene are associated with almost one in three patients not receiving ideal protection from ischemic events, when treated with standard doses of clopidogrel for PCI. Given how widely clopidogrel is used to treat patients with CVD, determination of the optimal antiplatelet treatment doses or regimens for individual patients is needed to tailor therapy appropriately. The total knowledge base on this topic now shows a definite increased risk of stent thrombosis and other cardiac events in carriers of CYP2C19 loss-of-function alleles. It is widely known that poor platelet function suppression is associated with poor outcomes.[18]

In order to customize antiplatelet therapy of the two most commonly used antiplatelet drugs (aspirin and clopidogrel), one needs to do the following studies. For aspirin prophylaxis, determine the platelet aggregation response to arachidonic acid, determine the ability of aspirin-treated platelets to generate thromboxane, or monitor urinary metabolites of thromboxane. For clopidogrel prophylaxis, determine the ADP-mediated platelet aggregation response, or determine CYP2C19 functional alleles. Alternately, use new clopidogrel (Plavix) point-of-care assay for rapid determination of antiplatelet activity (Bansal et al. J. Trauma. 2011;70:65-9). However, various guidelines published by major professional societies do not advocate such studies for optimization of standard of care with antiplatelet therapy. Lack of an easy-to-do assay for monitoring platelet function limits the validation/optimization of antiplatelet therapies. There is a great need for the development of a point-of-care assay to monitor the status of circulating blood in terms of its thrombotic state or otherwise similar to monitoring of the effect of anticoagulation therapy with international normalized ratios (INRs) (Rao GHR. Stroke. 2009;40:2271-72). We, at the University of Minnesota, have validated a platelet reaction–monitoring device, which uses shear-induced activation of platelets and clotting time (Rao GHR. New point-of-care methods for monitoring antiplatelet therapy. A symposium sponsored by Eli Lilly and Company: 21st Congress of the International Society on Thrombosis and Hemostasis. Geneva, Switzerland, 2007) (Fig. 10.4).

Based on the results of 11 clinical studies, an extensive guideline has been developed and published recently on duration of dual antiplatelet therapy (DAPT: aspirin plus $P2Y_{12}$ inhibitors: clopidogrel, prasugrel, or ticagrelor) in patients with CAD. Among $P2Y_{12}$ inhibitors, cilostazol, ticagrelor, and cangrelor are direct-acting drugs and prasugrel and

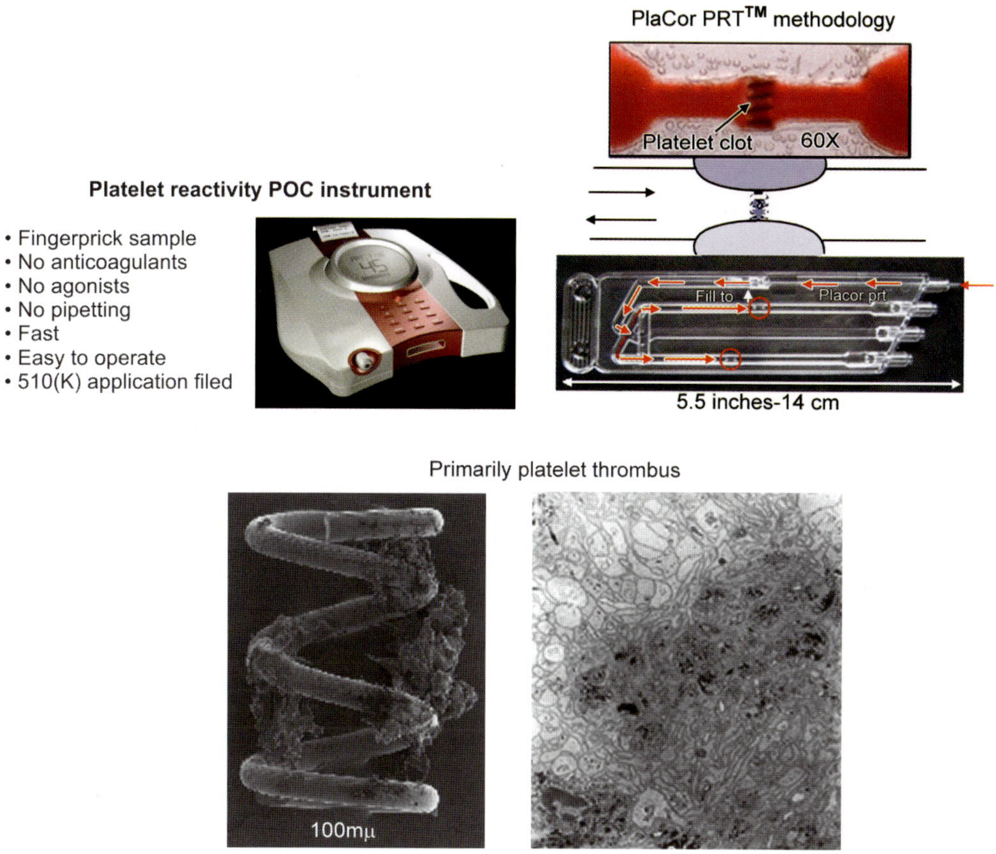

Fig. 10.4: Platelet reaction time testing.
Courtesy: Blood Biocompatibility Laboratory, University of Minnesota. (Presented at the symposium on New Point-of-Care Methods for Monitoring Antiplatelet Therapy by Prof Gundu HR Rao. (Symposium sponsored by Daichi-Sankyo and Eli Lilly Companies, at the XXI Congress of the International Society Thrombosis and Haemostasis (July 11, 2007, Geneva, Switzerland.)

clopidogrel are prodrugs. When it comes to clinical application of DAPT for studies of longer duration for an additional 18–36 months after drug-eluting stent (DES) placement, there was an absolute decrease in late stent thrombosis and ischemic complications.[36] As far as DAPT for coronary artery bypass graft (CABG) was concerned, it was associated with a significant lower vein graft occlusion at 1 year, versus antiplatelet monotherapy, but with no such improvement in arterial graft patency.[37] Of course, major bleeding was more frequent with DAPT compared to monotherapy. Aspirin remains the drug of choice for antiplatelet therapy with patients with acute coronary syndrome (ACS). DAPT recommendation beyond a minimum recommended period was associated with increased bleeding and thereby offsets the benefits of DAPT.[38,39] Therefore, careful monitoring of patients and customization of therapy is essential.

DAPT with aspirin and $P2Y_{12}$ inhibitors are the choice antiplatelet therapies worldwide for the care of ACS patients and those undergoing coronary interventional procedures such as PCI or CABG. These classes of antagonists inhibit only two specific pathways of platelet activation and minimally affect other pathways of platelet activation. These limitations may explain why even patients with DAPT experience recurrent ischemic events. In view of these observations, currently two oral thrombin receptor antagonists (PAR-1) are under clinical evaluation.[37,38] From time to time, several other agents that target various platelets' signaling pathways have been developed and evaluated in phase 1 and phase 2 trials. They include glycoprotein VI antagonist (6B4-Fab antibody), serotonin receptor inhibitor (sarpogrelate, APD791), prostaglandin E receptor antagonist (DG-041), nitric oxide donors (LA846, LA419), nitric oxide substrate, L-arginine, phosphatidylinositol 3-kinase inhibitors (TGX-221). Prostaglandin/thromboxane receptor antagonists such as GR32191, ifetroban, and sulotorban had disappointing results in phase 1 and phase 2 clinical trials. Antiplatelet drugs that are in preclinical studies include inhibitors of platelet adhesion: vWF (Mab, aptamer), GPIb/V/IX (peptide, MAB), GPVI (Mab, small molecule), collagen (protein) P13K inhibitors, intracellular targets: cytoplasmic tail of β_3-integrin, and tyrosine kinase inhibitors (Src, Syk). Dual antiplatelet therapy has become the standard care in the management of a variety of platelet-related clinical complications. However, emerging antiplatelet therapies are aimed at developing more potent novel drugs, which would offer better protection by reducing ischemic events, without increased bleeding. Currently, prasugrel, ticagrelor, cangrelor, oral thrombin antagonist SCH 530348, and elinogrel are undergoing extensive testing worldwide. We have made no attempt to review development of oral anticoagulants. Readers are urged to refer to recent reviews on this topic for additional information.[40-50] As mentioned in the introduction, this is not a comprehensive review on this subject. Readers are urged to refer to the current guidelines and reviews by the experts.[33-46, 51-57]

India has banned recently over 350 fixed-dose combinations (FDCs) as unsafe or ineffective. On the other hand, there are currently several ongoing clinical studies with various FDCs for the management of hypertension and type 2 diabetes. For treatment of hypertension, a combination of benazepril plus amlodipine or hydrochlorothiazide have been tested. For management of type 2 diabetes, the FDCs include metformin with sulphonylurea, thiazolidinedione, dipeptidylpeptidase-4 inhibitor, or meglitinide as well as thiazolidinedione–sulphonylurea. Professor Salim Yusuf of Population Health Research Institute of Ontario, Canada, has hypothesized that a combination of four drugs (aspirin, β blocker, a statin, and an angiotensin-converting enzyme inhibitor) could reduce CVD events by 75% in those with vascular disease.[51] Wald and Law have proposed a polypill containing three blood pressure (BP)-lowering drugs for different classes with each, at half doses, aspirin, a statin, and folic acid, for all individuals with established CVD and older than 55 years without CVD and have estimated that this approach will reduce CVD events by 88% and stroke by 80%.[53] Dr Reddy's Laboratory and Astra Zeneca have entered into a distribution agreement for Riax-M, an FDC of saxagliptin, a dipeptidyl peptidase-4 (DDP-4) inhibitor, and metformin. Various national and international health organizations like the World Health Organization (WHO), National Institutes of Health, the United States; National Heart, Lung and Stroke, the United Kingdom and Canada; and Centers for Disease Control and Prevention, the United States, have advocated development and validation of different FDCs.[51-54] For a comprehensive review on this, subject readers are urged to refer to the work of Yusuf and associates.[51] In their overview on this subject, they conclude, "On the basis of available data on the individual component drugs, the polypill could potentially be widely used in secondary prevention and in selected high-risk individuals without CVD (e.g. those with hypertension or diabetes with additional risk factors). We at the Nuwell Research and Innovations, Bengaluru, India, are planning to develop some special FDCs for better management of cardio-metabolic risks in South Asians.[58-60]

The role of platelets in the pathogenesis of inflammation, atherosclerosis, thrombosis, and stroke is well recognized. Variety of agonists, are capable of mediating platelet activation including shear force in the circulating blood.[11,58] Activation of platelets by agonists initiates a series of biochemical events leading to formation of second messengers, elevation of cytosolic calcium, shape change, contraction, release of proaggregatory components, and formation of hemostatic plug for the arrest of bleeding at the injured sites. Since the activation of GPIIb/IIIa receptors and fibrinogen binding is considered the common pathway for aggregation, thrombus formation and growth, several effective antiplatelet therapies have been developed related to this mechanism of activation. Similarly, antiplatelet therapies also have been developed using ADP receptor antagonists. As we have explained earlier, platelets are activated by a variety of external stimuli and as such there is a need to develop antiplatelet therapies that can offer better protection than these two inhibitory pathways and yet will not promote bleeding. There is a great window of opportunity for the development of novel antiplatelet therapies, including FDCs.

REFERENCES

1. Rao GHR (Ed). Handbook of Platelet Physiology and Pharmacology. Boston: Kluwer Academic Publishers; 1999.
2. Rao GHR, Kakkar VV (Eds). Coronary Artery Disease in South Asians: Epidemiology, Risk Factors, Prevention. New Delhi: Jaypee Medical Publishers; 2001.
3. Rao GHR, S Thanikachalam (Eds). Coronary Artery Disease: Risk Factors, Pathophysiology and Prevention. New Delhi: Jaypee Medical Publishers; 2005.
4. Rao GHR. Platelet hyperfunction as risk factor for chronic and acute coronary events. Toxicol Mech Methods. 2005;15:425-31.
5. Rao GHR (Ed). Diabetes Mellitus (Type-2): Epidemiology, Risk Management and Prevention. New Delhi: Jaypee Medical Publishers; 2007.
6. Rao GHR, Kalidoki E, Leong W, Fareed J. Clinical Handbook for the Management of Venous Thrombosis and Thromboembolism. New Delhi: Kontentworx; 2012.
7. Rao GHR. Handbook of Coronary Artery Disease. New Delhi: Macmillan Medical Communications; 2016.
8. Rao GHR. Role of cyclic AMP, cyclic GMP as modulators of platelet cytosolic calcium: a point of view. J Clin Prevent Cardiol. 2016;5(3):99-103.
9. Rao GHR, White JG. Disaggregation and reaggregation of irreversibly aggregated platelets: a method for more complete evaluation of antiplatelet drugs. Agents Actions. 1985; 16:425-34.
10. Rao GHR, Hill TD, John V, Vennerstrom JL, White JG, Holmes TJ. Inhibition of platelet aggregation by novel triphenylethylene analogs. Thromb Res. 1986;44:527-38.
11. Rao GHR. Influence of anti-platelet drugs on platelet-vessel wall interactions. Prostaglandins Leukot Med. 1987;30:133-45.
12. Rao GHR, Rao ASC, White JG. Aspirin in ischemic heart disease: an overview. Indian Heart J. 1993;45:73-9.
13. Rao GHR. Signal transduction, second messengers and platelet pharmacology. Pharmacol (Life Sci). 1994;13:39-44.
14. Rao GHR. Physiology and pharmacology of platelets. Int J Prog Cardiovas Sci. 1995;2:108-10.

15. Rao GHR. Physiology of blood platelet activation. Indian J Physiol Pharmacol. 1994;37: 263-75.
16. Rao GHR, Rao AT. Pharmacology of platelet inhibitory drugs. Indian J Physiol Pharmacol. 1994;38:69-84.
17. Rao GHR. Aspirin resistance: clinical significance. J Clin Prev Cardiol. 2012;1:118-29.
18. Rao GHR, Fareed J. Aspirin prophylaxis for the prevention of thrombosis: expectations and limitations. Thrombosis. 2012;2012:104707.
19. Kohil P, Whelton SP, Hus S, Yancy CW, Stone NJ, Chrispin J, et al. Clinicians guide to the updated ABCs of cardiovascular disease. J Am Heart Assoc. 2014;3:e001098.
20. Yusuf S, Hawken S, Ounpuu S, Dans T, Avezum A, Lanas F, et al. Effect of potentially modifiable risk factors associated with myocardial infarction in 52 countries (the INTERHEART study): case-control study. Lancet. 2004;364:937-52.
21. Antithrombotic Trialists' Collaboration. Aspirin in the primary and secondary prevention of vascular disease: collaborative meta-analysis of individual participant data form randomised trials. Lancet. 2009;373:1849-60.
22. Goff Dc, Lloyd-Jones DM, Bennett G, Coady S, D'Agostino RB Sr, Gibbons R, et al. 2013 ACC/AHA guidelines on the assessment of cardiovascular risk. J Am Coll Cardiol. 2014;63 (25 pt B):2935-59.
23. The EPIC Investigators. Use of monoclonal antibody directed against the platelet glycoprotein II B/III A receptor in a high-risk coronary angioplasty. N Engl J Med. 1994;330: 956-61.
24. The EPILOG Investigators. Platelet glycoprotein II B/III A receptor blockade and low-dose heparin during percutaneous coronary revascularization. N Engl J Med. 1997;336: 1689-96.
25. The IMPACT-II Investigators. Randomises placebo-controlled trial of effect of eptifibatide on complications of percutaneous coronary intervention. UMPCT-II. Lancet. 1997;349:1422-8.
26. The ESPRIT Investigators. Novel dosing regimen of eptifibatide in planned coronary stent implantation (ESPRIT): a randomized, placebo-controlled trial. Lancet. 2000;356:2037-44.
27. Armstrong PC, Peter K. GPIIb/IIIa inhibitors: from bench to bedside and back to bench again. Thromb Haemost. 2012;107:808-14.
28. Packham M, Rand M. Historical perspective on ADP-induced platelet activation. Purinergic Signal. 2011;7(3):283-92.
29. Herbert JM, Savi P. P2Y12, a new platelet ADP receptor, target of clopidogrel. Semin Vasc Med. 2003;3(2):113-22.
30. CAPRIE Steering Committee. A randomized, blinded, trial of clopidogrel versus aspirin in patients at risk of ischemic events (CAPRIE). Lancet. 1996;348:1329-39.
31. Antithrombotic Trialists Collaboration. Collaborative meta-analysis of randomised trials of antiplatelet therapy for prevention of death, myocardial infarction, and stroke in high-risk patients. BMJ. 2002;324:71-86.
32. Antiplatelet Trialists Collaboration. Collaborative overview of randomised trials of antiplatelet therapy. 1. Prevention of myocardial infraction and stroke by prolonged antiplatelet therapy in various categories of patients. BMJ. 1994;308:81-106.
33. Antiplatelet Trialists Collaboration. Collaborative overview of randomised trials of antiplatelet therapy—II. Maintenance of vascular graft or arterial patency by antiplatelet therapy. BMJ. 1994;308:159-68.
34. Antiplatelet Trialists Collaboration. Collaborative overview of randomised trials of antiplatelet therapy—III. Reduction in venous thrombosis and pulmonary embolism by antiplatelet prophylaxis among surgical and medical patients. BMJ. 1994;308:235-46.
35. Harker LA, Boissel JP, Pilgrim AJ, Gent M. Comparative safety and tolerability of clopidogrel versus aspirin: results from CAPRIE. CAPRIE Steering Committee and Investigators. Clopidogrel versus aspirin in patients at risk of ischaemic events. Drug Saf. 1999;21:325-35.
36. CURE Study Investigators. Effect of clopidogrel in addition to aspirin in patients with non-ST segment elevation acute coronary syndromes. N Engl J Med. 2001;345:492-502.
37. Levine GN, Bates ER, Bittl JA, Brindis RG, Fihn SD, Fleisher LA, et al. 2016 ACC/AHA Guideline Focused Update on Duration of Dual Antiplatelet Therapy in Patients with

Coronary Artery Disease: a report of the American College of Cardiology/American Heart Association Task Force on Clinical Practice Guidelines: an update of the 2011 ACCF/AHA/SCAI Guideline for Percutaneous Coronary Intervention, 2011, ACCF/AHA Guideline for Coronary Artery Bypass Graft Surgery, 2012; ACC/AHA/ACP/AATS/PCNA/SCAI/STS Guideline for the Diagnosis and Management of Patients With Stable Ischemic Heart Disease, 2013 ACCF/AHA Guideline for the Management of ST-elevation Myocardial Infarction, 2014 AHA/ACC Guideline for the Management of Patients with Non-ST-elevation Acute Coronary Syndromes, 2014, ACC/AHA Guideline on Perioperative Cardiovascular Evaluation and Management of Patients Undergoing Noncardiac Surgery. Circulation. 2016 Sep 6;134(10):e123-55. https://doi.org/10.1161/CIR.0000000000000404.
38. Ferreiro JL, Angiolillo DJ. New directions on antiplatelet therapy. Circ Cardiovasc Interv. 2012;5:433-45.
39. Tricoci P, Huang A, Held C, Moliterno DJ, Armstrong PW, Van de Werf F, et al. the TRACER Investigators. Thrombin-receptor antagonist vorapaxar in acute coronary syndromes. N Engl J Med. 2012;366:20-33.
40. Morrow DA, Braunwald E, Bonaca MP, Ameriso SF, Dalby AJ, Fish MP, et al. TRA2P-TIMI 50 Steering Committee and Investigators. Vorapaxar in the secondary prevention of atherothrombotic events. N Engl J Med. 2012;366:1404-13.
41. Wright RS, Anderson JL, Adams CD, Bridges CR, Casey DE Jr, Ettinger SM, et al. 2011 ACCF/AHA focused update of the guidelines for the management of patients with unstable angina/non-ST-elevation myocardial infarction (updating the 2007 guidelines): a report of the American College of Cardiology Foundation/American Heart Association Task Force on Practice Guidelines. Circulation. 2011;123:2022-60.
42. Levine GN, Bates ER, Blankenship JC, Bailey SR, Bittl JA, Cercek B, et al. 2011 ACCF/AHA/SCAI guidelines for percutaneous coronary intervention: a report of the American College of Cardiology Foundation/American Heart Association Task Force on Practice Guidelines and the society for cardiovascular angiography and interventions. Circulation. 2011;124:e574-651.
43. Hamm CW, Bassand JP, Agewall S, Bax J, Boersma E, Bueno H, et al. ESC guidelines for the management of acute coronary syndromes in patients without persistent ST-segment elevation. JAMA. 2002;288:2411-20.
44. Gaglia MA, Manoukian SV, Waksman R. Novel antiplatelet therapy. Am Heart J. 2010;160:595-604.
45. Kim L, Charitakis K, Swaminathan RV, Feldman DN. Novel antiplatelet therapies. Curr Atheroscler Rep. 2012;14:78-84.
46. Gupta AK, Arshad, Poulter NR. Compliance safety and effectiveness of fixed-dose combinations of antihypertensive agents: a meta-analysis. Hypertension. 2010;55:399-407.
47. Dickson M, Plauschinat CA. Compliance with antihypertensive therapy in the elderly: a comparison of fixed dose combination of amlodipine/benazepril versus component-based free-combination therapy. Am J Cardiovasc Drugs. 2008;8:45-50.
48. Jamerson K, Weber MA, Bakris GL, Dahlöf B, Pitt B, Shi V, et al. ACCOMPLISH Trial Investigators. Benazepril plus amlodipine or hydrochlorothiazide for hypertension in high-risk patients. N Engl J Med. 2008;359:2417-28.
49. Ahrens I, Peter K, Lip GY, Bode C. Development of clinical applications of novel oral anticoagulants. Part I. Clinically approved drugs. Discov Med. 2012;13(73):433-43.
50. Ahrens I, Lip GY. New oral anticoagulant drugs in cardiovascular disease. Thromb Haemost. 2010;104:49-60.
51. Ahrens I, Peter K Lip GY, Bode C. Development of clinical applications of novel oral anticoagulants. Part II. Drugs under clinical applications. Discov Med. 2012;13:445-50.
52. Lonn E, Bosch J, Teo KK, Pais P, Xavier D, Yusuf S. The polypill in the prevention of cardiovascular diseases: key concepts, current status, challenges and future directions. Circulation. 2010;122:2078-88.
53. Wald NJ, Law MR. A strategy to reduce cardiovascular disease by more than 80%. BMJ. 2003;326:1419-24.

54. Bailey CJ, Day C. Fixed-dose single tablet anti-diabetic combinations. Diabetes Obes Metab. 2009;11:527-33.
55. Wise J. Polypill holds promise for people with chronic disease. Bull World Health Organ. 2005;83:885-7.
56. Harrington RA, Hodgson PK, Larsen RL. Anti-platelet therapy. Circulation. 2003;108:e45-7.
57. Chassot P, Delabays A, Spahn DR. Perioperative use of anti-platelet drugs. Best Pract Res Clin Anaesthesiol. 2007;21:241-56.
58. Patrono C, Baigent C, Hirsh J, Roth G; American College of Chest Physicians. Anti-platelet drugs: American College of Chest Physicians evidence-based clinical practice guidelines (8th edition). Chest 2008;133: S199-S233.
59. Johnson GJ, Sharda A, Rao GHR, Ereth MH, Laxson DD, Owen WG. Measurement of shear-activated platelet aggregate formation: utility in evaluation of clopidogrel-aspirin-induced platelet function inhibition. Clin Appl Thromb Hemost. 2012;18:140-9.
60. Gowda K, Gandhi PG, Rao GHR. Development of specialty drugs for the management of cardiometabolic diseases. 2016. https://www.researchgate.net/profile/Gundu_Rao/contributions.

Reproduced with Permission from: Wolters Kluwer Permission Team (2017-02-02). Article published in the Journal of Clinical and Preventive Cardiology. 2016;5:130-137.

CHAPTER 11

Aspirin Resistance

INTRODUCTION

Aspirin as a therapeutic drug has been in use for over 100 years. Its use as an antiplatelet drug was recognized in the early 70s. For secondary prophylaxis of acute coronary syndromes (ACS), it is the most useful and cost-effective drug. Large number of clinical trials using aspirin has concluded that (low-to-medium dose of aspirin, 80–160 mg) at any given cardiovascular risk it is as effective as any other antiplatelet drugs of choice. However, in recent years, there are several studies in which aspirin resistance in patients with various vascular diseases has been demonstrated. Furthermore, some studies have suggested worst outcome in aspirin nonresponders. Studies from our laboratory (Thrombosis Research Laboratory, Lillehei Heart Institute, University of Minnesota) over three decades have not found any individuals, whose platelets are resistant to the action of aspirin. In other words, aspirin inhibited the cyclooxygenase (Cox-1) activity in platelets of all the individuals tested. Therefore, we feel that the confusion comes from the way people test platelet function for evaluating aspirin or clopidogrel resistance. Alternately, aspirin resistance may develop in nonresponders by as yet unknown mechanism. In this overview, we will discuss the expectations and limitations of aspirin as an antiplatelet drug.

Background

South Asians (Indians, Pakistanis, Bangladeshis, and Sri Lankans) have a very high incidence of coronary artery disease (CAD) compared to any other ethnic group in the world (www.sasat.org). According to the estimate of many professional societies, India ranks as the number one country, with the largest number of diabetics. China is closely competing for the number one position. Currently, India has over 65 million diabetics and an equal number of prediabetics. In view of this excess in cardiovascular risk, identification of "at-risk" population and management of the identified risks is crucial. In addition, we need to personalize therapies for this "at-risk" population. In this overview, we discuss in brief the observed phenomenon of aspirin resistance, methods used for monitoring this phenomenon, importance of developing specific assays for monitoring aspirin resistance, and stress the need for creating awareness of this problem and available solutions to the healthcare providers.

Role of platelets in the pathogenesis of atherosclerosis, thrombosis, and stroke is well documented.[1] Therefore, there is a great need for developing specific and effective drugs for modulating platelet function. A thorough understanding of the signaling mechanisms involved in the regulation of platelet function will facilitate the development of better antiplatelet drugs. Agonists interact with the platelet at specific receptor sites on the plasma membrane and initiate a series of signaling events.[2-10] In spite of the fact that there are very few drugs capable of modulating platelet function, there have been extensive clinical studies on those drugs that are commonly used for prophylaxis to demonstrate the beneficial effects of antiplatelet therapy. Several clinical studies have established the beneficial effect of antiplatelet therapy in reducing the risk of acute cardiovascular events. Data from large number of clinical studies done with aspirin have demonstrated that at any given cardiovascular risk, irrespective of the disease state, aspirin at low-to-medium concentration is as effective as any other antiplatelet drugs.[2-5]

Although ability of a plant bark (bark of willow, *Salix alba*) product to reduce fever was discovered 200 years ago, the mechanism of action of aspirin remained elusive till late 1900s.[6] Nobel laureate Sir John R Vane and his associates at the Royal College of Surgeons, in London, in 1971 proposed the first satisfactory mechanism as to how aspirin works.[7,8] Within a short period of time, extensive work was done by various groups to elucidate the mechanism of action of aspirin-like compounds.[8-20] At the same period, another Nobel laureate Bengt Samuelsson of the Karolinska Institute, Stockholm, Sweden, discovered that the prostaglandin synthase produced transient bioactive prostanoids like PGG_2/PGH_2 and thromboxane from the substrate arachidonic acid (AA).[10] These findings revolutionized the research in platelet physiology and pharmacology.[2-21]

PLATELET PHYSIOLOGY

Blood platelets interact with a variety of soluble agonists, such as epinephrine, adenosine diphosphate (ADP), thrombin, and thromboxane; many cell matrix components, including collagen, laminin, fibronectin, and von Willebrand factor (vWF); and biomaterials used for construction of invasive medical devices.[21-31] These interactions stimulate specific membrane-associated receptors and glycoprotein-rich domains (integrin and nonintegrin receptors) and initiate the activation of intracellular effector enzymes. Agonist-mediated activation of platelets stimulates phospholipase C (PLC) and induces the hydrolysis of phosphatidyl inositol 4, 5-bisphosphate, the formation of second messengers, such as 1, 2-diacylglycerol and inositol 1, 4, 5-trisphosphate. Diacylglycerol activates protein kinase, and inositol trisphosphate (IP_3) facilitates the mobilization of free calcium from the intracellular storage sites. The majority of regulatory events appear to require free calcium. Ionized calcium is the primary bioregulator, and a variety of biochemical mechanisms modulate the availability of free calcium. Elevation of cytosolic calcium stimulates phospholipase A_2 and liberates AA from the membrane phospholipids. Free AA is transformed to a novel metabolite thromboxane, a potent platelet agonist. This is one of the major metabolites of AA metabolism and plays an important role in platelet recruitment, granule mobilization, secretion of granule contents, and expression of activated GPIIb/IIIa ($\alpha_{IIb}\beta_3$) receptors. Upregulation of activation signaling pathways will increase the risk for clinical complications associated with thromboembolic episodes.

ARACHIDONIC ACID METABOLISM

AA is a 20-carbon polyunsaturated fatty acid (20:4w6) found in membrane phospholipids. Agonist-mediated activation mechanisms stimulate phospholipase A_2, which facilitates the release of AA from phospholipids. AA is converted to prostaglandin (PG) endoperoxides (PGG_2/PGH_2) by cyclooxygenase (prostaglandin G/H synthase; Cox-1). These transient metabolites are converted by thromboxane synthetase to thromboxane A_2, which is the major metabolite of this pathway in platelets.[10] In vascular tissues, the endoperoxides generated by Cox-1 enzymes are transformed by prostacyclin synthetase to prostacyclin (PGI_2). Thromboxane is a potent platelet agonist and a vasoconstrictor. Prostacyclin is an antiplatelet compound and exerts vasodilatory effects on vascular tissues. Thus from a single substrate AA, two pharmacologically opposing vasoactive prostanoids are generated by platelets and vascular tissues.[3] Aspirin selectively acetylates the hydroxyl groups of a single serine residue (position 529) in the prostaglandin G/H synthase and causes irreversible inhibition of the activity of this enzyme.[12,13] Inhibition of PG synthase results in the decreased conversion of AA to PG endoperoxides, PGG_2/PGH_2. Molecular mechanisms involved in aspirin-mediated inhibition of prostaglandin G/H synthase are well documented.[6-16]

However, little is known about how other nonsteroidal anti-inflammatory drugs inhibit this enzyme. To elucidate the mechanism by which this enzyme oxidizes AA, we developed a cell-free assay system.[31] This assay system used ferrous iron-induced oxidation of AA. Oxidation of the fatty acids by iron was followed by changes in the color of nitroblue tetrazolium.[31] Several drugs known to be inhibitors of this enzyme were used in this system to evaluate the affinity of these compounds to interact with ferrous iron. Results demonstrated that these compounds could form a complex with ferrous iron and inhibit AA metabolism.[32,33] Using a ferrous iron chelator, bipyridyl, we demonstrated the ability of this compound to inhibit prostaglandin synthesis and platelet function.[34] In a separate study, we showed that ibuprofen, a short-acting drug, interacted with the active site of PG synthase and blocked the ability of aspirin to acetylate the enzyme.[35] On the basis of these results and other studies, we concluded that aspirin-like compounds devoid of acetyl group interact with the heme part of the PG synthase and block AA oxidation. In platelets, AA also is converted by lipoxygenase to 12-hydroxyeicosatetraenoic acids. Aspirin does not inhibit this pathway of AA metabolism.

CLINICAL USE OF ASPIRIN

Earlier studies have demonstrated that a single oral dose of 10–100 mg of aspirin can significantly inhibit the platelet PG synthase activity.[36] The inhibitory effect is fast and probably occurs in the portal circulation. The half-life of aspirin is very short (15–20 minutes) but seems to be sufficient to inhibit PG synthase of circulating platelets. Since these cells lack DNA and the ability to resynthesize the enzyme, the dysfunction caused by aspirin cannot be overcome. Therefore, platelets exposed to aspirin lose the ability to make the prostanoids completely. However, one should keep in mind that once the aspirin is hydrolyzed to salicylic acid, ability to inhibit prostaglandin synthase is lost. Hence, the platelets produced from the bone marrow after the aspirin is hydrolyzed and will have active prostaglandin synthase. Approximately 10% of fresh platelets are added onto the circulating blood every day. Although aspirin-treated platelets do not make prostaglandins, they respond with aggregation to the stimulation by prostaglandin endoperoxides and thromboxane. Fresh platelets formed after the hydrolysis of aspirin can synthesize prostanoids and these newly formed metabolites of AA can cause aggregation of aspirin-exposed platelets. In view of the fact that aspirin irreversibly inhibits prostaglandin synthase, it is possible to take advantage of a daily low-dose aspirin to achieve a cumulative inhibitory effect on

Cox-1 enzymes and thereby on platelet function. Even doses as low as 30–50 mg aspirin taken daily will suppress platelet thromboxane synthesis significantly in 5–10 days.

Vascular tissues on the other hand have the ability to resynthesize prostaglandin G/H synthase.[36] Therefore, these cells can recover the enzyme activity following aspirin exposure. It is therefore possible to develop a strategy to promote the biochemical selectivity of aspirin in terms of inhibition of platelet prostaglandin synthase. This is done by modification of the drug delivery, so the amount of drug delivered is just enough to inhibit platelet enzymes in the peripheral circulation and spare the systemic effect on vascular endothelial cell enzymes.[37,38] Several studies have demonstrated the feasibility of this approach and various controlled-release or timed-release formulations have been developed for this novel therapy.[37-39] However, no such extended-release drug is commercially available at the time of this writing for prophylaxis.

As mentioned earlier, aspirin is metabolized rapidly and the major metabolite salicylic acid is a poor inhibitor of platelet prostaglandin synthase. Therefore, it is essential to develop appropriate strategies to maximize the beneficial effect of this novel drug. As low dose as 20 mg taken daily reduces the platelet thromboxane formation by more than 90%. However, it is generally believed that higher doses are essential for preventing thromboxane-dependent platelet activation. Studies by Wilson et al. demonstrated that maximal plasma concentration of 12 μmol/L could be achieved by a single oral 50 mg dose of enteric-coated aspirin.[17] This dose was found sufficient to cause significant inhibition of platelet function and daily ingestion of low-dose aspirin demonstrated a cumulative effect. In a separate study, McLeod et al. used doses ranging from 50 to 3,900 mg of aspirin and monitored platelet function, bleeding time, and concluded maximum dysfunction was obtained with daily doses of about 100 mg and no further changes were observed in these studies with higher doses.[18] Several workers have demonstrated the efficacy of low-dose oral aspirin in preventing platelet thromboxane production.[2-4,18] Indeed, one of these studies has demonstrated beneficial effect of a dermal aspirin preparation on selective inhibition of platelet prostaglandin synthase, sparing the prostacyclin biosynthesis.[38] However, no such transdermal aspirin preparations are commercially available for prophylaxis. Studies done with low-dose aspirin and the data generated by the two major clinical studies support the use of 80–160 mg of aspirin per day as a prophylactic drug for the primary prevention of clinical complications associated with platelet hyperfunction.[19,20]

The two major clinical trials on aspirin concluded that ingestion of 160 mg per day or 325 mg alternative day provided significant benefit in preventing fatal events associated with CAD.[20,21] It is very well established that 100 mg of aspirin per day is sufficient to significantly reduce the platelet thromboxane production.[2-4,20,21,40-42] Furthermore, studies by McLeod et al. have shown that dosages higher than 100 mg per day do not produce any greater inhibition of platelet function or enhance bleeding times.[18] Therefore, it is reasonable to conclude that 80–160 mg aspirin per day should be the choice for an ideal preventive protocol.[41] However, there is considerable room for improvement to maximize the benefits by better understanding the pharmacology of aspirin and platelet physiology.[2-4] It is possible to customize the aspirin treatment on the basis of the individual patient needs. One can monitor the platelet prostaglandin synthase activity following aspirin ingestion and recommend a dose that is appropriate.[34,41] It is possible to monitor the platelet response to agonists, such as ADP or arachidonate and determine the degree of inhibition by aspirin-like compounds.[18] In order to get maximum inhibition of platelet Cox-1 enzymes, continuous-release aspirin formulations can be developed and tested against currently available aspirin formulations. Platelets are produced and released constantly to the circulation. Therefore, a time-release aspirin, which would make available small amounts of aspirin into the circulation, may be more effective. For instance, a 100 mg formulation capable of releasing 10 mg acetyl salicylic acid per hour may be better than a preparation that releases all of its active principle in a short span of time. Using the strategy of slowing down the release of active principle, newer formulations could be used effectively to provide needed amounts of the drug into circulating blood at regular intervals. These novel formulations may also provide selectivity of aspirin action by preventing platelet thromboxane production and sparing the endothelial prostacyclin synthesis.

McLeod et al. studied the effect of various doses of aspirin (50, 100, 325, 1,000 mg) on platelet and vascular tissues.[43] They did not observe inhibition of urinary 6-keto-$PGF_1\alpha$ productions at low doses of 50 and 100 mg. They attributed these findings to the differential and selective inhibition of platelet Cox-1 enzymes and the sparring effect of vascular Cox-1 enzymes.[44] Sullivan and associates studied the effect of two different doses of aspirin on platelet function and TXA_2 production.[45] Platelet function in healthy volunteers was inhibited by both the doses (75 and 300 mg). Low dose failed to inhibit completely TXB_2 production 24 hours later, whereas 300 mg aspirin did.[46] Even alternate day regimen of these doses prevented platelet function and significantly inhibited the urinary levels of the 11-dehydro-TXB_2. In a separate study, in healthy volunteers, formation of thrombin [fibrinopeptide A (FPA)], α-granule release [β thromboglobulin (β-TG)], and thromboxane (TXB_2) were monitored in vivo in blood emerging from a template bleeding incision.[47] At the site of plug formation, significant platelet activation and thrombin generation was observed as indicated by 110-fold, 50-fold, and 30-fold increase in FPA, β-TG, and TXB_2 within the first minute. A low-dose regimen of aspirin (0.42 mg/kg/day for 7 days) caused greater than 90% inhibition of TXB_2 formation in both bleeding time and clotted blood in these studies suggesting critical role of platelet activation at the site of hemostatic plug formation. In a study to evaluate the effect of low-dose aspirin (0.5 and 15 mg/kg/day) on platelet and renal prostanoids, Wilson et al. monitored serum TXB_2 and urinary 6-keto-$PGF_1\alpha$.[47] Serum TXB_2 level was reduced to 3% of control by low dose and to 0.1% by the higher dose. Urinary TXB_2 was reduced only to 68% by low-dose aspirin and to 51% by high dose. Urinary 6-keto-$PGF_1\alpha$ was not reduced by either dose. Based on their observation, they concluded that low-dose aspirin could significantly affect platelet PG production without affecting stimulated release of PGI_2 production.

Several earlier studies evaluated the effect of low-dose aspirin on normal healthy volunteers as well as patients with various vascular diseases. However, earlier studies did not report prevalence of any aspirin resistance. Zucker et al. evaluated the effect of low-dose aspirin (0.45 mg/kg/day) and a high-dose aspirin (900 mg/day) in type II hyperlipoproteinemic subjects.[48] They found that low-dose aspirin effectively inhibited platelet function in these patients. Increased platelet thromboxane production has been described in several disorders, including type 2 diabetes and type IIa hypercholesterolemia. This increased production of TXB_2 in hypercholesterolemic patients is attributed to abnormal cholesterol levels in these patients. A low dose of aspirin, like 50 mg for 7 days, significantly reduced the production of 11-dehydro-TXB_2 metabolites in these hypercholesterolemic patients.[49] The effect of low-dose aspirin has been evaluated in patients with diabetes, coronary heart disease, myocardial infarction (MI), cerebrovascular disease (CVD), peripheral artery disease (PAD), and in patients undergoing a variety of surgical procedures. Diminno et al. studied the effect of single doses of 100 and 1,000 mg of aspirin for 1 month in normal volunteers and patients with diabetic angiopathy.[50] They found a dose schedule of aspirin, which may suffice in normal volunteers, was not effective in patients with diabetic angiopathy. Contrary to this observation, Terres et al. found that a low dose of aspirin (100 mg) caused significant inhibition of platelet function in both healthy subjects and patients with coronary heart disease.[51] Similarly, a low dose of aspirin (0.45 mg/kg/day) was found adequate for selective inhibition of TXA_2-mediated platelet activation in patients recovering from MI.[52] Looks like the results vary considerably depending on the type and stage of disease, dose of aspirin, and severity of procedure. In a study evaluating the effect of low-dose aspirin (100 mg) on hematological activity of left ventricular (LV) thrombus in anterior wall acute MI (AMI), Kupper et al. found that low dose of aspirin had no effect on the incidence of hematological activity and embolic potential of LV thrombosis in anterior wall AMI.[53] On the other hand, a low-dose aspirin (40 mg/day) daily was found to be as effective as higher doses in preventing platelet responses to agonists in patients who had recent cerebral ischemia.[54] Uchiyama et al. evaluated the effect of low-dose aspirin, ticlopidine, and a combination of both these drugs in patients with cerebral ischemia.[55] Aspirin alone markedly inhibited platelet aggregation induced by AA, partially inhibited aggregation induced by ADP, and did not inhibit aggregation by platelet-activating factor. Combination of these drugs inhibited aggregation by all agonists. Rao et al. demonstrated, in healthy volunteers, low doses of aspirin (40–80 mg) had no inhibitory effect on the response of platelets to ADP, epinephrine, and thrombin, but effectively inhibited the platelet response to threshold concentrations of AA. Epinephrine at concentrations too low to cause aggregation restored the sensitivity of aspirin-treated platelets to AA. This phenomenon, in which weak agonists restore the sensitivity of drug-induced refractory platelets to the action of other agonists, was described from our laboratory as "mechanism of membrane modulation."[56-64]

ASPIRIN RESISTANCE

Aspirin (acetyl salicylic acid) acetylates Cox enzymes at the serine residue and inhibits the enzyme irreversibly (Fig. 11.1).

Studies from our laboratory for the first time demonstrated that one could induce drug-mediated resistance in platelets to the

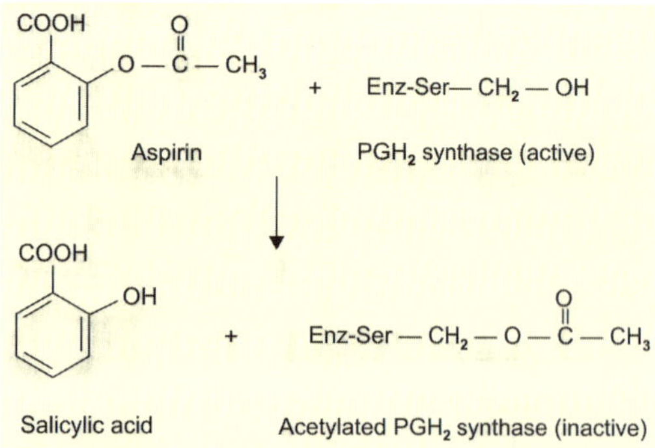

Fig. 11.1: Mechanism of action of aspirin.

action of aspirin.[35] In this study, the subjects were given a short-acting inhibitor of Cox-1 enzymes, ibuprofen. This was followed by administration of a full-strength (325 mg) aspirin. Ibuprofen-mediated inhibition of Cox-1 enzyme lasts for a short time, whereas, aspirin-induced inhibition is irreversible. Ibuprofen-treated platelets recovered their sensitivity to the action of AA by 24 hours, whereas, aspirin-treated platelets failed to respond to the action of AA even after 24 hours. In those subjects who had ingested aspirin after taking ibuprofen first, aspirin failed to inhibit irreversibly the Cox-1 enzymes, suggesting ibuprofen molecules effectively prevented the acetylation of Cox-1 enzymes. One of the earliest work describing "nonresponders" and "responders" evaluated the effect of low-dose aspirin and a thromboxane synthetase inhibitor dazoxiben (UK3724B) in healthy subjects.[56] These studies demonstrated that low-dose aspirin and ingestion of two dazoxiben tablets prevented the release of granules from platelets in response to AA in some individuals (responders) and not in others (nonresponders). These subtle differences in response of platelets to various drugs as well as differences in response to various agonists may be critical when considering the outcome of acute vascular events. For instance, collagen seems to exert its effect by multiple mechanisms. In a study, using aspirin, monoclonal antibodies to IIb\IIIa receptor and fibrinogen, it was demonstrated that there exist at least three mechanisms by which collagen activates platelets: (1) GPIIb\IIIa-associated activation, (2) prostaglandin-dependent pathway, and (3) alternate pathway responsible for 20–30% platelet aggregation.[65]

Although it is well known that there are individual differences in response to drugs as well as agonists, this subject has not been studied thoroughly. Therefore, the time has come for an in-depth study to look at the response of patients under antiplatelet therapies. There is a need to explain why the protection offered to patients is not complete, although multiple antiplatelet drugs are used. Furthermore, several recent studies have demonstrated variable degree of aspirin resistance that exists in patients with a variety of cardiovascular diseases. This subject currently is a very hot topic and has made national headlines. Andrew Pollack published an article in July of 2004 in New York Times on this subject titled "For Some, Aspirin May Not Help Hearts."[66] According to this article, 5–40% of aspirin users are nonresponders or resistant to the medicine. In the same article, he cites the opinion of Dr Daniel I Simon, which reads as follows: "They are taking it for stroke and heart attack prevention and it's not going to work". He also supports the opinion of Dr Michael J Domanski, head of clinical trials unit at the National Institutes of Health (NIH). In his opinion, the nonresponders may represent a huge number of patients. According to Dr Deepak L Bhatt, Professor, Executive Director, Interventional Cardiovascular Program, Brigham and Women's Hospital Heart and Vascular Center, Boston, Massachusetts. Dr Eric Topol, Cardiologist, Executive VP and Professor of Molecular Medicine, The Scripps Research Institute, LaJolla, California, states "Aspirin resistance carries high risk, with over 20 million Americans taking aspirin to prevent heart attacks or strokes, it is important that further work need to be done to confirm our findings and develop a rapid detection method. He also assures that for individuals with aspirin resistance, there are excellent alternatives." Not much is done to develop specific simple assays to determine aspirin resistance in patient population. Not much progress has been made to determine "at-risk" population, so that they can be monitored better. Pharmaceutical companies have not found any substitute for simple cost-effective aspirin.

These observances from healthcare providers and researchers raise number of issues. Do we know enough about aspirin resistance? What causes this resistance to develop in patient populations? Are there specific, rapid, cost-effective tests available? What alternative long-term treatments are available, if patients are resistant to common antiplatelet drugs, such as aspirin and clopidogrel, should the doses of these drugs used for therapy be increased? Should we drop the use of these drugs in nonresponders? We need to find answers to these and other emerging questions soon. We have initiated studies in the Cardiovascular Division of JSS Hospitals, Mysore and at Division of Clinical and Preventive Cardiology, Medanta Hospital, The Medicity, New Delhi to address these issues. In the next few paragraphs, a brief overview of what is known about the prevalence of aspirin resistance, clinical findings, and methodologies available will be discussed.

The first and foremost need at the time of this revision is to standardize a definition of aspirin resistance. The mechanism of action of aspirin is very well documented.[7-13] The drug acetylates the platelet Cox-1 enzyme and irreversibly inhibits its ability to convert AA to PG endoperoxides.[12,13] In the absence of this pathway, platelets do not respond to AA stimulation with aggregation. Weak agonists, such as ADP and epinephrine depend on the formation of PG endoperoxides to initiate secondary wave of aggregation and promote release of platelet granule contents. Therefore, weak agonists fail to induce platelet aggregation and release of granules from aspirin-treated platelets. Failure of AA, ADP, and epinephrine to cause aggregation of platelets more or less establishes drug-induced platelet dysfunction. If platelets obtained from individuals who have ingested a full-strength aspirin respond with aggregation to the action AA, ADP, and epinephrine and release their granule contents, then one can safely conclude that these platelets are resistant to aspirin action. Real proof for aspirin resistance of platelets can be provided by studying AA metabolism by aspirin-treated platelets, monitoring serum TXB_2 levels, or urinary levels of TXB_2 or its metabolite, 11-dehydro-TXB_2.

PREVALENCE OF ASPIRIN RESISTANCE

Aspirin resistance has been poorly defined; variety of nonspecific methods have been employed to monitor the aspirin resistance and conflicting reports have been published on the rates, prevalence, and outcome of continuing this therapeutic modality.[67-69] Aspirin resistance has been reported in patients with cardiovascular, cerebrovascular, and peripheral vascular disease.[70] Because of the differences in methodologies used to monitor this phenomenon and lack of a specific assay to determine the true aspirin resistance, there is considerable confusion and the true significance of this observation remains obscure.[69,70] It also raises the question as to how we missed this phenomenon all these years. Large numbers of clinical trials have demonstrated the beneficial effects of aspirin therapy irrespective of the disease state.[40] Is it possible that these earlier trials missed nonresponders? Is it possible that only responders got the benefit of this therapy? These questions need to be readdressed.

Studies in our laboratory over three decades have failed to show any aspirin resistance in normal healthy subjects. The only subject whose platelets failed to aggregate in response to arachidonate stimulation was found to be deficient in platelet Cox-1 enzymes.[59] Platelets obtained from this subject responded with aggregation when stirred with epinephrine and arachidonate suggesting PG endoperoxides and TXA_2 are not essential to induce irreversible aggregation of platelets. There is not much data on the prevalence of aspirin resistance in general healthy subjects. In patients with various cardiovascular diseases, the rate of nonresponders reported varies between less than 2% and over 60%. Since the methods used to monitor aspirin resistance in these reports are not specific, the prevalence rate published is debatable.

Hurlen et al. used the method of Wu and Hoak to determine the platelet aggregation ratio as a marker for assessing platelet function and evaluated the effect of aspirin (160 mg/day) in 143 patients, who had survived MI.[71,72] Based on their definition, they could only identify two subjects as primary nonresponders. Gum et al. on the other hand from Cleveland Clinic studied 326 stable cardiovascular subjects on aspirin (325 mg/day) and tested aspirin sensitivity by platelet response to aggregating agents, such as ADP and AA. They found 5.5% as nonresponders to aspirin and 24% as semiresponders.[73] Gum et al. used the platelet function assay (PFA-100), a method that is supposed to measure platelet function, to determine aspirin resistance in their patient population.[74] On the basis their studies with this methodology, they found 9.5% to be nonresponders to aspirin action.

Some studies have reported as high as 30–40% nonresponders in stroke or cardiovascular disease patients and predicted more than 80% increased risk for a repeat acute vascular event during a 2-year follow-up period.[75-78] Eikelboom et al. analyzed baseline urinary levels of TXB_2 metabolites 11-dehydro-TXB_2 in 5,529 patients enrolled in the Heart Outcomes Prevention Evaluation (HOPE) Study.[79] Of these subjects, 488 were on aspirin regimen. On the basis of their findings, they concluded that in aspirin-treated patients, increased levels of urinary metabolite of TXB_2 predicted future risk of MI or cardiovascular death. The patients with the highest levels of TXB_2 metabolite had three- to five-fold higher risk of cardiovascular death compared to those in the lowest quartile. Another study reporting clinical outcomes of aspirin resistance is from Austria.[78,80,81] In this study, patients undergoing arterial angioplasty were on 100 mg aspirin per day. Platelet function was assessed by whole blood aggregometry. This study demonstrated that reocclusion at the sites of angioplasty occurred only in men for whom platelet dysfunction was evident by aggregometry.[78] Zimmerman et al. identified aspirin nonresponders as those who had greater than 90% inhibition of TXB_2 formation in presence of 100 μmol/L aspirin and 1 mmol/L arachidonate.[82] In patients who had undergone coronary artery bypass surgery (CABG), AA and collagen-stimulated formation of TXB_2 was same before and after CABG indicating oral aspirin did not significantly inhibit platelet Cox-1 enzymes. Collagen-mediated platelet aggregation does not depend on the prostaglandin availability. If they had used AA as agonist, they would have found the real answer. However, their in vitro studies with 100 μmol/L aspirin on blood obtained from these subjects showed decreased TXB_2 (>10%) in most samples studied confirming our prediction. In spite of this observation, they concluded that platelet inhibition by aspirin is compromised for several days after CABG, probably due to an impaired interaction between aspirin and platelet Cox-1 enzymes. This observation indicates how complex the issues are, when evaluating the effect of antiplatelet drugs during and after interventional procedures. Sane et al. evaluated the effect of aspirin (325 mg/day/month) in patients suffering from congestive heart failure (left ventricular ejection fraction <40%).[83] They used whole blood aggregometry (Chronolog, Chronolog Corp., Havertown, PA) platelet receptor expression by flow cytometry and PFA-100. Patients were considered nonresponders when four of the five parameters assayed were observed. Using this complex rating, persistent platelet activation was observed in 50 of the 88 (56.8%) patients. These observations remind us of the inadequacy of the existing methods to detect what truly represents aspirin resistance.

Methodologies

Researchers have used a variety of methods to assess the aspirin and clopidogrel resistance.[84-98] In spite of the inherent problems associated with platelet aggregometry, it still is the gold standard for determining aspirin resistance of platelets. Studies from our laboratory and that of others have shown that even low-doses (40–80 mg) of aspirin effectively inhibit arachidonate-mediated platelet aggregation. In the absence of any other specific rapid point-of-care assay systems for detecting the sensitivity of platelets to aspirin or lack of aspirin sensitivity, it is preferable to use optical aggregometry to validate the results obtained by other methods. Hurlen et al. used platelet aggregate ratio (PAR) to evaluate the effect of aspirin in post-MI patients. Basically, the method developed by Wu and Hoak uses a ratio of platelets obtained with ethylenediaminetetraacetic acid (EDTA)/formalin as anticoagulants and compares the counts of platelets obtained with EDTA alone. In the presence of platelet aggregates the ratio is less than 1. Using this method, they found two individuals as primary nonresponders and 14 patients as secondary nonresponders.

Several researchers have used PFA-100 (Dade International Inc., Miami, FL) to evaluate aspirin resistance in patients with various cardiovascular diseases. This analyzer measures platelet function as their ability to occlude a membrane coated with collagen and epinephrine or collagen and ADP under high shear stress. Sambola et al. evaluated the effect of low-dose aspirin (100 mg/day/month, 6 months) in 100 patients with ACS. At 1-month post-aspirin therapy, they found 49 patients to have suboptimal response to aspirin (SASAR), whereas only 25 of them showed SASAR by conventional aggregometry. Anderson et al. evaluated the effect of 75 mg aspirin in patients (n = 202) with MI. In patients on aspirin alone they found 25/71 as nonresponders with the epinephrine cartridge. They did not find a significant difference between epinephrine cartridge and ADP cartridge. Gum et al. evaluated the phenomenon of aspirin resistance in 325 stable cardiac patients. They found 5% were nonresponders and 23% semiresponders by optical aggregometry. Whereas, using PFA-100, they found 9.5% as aspirin resistant. This detection system does not seem to detect difference between the effects of low- and high-dose aspirin on platelet function. Since it evaluates the synergistic effect of a combination of two agonists on platelet function, the results obtained or similar to that obtained in our aggregation studies. In a series of studies, we have demonstrated that a combination of two agonists overcomes the inhibition by aspirin and other drugs.[35,57-60,62-64] Studies by Kawasaki et al. have demonstrated increased sensitivity to collagen in individuals who are resistant to low-dose aspirin.

Malinin et al. used THE Ultegra RPFA-ASA (VerifyNow; Accumetrics, Inc., San Diego, CA) to monitor the effect of a single dose of aspirin

(325 mg) in subjects with multiple risk factors.[91] This system uses turbidimetric optical detection system. It uses a test cartridge that contains lyophilized preparation of human fibrinogen-coated beads, platelet agonist, and buffer. Fibrinogen-coated beads bind available receptor on platelet membrane. A cationic agonist, propyl gallate, is used to obtain complete activation of platelets. It uses citrated whole blood for assays. The results are expressed in aspirin response units (ARU). Of the 14 subjects studied, only one was found to be nonresponsive by aggregometry, whereas they found 10 subjects as nonresponders by RPFA-ASA. They concluded that this system was a sensitive device for measuring antiplatelet responsiveness. Newly introduced "VerifyNow" kit includes AA as an agonist for activating platelets. Inclusion of this agonist instead of propyl gallate has considerably improved the performance of this system. In our hands, this system is as good as whole blood aggregometry in identifying aspirin nonresponders to the action of aspirin.

A variety of assays, including platelet aggregometry, PAR, PFA-100, RPFA-ASA, plasma, serum, urinary TXB_2, and urinary 11-dehydro-TXB_2 could monitor aspirin resistance. We used majority of these methods to validate data in our efforts to develop a rapid, specific point-of-care assay system for monitoring platelet function. Majority of these methods are labor intensive, time consuming, and expensive. Technologies are available to develop a rapid and specific assay system, which can monitor platelet function. Specific fluorescent antibodies can be used to detect platelet-bound fibrinogen, P-selectin, or released granule products, such as β thromboglobulin, platelet factor 4, and soluble P-selectin. Furthermore, ATP release or thromboxane generated also could be easily monitored. All the available methods use large quantities of blood and take considerable amount of time. It is possible to device methods that use only small quantities of blood obtained from a fingerstick. Using this approach, we are trying to develop lab-on-a-chip assay for monitoring aspirin resistance with German Collaboration (www.loac-hsg-ismit.de). By using state-of-the-art detectors, one could detect the luminescence (ATP) or fluorescence (specific antibodies) in minutes and develop needed software to standardize the results. If the assay uses AA as standard platelet agonist, then specificity could be built into this system for monitoring aspirin sensitivity. Similarly, by using ADP as agonist, one can build the needed specificity to monitor nonresponders to clopidogrel. The limiting factors for nonavailability of such a system are lack of funds and the assumption that currently available methods detect platelet sensitivity or otherwise to antiplatelet drugs effectively. We feel strongly that there is a great need for creating awareness of this need, to detect at-risk patients to the health care providers, so that those at risk could be offered personalized therapies.

Discussion

Aspirin is the most effective, widely used, relatively inexpensive antiplatelet drug currently available. In the developing world, aspirin is the most cost-effective drug for primary as well as secondary prophylaxis for platelet-mediated cardiovascular complications.[3-5] The mechanism by which it inhibits platelet function is well documented.[7-14] Many large clinical trials have established beyond any doubt that aspirin therapy significantly reduces the incidence of acute events in a variety of vascular diseases.[40] Recent studies have provided evidence to suggest that some subpopulation of patients on aspirin therapy may have developed resistance to the action of aspirin.[66-89] These observations have raised alarm in the public as to who is getting benefited and who is not? Since there is no simple test that can be performed at the doctor's office to detect such a condition, there is some panic in the patient population. Furthermore, there is still lack of awareness of this problem in the medical community at the time of this writing. There are only two major studies, which have described adverse outcome in those patients who are defined as nonresponders to the action of aspirin.[74,78]

Based on methods, which still are not very specific, researchers have identified a subpopulation of patients who are considered nonresponders and another group as semiresponders to the action of aspirin.[73-89] Although the majority of methods used for monitoring this phenomenon lack specificity, it is important to recognize that the problem exists. If these patients for whatever reason are not getting appropriate protection, there is an immediate need to identify them and change their therapeutic regimen. It is equally important to recognize that even those who are considered responders may need additional protection to prevent adverse outcomes if they have hyperresponsive platelets or hyperresponsive coagulation pathways.

Subject of aspirin resistance has received lot of attention in the press and scientific publications.[66-89] However, the practising physicians and the public are not fully aware of the problem. Therefore, there is an immediate need for the development of awareness programs to educate the healthcare providers as well as the public who receive health care. Since there is considerable interest in this subject in the research community, a number of reviews have been published on this subject.[66-89] No attempt has been made in this article to extensively review this subject. Focus of this article has been to bring into discussion three specific areas of concern. First and foremost is the molecular mechanism involved in the initiation of thrombosis and stroke. Basically, two major pathways play a role in the pathophysiology of this process. Therefore, there is a need to identify the hyperresponsiveness of individuals to both these pathways and develop appropriate combination therapy. Secondly, inhibitors of Cox-1 enzymes block only one of the many mechanisms modulating platelet activation. Therefore, there is an immediate need to develop appropriate drugs or drug combinations to prevent the common pathway of platelet activation. Since fibrinogen binding to activated GPIIb/IIIa receptor promotes thrombus formation and growth, drugs should be designed and developed to modulate these mechanisms. In other words, we should develop a synthetic substitute for ReoPro-like antagonist. We are trying to develop a robust screening program for developing synthetic molecules that can prevent fibrinogen binding to platelet GPIIb/IIIa receptor (www.lgcpromochem.com). Thirdly, there is a great need for the development of better point-of-care assays, which can profile the coagulation pathway as well as platelet activation mechanisms. Such an assay system could be effective in identifying nonresponders to commonly used antiplatelet drugs, as well as semiresponders or hyperresponsive individuals and those with hypercoagulable states. Since there is no such detection system, a lot of individuals *at risk* are not getting appropriate treatment for prophylaxis against acute vascular events.

In the early 80s, based on our extensive studies, we concluded that aspirin and other antiplatelet drugs do not prevent platelet activation under a variety of experimental conditions.[35,57-64] Aspirin only inhibits one of the many platelet activation mechanisms. Furthermore, it does not prevent platelet interaction with vessel wall. However, in large number of clinical studies, it has been shown to offer significant beneficial effect to patients with various vascular diseases. Several recent studies have demonstrated that there exists some degree of nonresponders in the patient population undergoing antiplatelet therapy to the action of aspirin.[66-89] Therefore, it is of great importance to thoroughly examine this issue and determine the prevalence of true "aspirin resistance" among the patients and provide them alternate therapies. Since our studies have clearly demonstrated epinephrine, norepinephrine, and ADP can potentiate the action of other agonists on platelets, we may as well screen those who are hyperresponsive to various agonists so that these individuals also could be provided appropriate therapeutic regimen. There are reports suggesting those who are nonresponders to the action of aspirin may be more responsive to the action of agonists, such as ADP or collagen. Studies should take into consideration the fact that platelets can be stimulated by a variety of soluble agonists as well as cell matrix components and even increased shear stress.

In spite of the fact several attempts have been made to explain the mechanisms involved in aspirin resistance, there exists no clear explanation. Serious attempts have to be made to understand the mechanism by which an individual develops resistance to these drugs. Since platelets lack DNA, it is highly unlikely that they resynthesize Cox-1 enzyme. Since many of these patients are on long-term aspirin therapy, the effect of aspirin on megakaryocytes is poorly understood. Platelets are formed from megakaryocytes and these cells do have DNA, hence studies are warranted to explore the effect of aspirin on bone marrow megakaryocytes. Majority of patients with vascular disease also will be taking many other drugs. As such, some amount of drug–drug interaction cannot be ruled out. Whatever may be the mechanism by which individuals with vascular disease develop resistance to aspirin, a better understanding of the molecular mechanisms involved in the platelet activation pathways will facilitate the development of newer antiplatelet drugs and appropriate therapeutic regimen.[97-99]

Major class of antiplatelet drugs includes cyclooxygenase inhibitors, ADP receptor antagonists, and IIb/IIIa antagonists. ReoPro (abciximab) as IIb/IIIa antagonist has been quite useful (www.abciximab.com). However, it is primarily used for preventing acute vascular events. A synthetic small molecule to substitute ReoPro will be very useful. Low-dose aspirin and low-dose clopidogrel are the choice of drugs from primary as well as secondary prevention of acute vascular events.[100-103] However, new drugs, such as cilostazol, prasugrel, and ticagrelor are being evaluated for safe and effective antiplatelet therapy. Dual antiplatelet therapy is important in the treatment of ACS. Newer antiplatelet drugs, such as $P2Y1_2$ inhibitors, ticagrelor, and prasugrel have been investigated compared to clopidogrel in reduction of vascular events with positive outcomes.[103,104] Having said that, even with dual antiplatelet therapy, significant protection is limited, because of multiple mechanisms of platelet activation. Several individual pharmacological agents, such as antiplatelet drugs, β blockers, angiotensin-converting enzyme (ACE) inhibitors, and lipid-lowering agents, have proven efficacy in reducing mortality in patients with ACS. However, the impact of the combination of these agents on clinical outcomes has not been studied or documented in India before. It is high time we initiate some studies and develop evidence-based therapeutic regimens.

Since this review is written primarily for South Asian audience, it is important to discuss the opportunities and challenges for developing an effective antiplatelet therapy. At the time of this writing in India more than 60 fixed drug combinations (FDCs) are available for testing. Majority of them are combinations of aspirin (75–150 mg) and clopidogrel (75 mg). Some of them have included atorvastatin (Lipitor: 10–20 mg). It is possible to initiate a thorough evaluation of these drug combinations to find out if one can develop customized therapy with FDCs. When considering discussions about dual and three-drug combinations, it is worth discussing beneficial effects of polypills as well, since there is considerable interest in these drug formulations. Different polypills have different formulations. Basically, they contain a statin to lower blood cholesterol, aspirin for prevention of thrombosis, and an ACE inhibitor to treat hypertension, and a β blocker to manage cardiac arrhythmias. The Red Heart Pill (British Heart Foundation and Welcome Trust, UK) was a polypill that underwent a large clinical trial. Salim Yusuf and Prem Pais did Indian Polycap Study in which they used a polypill with five constituents: simvastatin, aspirin, and three blood pressure drugs: thiazide (diuretic), atenolol (a β blocker), and ramipril (an ACE inhibitor). This study showed that giving individuals a polypill was as effective as giving combination therapy with single drugs.[105] However, one of the main ideas behind the development of a polypill is that it consists of low-cost ingredients, making it a potentially affordable drug for treating people all over the world, even in the third-world countries. In India, 80% of healthcare costs are paid out of pocket, and some heart disease medications are not affordable to the majority of the people. Therefore, it is possible to work on this concept and develop polypill for cardiovascular and antihyperglycemia management applications. We can further stretch this imagination to include development of affordable polypills with known phytochemicals used in Ayurveda and Herbal medicine.

What other choices we have for better management of ACS patients? Triflusal (Aflen, Disgren, Tecnosal, Triflux; Urechia Labs, Spain) is an antiplatelet drug that is chemically similar to aspirin and seems to be better tolerated by patients.[106] Several studies from Spain have demonstrated that major systemic hemorrhages were significantly lower with triflusal administration compared to aspirin. Triflusal and its metabolite 2-hydroxy-4-(trifluoromethyl) benzoic acid (HTB) inhibit Cox-1 enzymes. It also inhibits cyclic adenosine monophosphate (cAMP) phosphodiesterase thereby preventing breakdown of cAMP. There is some speculation that it selectively inhibits platelet Cox-1 enzymes relative to endothelial Cox-2 enzymes. SASAT (www.sasat.org) under Dr Rao's leadership did a small clinical study on triflusal supported by Glenmark Pharmaceuticals Company at Chennai. These studies demonstrated that this drug indeed lowers TXA_2 and promotes elevation of cAMP. Further large-scale trials are needed to support these preliminary observations.

When we are considering alternate therapies for nonresponders to aspirin or clopidogrel, we will have to think of other novel approaches to manage ACS patients. One such approach is the use of omega-3 fatty acids. Omega-3 fatty acids are currently recommended by American Heart Association, American College of Cardiology, and European Society of Cardiology for reducing risk of coronary heart disease and for management of post-MI patients.[107] In addition, we have a window of opportunity to test and develop some novel therapies based on evidence from traditional medical system. It is worth considering complementing the present therapeutic regimens with a holistic approach, including yoga and lifestyle changes. Studies conducted by SASAT as well as other organizations have demonstrated beneficial effects of diet, exercise, and lifestyle changes in reducing cardiometabolic diseases.[108] Indians are beneficiary for an ancient art and science of healing (ayurveda and yoga). Indians also have access to a huge resource in terms of herbal products developed as supplements. Even National Institute of Health (NIH), USA has found that 80% of the ayurvedic products tested (out of 192 tested) were relatively free of toxic components. It is high time that we take advantage of the observation based on ancient knowledge of traditional medicines and develop a robust integrative approach to health care.[109,110]

CONCLUSION

Platelets play a very important role in the pathogenesis of atherosclerosis, thrombosis, and stroke. Aspirin, even at a low-to-medium dose (80–120 mg/day) has been shown to offer significant protection to individuals from developing acute vascular events. Aspirin is the most cost-effective drug available for the secondary prophylaxis of cardiovascular diseases. In view of these earlier observations, expectations of clinicians on the beneficial effect of aspirin therapy were very high. However, from the available evidence, both experimental and clinical, it is reasonable to conclude that significant number of patients are not getting full protection from the use of aspirin. Even those who are considered responders to aspirin therapy may need additional protection if their platelets are hypersensitive or have a hyperresponsive coagulation pathway. Therefore, there are some limitations in the benefit derived from currently available antiplatelet therapy. Since currently available methods to assess aspirin sensitivity are not specific, labor intensive, and time consuming, efforts should be made to develop specific rapid detection methods. Serious attempts should be made to develop state-of-the-art, point-of-care assay systems, which are capable of detecting hyperresponsiveness to both platelet and coagulation activation mechanisms. In addition, efforts should be made to develop better and effective antiplatelet drugs. Prevention is a better choice than any therapeutic approach. Hence, we should develop holistic integrative preventive approaches for better health care.

REFERENCES

1. Sherry S, Scriabine A. Platelets and Thrombosis. Cambridge University Press, Cambridge, Mass. USA; 1999. p. 309.
2. Suldow C, Baigent C. Randomized trials of antiplatelet therapy. In: Rao GHR (Ed). Handbook of Platelet Physiology and Pharmacology. USA: Kluwer Academic Publishers, Boston; 1999. pp. 526-49.
3. Rao GHR, Rao AT. Pharmacology of platelet inhibitory drugs. Indian J Physiol Pharmacol. 1994;38:69-84.
4. Rao GHR, Rao ASC, White JG. Aspirin in ischemic heart disease—an overview. Indian Heart J. 1993;45:73-9.
5. Rao GHR. Aspirin and coronary artery disease. In: Rao GHR, Kakkar VV (Eds). Coronary Artery Disease in South Asians: Epidemiology, Risk Factors and Prevention. India: Jaypee Brothers Medical Publishers; 2001. pp. 263-78.
6. Weisman G. Aspirin. Sci Am. 1991;264:84-91.
7. Vane JR. Inhibition of prostaglandin synthesis as a mechanism of action of aspirin-like drugs. Nature. 1971;231:232-5.
8. Vane JR, Flower RJ, Botting RM. History of aspirin and its mechanism of action. Stroke. 1990;21:IV12-23.
9. Ferreira SH, Vane JR. Newer aspects of the mode of action of non-steroidal anti-inflammatory drugs. Ann Rev Pharmacol. 1974;14:57-73.
10. Hamberg M, Svensson J, Samuelsson B. Thromboxanes: a new group of biologically active compounds derived from prostaglandin endoperoxides. Proc Natl Acad Sci U S A. 1975;72:2994-8.

11. Marcus AJ. Aspirin as an anti-thrombotic medication. N Engl J Med. 1983;309:1515-7.
12. Roth JG, Caverley DC. Aspirin, platelets and thrombosis: theory and practice. Blood. 1994;83:885-98.
13. Roth JG, Stanford N, Majerus PW. Acetylation of prostaglandin synthetase by aspirin. Proc Natl Acad Sci U S A. 1975;72:3073-6.
14. Meade EA, Smith WL, Dewitt DL. Differential inhibition of prostaglandin endoperoxide synthase (cyclooxygenase) iso-enzymes by aspirin and other non-steroidal anti-inflammatory drugs. J Biol Chem. 1993;268:6610-4.
15. Burch JW, Stanford N, Majerus PW. Inhibition of platelets prostaglandin synthetase by oral aspirin. J Clin Invest. 1978;61:314-9.
16. Reilly IA, FitzGerald GA. Aspirin in cardiovascular disease. Drugs. 1988;35:154-76.
17. Wilson KM, Siebert DM, Duncan EM, Somogyi AA, Lloyd JV, Bochner F. Effect of aspirin infusions on platelet function in humans. Clin Sci (Lond). 1990;79:37-42.
18. McLeod LJ, Roberts MS, Cossum PA, Vial JH. The effects of different doses of some acetyl salicylic acid formulations on platelet function and bleeding times in healthy subjects. Scand J Haematol. 1986;36:379-84.
19. Masptti G, Galanti G, Pogessi L, Abbate R, Neri Serneri GG. Differential inhibition of prostacyclin production and platelet aggregation by aspirin. Lancet. 1972;2:1213-7.
20. Steering Committee of the Physicians Health Study Research Group. Preliminary Report: Findings from the aspirin component of the ongoing physicians' health study. N Engl J Med. 1988;318:262-4.
21. Steering Committee of the Physicians Health Study Research Group. Final report. N Engl J Med. 1989;321:129-35.
22. Hallam TJ, Sanchez A, Rink TJ. Stimulus response coupling in platelets. Biochem J. 1984;218:819-27.
23. Zucker MB, Nachmias VT. Platelet activation. Arteriosclerosis. 1985;5:2-18.
24. Edridge MJ. The molecular basis of communication within the cells. Sci Am. 1985;253: 142-52.
25. Holmsen H. Platelet metabolism and activation. Semin Hematol. 1985;22:219-40.
26. Seiss W. Molecular mechanism of platelet activation. Physiol Rev. 1990;70:115-64.
27. Rao GHR. Physiology of blood platelet activation. Indian J Physiol Pharmacol. 1993;37:263-75.
28. Rao GHR. Signal transduction, second messengers and platelet function. J Lab Clin Med. 1993;121:18-21.
29. Rao GHR. Signal transduction, second messengers and platelet pharmacology. Pharmacol. 1994;13:39-44.
30. Packham MA. Role of platelets in thrombosis and hemostasis. Can J Physiol Pharmacol. 1993;72:278-84.
31. Rao GHR, Gerrard JM, Eaton JW, White JG. The role of iron in prostaglandin synthesis: ferrous iron mediated oxidation of arachidonic acid. Prostaglandins Med. 1978;1:55-70.
32. Peterson DA, Gerrard JM, Rao GHR, Mills EL, White JG. Interaction of arachidonic acid and heme iron in the synthesis of prostaglandins. Adv Prostaglandin Thromboxane Res. 1980;6:157-61.
33. Peterson DA, Gerrard JM, Rao GHR, White JG. Inhibition of ferrous iron induced oxidation of arachidonic acid by indomethacin. Prostaglandins Med. 1979;2:97-108.
34. Rao GHR, Cox AC, Gerrard JM, White JG. Effects of 2,2‘ dipyrydil and related compounds on platelet prostaglandin synthesis and platelet function. Biochim Biophys Acta. 1980;628:468-479.
35. Rao GHR, Johnson GJ, Reddy KR. Ibuprofen protects cyclooxygenase from irreversible inhibition by aspirin. Arteriosclerosis. 1983;3:383-8.
36. Patrono C. Aspirin as an antiplatelet drug. N Engl J Med. 1994;330:1287-94.
37. Hanley SP, Cockbill SR, Bevan J, Heptinstall S. Differential inhibition by low-dose aspirin of human venous prostacyclin synthesis and platelet thromboxane synthesis. Lancet. 1981;2:969-71.
38. Keimowitz RM, Pulvermacher G, Mayo G, Fitzgerald DJ. Transdermal modification of platelet function: a dermal aspirin preparation selectively inhibits platelet cyclooxygenase and preserves prostacyclin biosynthesis. Circulation. 1993;88:556-61.
39. Clarke RJ, Mayo G, Price P, FitzGerald GA. Suppression of thromboxane A_2 but not systemic prostacyclin by controlled release aspirin. N Engl J Med. 1991;325:1137-41.

40. Antiplatelet Trialists' Collaboration. The aspirin papers. BMJ. 1994;308:71-2, 81-106.
41. Fuster V. Dyken ML, Vokomas PS. Aspirin as a therapeutic agent in cardiovascular disease. Circulation. 1993;87:659-675.
42. Rao GHR, Reddy KR, White JG. Low-dose aspirin, platelet function and prostaglandin synthesis: influence of epinephrine and alpha-adrenergic receptor blockade. Prostaglandins Med. 1981;6:485-94.
43. McLeod LJ, Roberts MS, Seville PR. Selective inhibition of platelet cyclooxygenase with controlled release low dose aspirin. Aust N Z J Med. 1990;20:652-6.
44. Rao GHR, Radha E, Johnson GJ, White JG. Enteric coated aspirin, platelet cyclooxygenase activity and platelet function. Prostaglandins Leukot Med. 1984;13:3-12.
45. Sullivan MH, Zosmer A, Gleeson RP, Elder MG. Equivalent inhibition of in vivo platelet function by low dose and high dose aspirin. Prostaglandins Leukot Essent Fatty Acids. 1990;39:319-21.
46. Kyrle PA, Eichler HG, Jager U, Lechner K. Inhibition of prostacyclin and thromboxane A2 generation by low dose aspirin at the site of plug formation in man in vivo. Circulation. 1987;75:1025-9.
47. Wilson TW, McCauley FA, Wells HD. Effects of low dose aspirin on responses to Furosemide. J Clin Pharmacol. 1986;26:100-5.
48. Zucker Ml, Trowbridge C, Woodroof J, Chernoff SB, Reynoso L, Dujovne CA. Low-vs. high-dose aspirin. Effects on platelet function in hyper-lipoproteinemic and normal subjects. Arch intern Med. 1986;146:921-5.
49. Davi G, Averna M, Catalano I, Barbagallo C, Ganci A, Notarbartolo A, et al. Increased thromboxane biosynthesis in type 11a hypercholesterolemia. Circulation. 1992;85:1792-8.
50. Diminno G, Silver MJ, Cerbone AM, Murphy S. Trial of repeated low-dose aspirin in diabetic angiopathy. Blood. 1986;68:886-91.
51. Terres W, Schuster O, Kupper W, Bleifeld W. Effects of low-dose acetylsalicylic acid on thrombocytes in healthy subjects and in patients with coronary heart disease. Dtsch Med Wochenschr 1989;18:1231-6.
52. De Caterina R, Giannessi D, Bernini W, Gazzetti P, Michelassi C, L'Abbate A, et al. Low-dose aspirin in patients recovering from myocardial infarction. Evidence for a selective inhibition of thromboxane-related platelet function. Eur Heart J. 1985;6:409-17.
53. Kupper AJ, Verheugt FW, Peels CH, Galema TW, den Hollander W, Roos JP. Effect of low dose acetylsalicylic acid on the frequency and hematologic activity of left ventricular thrombus in anterior wall acute myocardial infarction. Am J Cardiol. 1989;63:917-20.
54. Weksler BB, Kent JL, Rudolph D, Scherer PB, Levy DE. Effects of low dose aspirin on platelet function in patients with recent cerebral ischemia. Stroke. 1985;16:5-9.
55. Uchiyama S, Sone R, Nagayama T, Shibagaki Y, Kobayashi I, Maruyama S, et al. Combination therapy with low-dose aspirin and ticlopidine in cerebral ischemia. Stroke. 1989;20:1643-7.
56. Jones EW, Cockbill SR, Cowley AJ, Hanley SP, Heptinstall S. Effects of dazoxiben and low-dose aspirin on platelet behavior in man. Br J Clin Pharmacol. 1983;15:S39-S44.
57. Rao GHR, White JG. Epinephrine-induced platelet membrane modulation. Myers KM, Barnes CD (Eds). The Platelet Amine Storage. Roca Baton: CRC Press; 1992. pp. 117-49.
58. Rao GHR, Johnson GJ, White JG. Influence of epinephrine on the aggregation response of aspirin-treated platelets. Prostaglandins Med. 1980;5:45-58.
59. Rao GHR, White JG. Epinephrine potentiation of arachidonate-induced aggregation of cyclooxygenase deficient platelets. Am J Hematol. 1981;11:355-66.
60. Rao GHR, White JG. Role of arachidonic acid in human platelet activation and irreversible aggregation. Am J Hematol. 1985;19:339-47.
61. Rao GHR, White JG. Aspirin, PGE1 and Quin-2 AM induced platelet dysfunction. Restoration of function by norepinephrine. Prostaglandins Leukot Essent Fatty Acids. 1990;39:141-6.
62. Rao GHR, Escolar G, White JG. Epinephrine reverses the inhibitory influence of aspirin on platelet vessel wall interaction. Thromb Res. 1986;44:65-74.
63. Rao GHR, Escolar G, Zavrol J. Influence of adrenergic receptor blockade on aspirin-induced inhibition of platelet function. Platelets. 1990;1:145-50.
64. Rao GHR, Reddy KR, White JG. Modification of human platelet response to sodium

arachidonate by membrane modulation. Prostaglandins Med. 1981;6:75-90.

65. Connelan JM, Thurlow PJ, Barlow B, Lowe M, McKenzie IF. Investigation of alternative mechanisms of collagen-induced platelet activation using monoclonal antibodies to glycoprotein IIb-IIIa and fibrinogen. Thromb Haemost. 1986;55:153-7.
66. Pollack A. For Some, Aspirin May Not Help Hearts. New York Times. 2004, July.
67. Weber AA, Przytuski B, Schanz A, Hohlfeld T, Schrör K. Towards a definition of aspirin resistance: a typological approach. Platelets. 2002;13:37-40.
68. Yilmaz MB, Balbay Y, Korkmaz S. Aspirin resistance. Anadolu Kardiyol Derg. 2004;4:59-62.
69. Patrono C, Coller B, FitzGerald GA, Hirsh J, Roth G. Platelet-active drugs: the relationships among dose, effectiveness, and side effects: the Seventh ACCP Conference on Antithrombotic and Thrombolytic Therapy. Chest. 2004;126:2348-645.
70. Howard PA. Aspirin resistance. Ann Pharmacother. 2002;36:1620-4.
71. Hurlen M, Seijeflot I, Arnesen. The effect of different regimens on platelet aggregation after myocardial infarction. Scand Cardiovasc J. 1998;32:233-7.
72. Wu KK, Hoak JC. A new method for the quantitative detection of platelet aggregation in patients with arterial insufficiency. Lancet. 1974;11:924-6.
73. Gum PA, Kottke-Marchant K, Poggio ED, Gurm H, Welsh PA, Brooks L, et al. Profile and prevalence of aspirin resistance in patients with cardiovascular disease. Am J Cardiol. 2001;88:230-5.
74. Gum PA, Kottke-Marchant K, Welsh PA, White J, Topol EJ. A prospective, blinded determination of the natural history of aspirin resistance among stable patients with cardiovascular disease. J Am Coll Cardiol. 2003;41:961-7.
75. Deliargyris E, Boudoulas H. Aspirin resistance. Hellenic J Cardiol. 2004;45:1-5.
76. Grotemeyer KH. Effects of acetyl salicylic acid in stroke patients; evidence of nonresponders in a subpopulation of treated platelets. Thromb Res. 1991;63:587-93.
77. Grotemeyer KH. Two-year follow-up of aspirin responder and aspirin non-responder: a pilot-study including 180 post-stroke patients. Thromb Res. 1993;71:397-403.
78. Mueller MR, Salat A, Stangi P, Murabito M, Pulaki S, Boehm D, et al. Variable platelet response to low-dose ASA and the risk of limb deterioration in patients submitted to peripheral arterial angioplasty. Thromb Haemost. 1997;78:1003-7.
79. Eikelboom JW, Hirsh J, Weitz JI, Johnston M, Yi Q, Yusuf S. Aspirin-resistant thromboxane biosynthesis and the risk of myocardial infarction, stroke, or cardiovascular death in patients at high risk for cardiovascular events. Circulation. 2002;105:1650-5.
80. Smout J, Stansby G. Aspirin resistance. Br J Surg. 2002;89:4-5.
81. Helgason CM, Bolin KM, Hoff JA, Winkler SR, Mangat A, Tortorice KL, et al. Development of aspirin resistance in persons with previous ischemic stroke. Stroke. 1994;25: 2331-6.
82. Zimmerman N, Wenk A, Kim U, Kienzle P, Weber AA, Gams E, et al. Functional and biochemical evaluation of platelet aspirin resistance after coronary artery bypass surgery. Circulation. 2003;108:542-7.
83. Sane DC, McKee SA, Malinin AI. Frequency of aspirin resistance in patients with congestive heart failure treated with antecedent aspirin. Am J Cardiol. 2002;90:893-5.
84. Muller I, Besta F, Schulz C, Massberg S, Schönig A, Gawaz M. Prevalence of clopidogrel non-responders among patients with stable angina pectoris scheduled for elective coronary stenting. Thromb Haemost. 2003;89:783-7.
85. Lau WC, Grubel PA, Watkins PB, Neer CJ, Hopp AS, Carville DG, et al. Contribution of hepatic cytochrome P450 3A4 metabolic activity to the phenomenon of clopidogrel resistance. Circulation. 2004;109:166-71.
86. Angiolilo DJ, Fernandez-Ortiz A, Bernardo E. High clopidogrel loading dose during coronary stenting: effect on drug response and inter-individual variability. Eur Heart J. 2004;25:1903-10.
87. Serebruany VL, Steinhubl SR, Berger PB, Malinin AI, Bhatt DL, Topol EJ. Variability in platelet responsiveness to clopidogrel among 544 individuals. J Am Coll Cardiol. 2005;45:246-51.

88. Patrono C. Aspirin resistance, mechanisms and clinical readouts. J Thromb Haemost. 2003;1:1710-3.
89. Altman R, Luciardi HL Muntaner J, Herrera RN. The antithrombotic profile of aspirin, aspirin resistance or simply failure? Thromb J. 2004;2:1-8.
90. De Gaetano G, Cerletti C. Aspirin resistance: a revival of platelet aggregation tests? J Thromb Haemost. 2003;1:2048-61.
91. Malinin A, Spergling M, Muhlestein B, Steinhubl S, Serebruany V. Assessing aspirin responsiveness in subjects with multiple risk factors for vascular disease with a rapid platelet function analyzer. Blood Coagul Fibrinolysis. 2004;1:295-301.
92. Sambola A. Heras M, Escolar G, Lozano M, Pino M, Martorell T, et al. The PFA-100 detects sub-optimal antiplatelet responses in patients on aspirin. Platelets. 2004;15(7):439-46.
93. Coleman JL, Wang JC, Simon DI. Determination of individual responses to Aspirin therapy using the Accumetric Ultegra. The J Near-Patient Testing and Technol. 2004;3:77-82.
94. Feuring M, Hasseroth K, Janson CP, Falkenstein E, Schmidt BM, Wehling M. Inhibition of platelet aggregation after intake of acetylsalicylic acid detected by a platelet function analyzer (PFA 100). Int J Clin Pharmacol Ther. 1999;37:584-8.
95. Andersen K, Hurlen M, Arnesen H, Seljeflot I. Aspirin-responsiveness as measured by a PFA 100 in patients with coronary artery disease. Thromb Res. 2002;108:37-42.
96. Christiaens L, Allal J, Corbi C. Impact of ABO blood group on the detection of aspirin resistance with the Platelet Function Analyzer PFA-100. Thromb Res. 2003;108:115-9.
97. Singh S, Kothari SS, Bahl VK. Aspirin resistance: myth or reality? Indian Heart J. 2003;55:1-8
98. McKee SA, Sane DC, Deliagyris. Aspirin resistance in cardiovascular disease: a review of prevalence, mechanisms, and clinical significance. Thromb Haemost. 2002;88:711-5.
99. Eikelboom JW, Hankey GJ. Aspirin resistance: a new independent predictor of vascular events? J Am Coll Cardiol. 2003;41:966-8.
100. Rao GHR. Aspirin resistance: a fact or a myth? Exp Clin Cardiol. 2005;10:17-20.
101. Rao GHR, Fareed J. Aspirin prophylaxis for the prevention of thrombosis: expectations and limitations. Thrombosis. 2012;2012:104707.
102. Divani A, Zentek ND, Haghighi A, Rao GHR. Antiplatelet therapy: aspirin resistance and all that jazz. J Clin Appl Thromb Hemost. 2013;19:5-18.
103. Wiviotk SD, Braunwald E, McCabe CH, Montalescot G, Ruzyllo W, Gottlieb S, et al. Prasugrel vs clopidogrel in patients with acute coronary syndrome. N Engl J Med. 2007;357:2001-15.
104. Wallutin L, Backer RC, Budaj J. Ticagrelor vs clopidogrel in patients with acute coronary syndrome. N Engl J Med. 2009;361: 1045-57.
105. Lonn E, Bosch J, Teo KK, Pais P, Xavier D, Yusuf S. The polypill in the prevention of cardiovascular diseases: key concepts, current status, challenges and future directions. Circulation. 2010;122:2078-88.
106. Anninos H, Andrikopoulos G, Pastromas S, Sakellariou D, Theodorakis G, Vardas P. Triflusal: an old drug in modern antiplatelet therapy. Review of it is action, use safety and effectiveness. Hellenic J Cardiol. 2009;50:199-207.
107. Harris W, Von Schacky. Omega-3 fatty acids, acute coronary syndrome and sudden death. 2008;2:161-6.
108. Rao GHR, Nagendra HR. Holistic approach for prevention of heart disease and diabetes. J Prev Cardiol. 2013;2:231-8.
109. Rao GHR, Gandhi PG. Integrative medicine: global perspective. J Homeop Ayurv Med. 2014;3:150.
110. Patwardhan B, Mutalik G, Tillu G. Integrative Approach for Health: Bio Medical Research, Ayurveda and Yoga. The Netherlands: Elsevier Publications; 2015.

Platelet Dysfunctions Associated with Diabetes Mellitus

CHAPTER 12

INTRODUCTION

Indians have a very high incidence of vascular complications, such as hypertension, atherosclerosis, coronary artery disease (CAD), and stroke, compared to any other ethnic group in the world.[1-4] They also have a very high incidence of multiple metabolic diseases, including diabetes.[5,6] Elevated levels of known risk promoters in this population for CAD do not adequately explain the significant increase in the vascular disease burden in this population. There is some speculation that genetic predisposal may account for this increased incidence in vascular diseases. Functional and structural changes in the arterial wall precede the development of clinical complications, such as endothelial dysfunction, hypertension, atherosclerosis, hyperfunction of platelets, and coagulation pathways.[7,8] Vascular dysfunction, therefore, is the major contributor for the pathogenesis of hypertension, atherosclerosis, diabetes, thrombosis, and stroke. Alterations in the balance between platelet associated vasoconstrictors and endothelial-derived vasodilators result in the vascular dysfunction. Blood platelets play a very important role in the pathogenesis of hypertension, atherosclerosis, diabetes-related clinical complications, thrombosis, and stroke. These cells interact with a variety of soluble and insoluble cell matrix-associated agonists. Such interactions lead to the activation of intracellular effector enzymes. Ionized calcium is the primary bioregulator and a variety of signaling mechanisms modulate the cellular physiology and functions.[9] Activated platelets promote the formation of thrombin and initiate coagulation cascade. They also interact with circulating blood cells and facilitate inflammatory response.[10-12] Similar to atherosclerosis, pathogenesis of vascular complications in diabetes is also complex and is mediated by a variety of factors. Contributions of atherosclerosis, vascular dysfunction, inflammation, and platelet hyperfunction to the pathogenesis of vascular complications are well documented.[13-18] In this chapter, we provide a brief overview on platelet physiology, platelet hyperfunction, oxidative stress, and the role of blood cells and blood components on platelet-related clinical complications in diabetes mellitus.

PLATELET PHYSIOLOGY

Blood platelets interact with a variety of soluble agonists such as epinephrine and adenosine diphosphate (ADP), many insoluble cell matrix components including collagen, laminin, and biomaterials used for construction of invasive medical devices.[9] These interactions stimulate specific receptors and glycoprotein-rich domains (integrin and nonintegrin domains) on the plasma membrane and lead to the activation of intracellular enzymes.[19,20] The majority of the regulatory events appear to require free calcium.[21,22] Major enzymes that regulate the free calcium levels via second messengers include phospholipase C, phospholipase A_2, and phospholipase D together with adenylyl and guanylyl cyclases. Activation of phospholipase C results in the hydrolysis of phosphatidyl inositol 4,5-bisphosphate and formation of second messengers 1, 2 diacylglycerols and inositol 1,4,5-trisphosphate (IP_3). Diglyceride induces activation of protein kinase C, whereas IP_3 mobilizes calcium from internal membrane stores.[21-26] Elevation of cytosolic calcium stimulates phospholipase A_2 and liberates arachidonic acid (AA). Free AA is transformed to a novel metabolite, thromboxane A_2, by fatty acid synthase (Cox-1, cyclooxygenase). Thromboxane A_2 is the major metabolite of this pathway and plays a critical role in platelet recruitment, granule mobilization, and secretion of granule contents.[27] Secretory granules contain a variety of growth factors, mitogens, and inflammatory mediators. Secretion of granules promote P-selectin (adhesive molecule) expression on the platelet membrane. Furthermore, activation also promotes the expression of acidic lipids and tissue factor on the membrane, thus making these cells procoagulant. Fully activated platelets can modulate the function of other circulating blood cells such as leucocytes, monocytes, macrophages, as well as vascular endothelial cells.[12,28] Agonist-mediated stimulation of platelets promotes the expression of an epitope on glycoprotein IIb/IIIa receptors. Activation of this receptor is essential for the binding of circulating fibrinogen. Fibrinogen forms a bridge between individual platelets and facilitates the thrombus formation and its growth. von Willebrand factor (vWF) binds platelet GPIb-IX complex only at high shear rate unlike fibrinogen, which can bind platelets at low shear. Upregulation in signaling events will increase the risk for clinical complications associated with acute coronary events. Downregulation of signaling pathways may precipitate bleeding diathesis or hemorrhagic stroke.

ARACHIDONIC ACID METABOLISM

Arachidonic acid (AA) is a 20-carbon polyunsaturated acid (20:4w6) found in membrane phospholipids.[27] Cell activation stimulates phospholipase A_2, which facilitates the release of this fatty acid from membrane phospholipids. AA is converted to prostaglandin (PG) endoperoxides (PGG_2/PGH_2) by cyclooxygenase (prostaglandin GH synthase; Cox-1) (Fig. 12.1). These transient metabolites are converted to thromboxane A_2, which is the major metabolite of this pathway in platelets.[27,29-32] Whereas, in vascular tissues, the endoperoxide generated by Cox-1 is converted by prostacyclin synthase to prostacyclin (PGI_2). Thromboxane is a potent platelet agonist and vasoconstrictor. Prostacyclin is an antiplatelet compound and exerts vasodilatory effects on vascular tissues.[30] Thus from a single substrate (AA) two pharmacologically opposing prostanoids are generated by platelets and vascular tissues.[30,33] Aspirin selectively acetylates the hydroxyl groups of a single serine residue (position 529) in the prostaglandin synthetase enzymes, which results in the irreversible inhibition of this key enzyme and decreased conversion of AA to PG endoperoxides, PPG_2/PGH_2. Molecular mechanisms involved in aspirin-mediated inhibition of prostaglandin GH synthase are well documented.[27,29-33]

PLATELET HYPERFUNCTION

There is increasing evidence suggesting that the inflammatory mediators play a pathogenic role in the atherogenesis as well as in acute

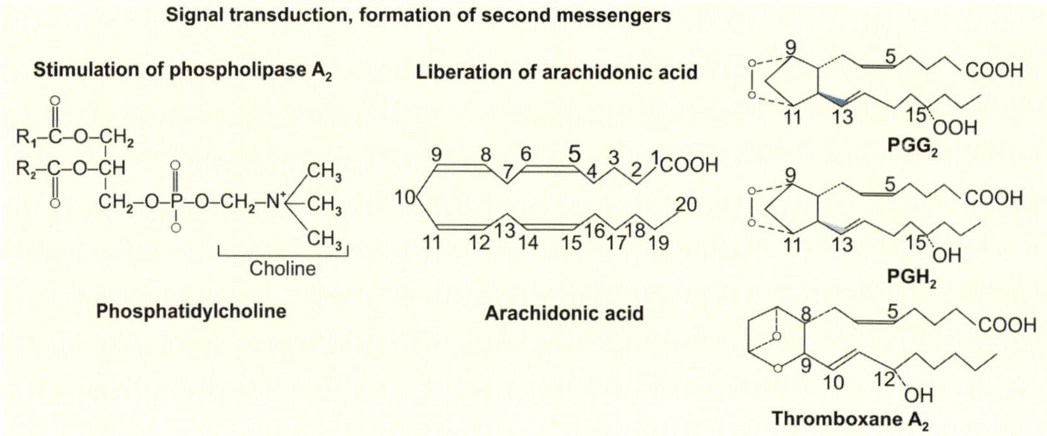

Fig. 12.1: Arachidonic acid metabolism in platelets.

coronary syndromes. Several recent studies suggest that inflammatory cytokines such as tumor necrosis factor (TNF-α), interleukin (IL-1), and various chemokines (IL-8) may activate matrix metalloproteinase and induce degradation of connective tissue and promote apoptosis of cells in the atherosclerotic lesion, thus promoting plaques' destabilization and rupture. There is considerable evidence to show that platelets contribute significantly to the pathogenesis of acute coronary syndromes by facilitating thrombus formation. They may also trigger acute coronary events by other mechanisms including stimulation of an inflammatory response within the atherosclerotic plaque. They secrete a wide range of growth factors and inflammatory mediators. In addition, they activate other cells such as monocytes and macrophages and promote the expression of tissue necrosis factor and tissue factor. They also modulate the function of leucocytes and promote the expression of chemotactic and adhesive properties of endothelial cells as well as IL-1 production in smooth muscle cells. Increased leucocyte-platelet aggregation has been demonstrated in acute myocardial infarction (MI) and cerebral infarction. It has been shown that release of CC-chemokines RANTES by platelets triggers the arrest of monocytes on inflamed atherosclerotic endothelium.

Furthermore, in vulnerable plaque, significant amounts of tissue factor expression also have been demonstrated. It is clear from the available evidence that several platelet-derived factors, both membrane-bound (P-selectin, pCD40L) and soluble (S-selectin, sCD40L), are involved in the inflammatory response mediated by the activation of platelets, leucocytes, monocytes, macrophages, and endothelial cells. Some studies have demonstrated the presence of platelet activation markers such as P-selectin and CD40 in patients with MI. There is some evidence to suggest that overexpression of CD40L on platelets is correlated with the need for reangioplasty. Expression of this protein promotes the expression of adhesion molecules, chemokines and inflammatory cytokines, and recruitment of leucocyte within the vulnerable plaque. Levels of circulating markers of inflammation, C-reactive protein (CRP) has been found to be higher in patients with unstable coronary syndromes. Furthermore, according to Harvard researchers, persistent elevation of CRP in patients with unstable angina seems to be a good predictor of future coronary events such as ischemia and MI.

Contribution of circulating blood platelets to the pathogenesis of atherosclerosis, progression of vascular complications related to diabetes is well documented.[17] Patients with type 2 diabetes seem to have a two- to fourfold increased risk of morbidity and mortality due to CAD.[34,35] Platelets obtained from diabetic subjects show increased adhesiveness, hyperfunction both spontaneous and in response to agonists. These observed hyperfunctions are attributed to increased expression, activation or abundance of surface membrane receptors for agonists as well as cell matrix components, increased binding to fibrinogen, altered membrane fluidity, changes in activation mechanisms and signaling pathways. Several earlier studies (both in animal models and human subjects) have demonstrated platelet hyperfunction-associated hyperglycemia.[11] In early 60s, Bridges et al. showed both in vitro as well as in vivo administration of glucose on increased platelet stickiness.[36] Studies by Kwaan et al. demonstrated that plasma from diabetic patients can enhance the response of normal platelets to the action of agonists.[37]

With the discovery of prostanoids (prostaglandin endoperoxides thromboxanes and prostacyclin), there was considerable interest in showing a definite role for these lipid mediators in the diabetes-related clinical complications.[30] In the early 80s, we explored the mechanism involved in platelet hyperfunction in a rat model.[38] In this novel study, drug (streptozotocin)-induced diabetic condition increased the ability of platelets to produce significantly higher levels of thromboxane upon stimulation. Whereas, stimulation of vascular tissues obtained from diabetic animals generated much lower quantities of prostacyclin compared to the tissue from normal animals. We speculated that such an imbalance in the production of vasoactive metabolites will create a prothrombotic condition in diabetic subjects. However, in what turned out to be a novel experiment, pancreatic islet cell transplantation restored the normal functional response of both the platelets and vascular tissues.[38]

Mandal et al. using whole blood aggregometry showed that platelets' hyperaggregation was present even at the time of diagnosis in patients with diabetes mellitus, even in the absence of any vascular complications. Various platelet activation markers such as CD62, CD63, PAXC-1, annexin V, and platelet-derived microparticles (PDMP) have been used to follow the state of platelet activation in diabetic subjects. Some studies have suggested that PDMP may contribute to the development of atherosclerosis.[39,40] Whereas, a study from Germany demonstrated that in diabetes, increased number of large platelets circulate in an activated state mostly in patients with angioplasty.[41] Based on the results of their studies, they suggested three different mechanisms by which activated platelets modulate the prothrombotic state in the diabetic population: (1) microembolization of the capillaries, (2) local progression of preexisting vascular lesions, and (3) trigger of the arterial thrombotic event.[42] Therefore, there is a reason to believe that activated platelets as well PDMP may contribute significantly to the prothrombotic state in the diabetes mellitus. Fattah et al. evaluated hemostatic parameters such as prothrombin time, partial thromboplastin time, thrombin time, coagulation factors II, VII, IX, and plasma fibrinogen, α-2-antiplasmin, plasminogen activator inhibitor (PAI), and lower levels of protein C.[43] They concluded that altered state of these hemostatic parameters could lead to prothrombotic tendency in diabetic patients.[41] Studies by Deepa and Mohan at the Madras Diabetes Research Foundation, Chennai, India, demonstrated elevated PAI-1 and tissue plasminogen activator (t-PA) antigen levels in subjects with CAD and not so significantly in diabetic subjects.[44]

Although several studies have suggested that hypersensitivity of platelets as well as hyperfunction of coagulation cascade predispose diabetic subjects to a prothrombotic state, there is not much of direct evidence to suggest that such conditions induce acute vascular events.[45] Studies by Kawamori et al. demonstrated a relationship between progression of atherosclerosis and in vivo platelet activation. They concluded from their studies that the progress of atherosclerosis in diabetes mellitus is associated with in vivo platelet activation and platelet activation does not occur in diabetics without carotid atherosclerosis.[46] Nakajima et al. using the thrombotic status analyzer (TSA) found that elderly male subjects had prothrombotic state not because of platelet hyperaggregability but because of suppressed thrombolytic activity.[47] Carr et al. showed that both platelet function and clot structure may be altered in diabetes.[48] They observed increased platelet contractile force as well as clot elastic modulus in diabetic patients with chest pain. Hyperglycemia spikes seem to play a role in vascular complications. Gresele et al. demonstrated that shear stress-induced platelet activation, P-selectin and LIMP expression on platelets in the bleeding time blood, and urinay-11-dehyro-TXB_2 excretion were increased after hyperglycemic clamping and not after euglycemic clamping.[49]

Diabetes mellitus is associated with increased risk for atherosclerosis and stroke. Several earlier studies have demonstrated a critical role for platelets in diabetes-related clinical complications.[17,44] Platelets of patients with diabetes have shown to be sticky, hypertensive to the action of agonists, possess increased number of surface membrane receptors for binding fibrinogen as well as cell matrix components, enhanced arachidonate pathway, and increased phosphoinositol turnover leading to production of second messengers, and calcium mobilization and protein phosphorylation. Furthermore, activated coagulation pathway also has been demonstrated in the diabetic subjects. Further studies are needed to evaluate the specific role of platelet hyperfunction and hypercoagulation in the pathogenesis of thrombosis and stroke.

OXIDATIVE STRESS

Diabetes mellitus is associated with multiple abnormalities and the most common major diagnostic parameter is hyperglycemia as measured by fasting blood glucose levels or glycosylated hemoglobin A_{1c} (HbA_{1c}). Reversible glycosylation of amino groups or glycation is the basis for the formation of HbA_{1c}, the known marker for diabetes. Final end product of this reaction is the formation of irreversible oxidation or glycoxidation to yield advance glycation end products (AGEs). Although the exact mechanism by which this increased state of blood glucose initiates the various clinical complications associated with diabetes is not known, there is considerable interest in its role in oxidative stress. Role of lipid peroxidation in the pathogenesis of atherosclerosis and promotion of the disease of the vessel wall is well documented.[50,51] Studies by Nomura et al. showed that activated platelets, platelet-derived microparticles, and oxidized low-density lipoprotein (LDL) promote endothelial cell membrane vesiculation and microparticle formation.[51] Several studies have demonstrated increased levels of thiobarbituric acid reactive substances and lipid hydroperoxides in plasma of diabetic subjects as an index of oxidative stress–related oxidation of lipids. There is considerable interest in the role of reactive oxygen and nitrogen species in the pathogenesis of diabetes-related clinical complications. In a recent review on this subject, the authors suggest that chemical modifications of proteins, carbohydrates, and lipids in diabetes may be viewed as a result of carbonyl stress mediated by reactive carbonyl precursors.[52]

Recently, a novel class of prostanoids-like compounds known as F2-isoprostanes has been described as reliable markers for monitoring oxidative stress.[53] Studies by Gopaul et al. have demonstrated that plasma level of 8-epi $PGF_2\alpha$ are threefold higher in diabetic subjects than in normal subjects.[54] In a separate study, it was shown that the increase of this AA metabolite was correlated well with the increase in thromboxane levels.[55] Furthermore, they demonstrated that improved metabolic control as well as vitamin E supplementation lowered the levels of these AA metabolites. De Cristofaro et al. monitored carbonyl activation of plasma urinary lipid oxidation product (8-iso-prostaglandin $F_2\alpha$), platelet activation (urinary 11-dehydro-TXB_2), and plasma prothrombin F_{1+2} levels in diabetic subjects and showed that all these parameters were significantly higher in these patients, compared to the control subjects.[56]

Altered platelet function has been implicated in many of the complications associated with diabetic micro- and macroangiopathies. Yamagashi et al. studied hyperglycemia-mediated reactive oxygen species formation in human platelets and showed an additive effect of this on platelet response to collagen stimulation.[57] They used an inhibitor of electron transport chain and an uncoupler of oxidative phosphorylation to show that the source of the superoxide radicals was from platelet mitochondria. Increased oxidative stress may not only lead to the activation of platelets but also to the depletion of antioxidants. Vericel et al. demonstrated that basal thromboxane levels were increased in both types 1 and 2 diabetic subjects. Furthermore, both vitamin E and cytosolic glutathione levels were lower in platelets from diabetic patients compared with respective control subjects.[58]

Role of free radicals and antioxidants in platelet physiology and function is poorly understood.[59] Several researchers have worked on this subject. Reduced glutathione and GDSH-related enzymes play a key role in defense against oxygen-free radicals. In addition, platelets have several other free radical scavengers, such as ascorbic acid, serotonin, and taurine. In the 80s, studies from our laboratory demonstrated that glutathione levels in human platelets display a circadian rhythm in vitro.[60] Values fell steadily during first few hours and then rose to a new peak at midnight. To better understand the role of glutathione and its peroxidase, we performed in vitro studies using appropriate drugs, capable of depleting this compound. Agents used in these studies included diamide, N-ethylmaleimide (NEM), and 1-chloro-2,4-dinitrobenzene (CDNB). In addition to lowering GSH levels, these agents also inhibited the GSH-peroxidase activity. In GSH-depleted cells, total conversion of AA was reduced by the lipoxygenase; however, there was significant increased conversion of AA to proaggregatory metabolites by the Cox-1 enzymes.[61] AA induced platelet aggregation and secretion was attenuated in platelets depleted of GSH by diamide or NEM.[62]

Whereas, platelets treated with CDNB responded with irreversible aggregation to low doses of AA.[63]

Our own studies as well as that of others have showed influence of peroxides on AA-mediated activation of platelets. We also demonstrated in these studies that inhibition of lipoxygenase by 4,7,10,13-eicosatetraenoic acid also potentiated AA-mediated platelet aggregation.[64] These results suggest that at least three modes of treatment share a common mechanism of increasing AA metabolism to biologically active prostaglandins and thromboxane through alterations in cyclooxygenase kinetics and available substrate levels. Studies by Simplicio et al. demonstrated that mean effective dose of AA required to cause platelet activation was on an average significantly lower in diabetic subjects as compared with age, gender-matched control subjects.[65] Franconi and associates have done extensive studies on the role of glutathione utilizing enzymes thioltransferase and various endogenous antioxidants in platelet physiology and function.[64-69] They demonstrated that in diabetic subjects with increased urinary albumin, a marked decrease was observed in thioltransferase activity. Furthermore, they also demonstrated a significant decrease in plasma and platelet content of taurine, a prooxidant substance, whereas after taurine supplementation values equaled the mean value for healthy control subjects.[66] Ascorbate is another powerful antioxidant. Sinclair et al. found that patients with microangiopathy had lower ascorbic acid concentrations than those without microangiopathy and control subjects.[70] Supplementation of 1 g ascorbate per day for 6 weeks raised dehydroascorbate levels significantly in all the groups tested.[70]

In spite of the fact that there is ample evidence to suggest that diabetic subjects demonstrate telltale signs of oxidative stress, the source of this stress has been elusive. Both plasma and urinary isoprostane levels are increased in diabetic subjects. Furthermore, urinary excretion of thromboxane has also been well documented in the case of diabetic subjects. Davi and associates have demonstrated that vitamin E supplementation significantly lowers the urinary isoprostanes as well as thromboxane metabolites, products of AA metabolism.[71] Further evidence in support of the hypothesis that hyperglycemia is the major source of oxidative stress comes from the work of Pieper et al. using drug-induced animal model for diabetes.[72] In their novel study, they have demonstrated that improved glycemic control by pancreatic islet cell transplantation reduces vascular oxidative stress and reverses antioxidant enzyme regulation. In an earlier work in the 80s, our laboratory at the University of Minnesota had demonstrated similar reversal of altered prostaglandin metabolism in platelets and vessel wall after pancreatic islet cell transplantation in a drug-induced diabetic rat model.[73]

VASCULAR DYSFUNCTION

Functional and structural changes in the arterial wall precede the development of atherosclerosis, obstructive coronary disease, and may even serve as an early marker for the hypertensive disease.[74,75] Function and structural changes of vascular endothelial cells (ECs) are modulated by a variety of thrombogenic factors as well as antithrombogenic factors.[75] Some of the vasoactive compounds released by the ECs include vasodilatory compounds such as adenosine, prostacyclin, and nitric oxide (NO), and vasoconstrictory molecules like cyclooxygenase-derived endothelium-dependent constrictor factor (EDCF), hypoxia-induced EDCF, and endothelin. Lipid peroxides, oxidized lipids, and lipoproteins promote the formation of vasoconstrictors by platelets.[76] These lipid mediators inhibit enzymes that promote the formation of vasodilators by the healthy endothelium and lower endogenous production of vasodilators. Alterations in the balance between platelet associated vasoconstrictors and EC-derived vasodilators result in vascular dysfunction.[77,78] This is probably the earliest stage at which one can detect the manifestation of the arterial dysfunctions, hypertension, and atherosclerosis. Indeed, one can classify the risk according to the level of EC dysfunction and additional CAD risk factors present. One can use acetylcholine, L-arginine, and nitric oxide synthase inhibitor, LNNMA, and monitor the flow response to determine the degree of endothelial dysfunction.[79-82] Alternatively, one can use CV-profiler (DO-2020, Hypertension Diagnostics, Egan, MN) of the Periscope (Genesis Medical Systems, Hyderabad, India) and monitor pulse pressure waveforms of the small arteries.[82,83] Several earlier studies have shown that there are alterations in the pulse flow of the blood in the diabetic subjects indicating the pathogenesis of vascular dysfunctions and arterial stiffness. Studies by Rema et al. as part of the CURE project have demonstrated that diabetic retinopathy is associated with internal media thickness and arterial stiffness, suggesting these vascular alterations might predispose diabetics to micro- and macroangiopathies.[84]

Several earlier studies have demonstrated that hyperglycemia, oxidative stress, and platelet activation might predispose diabetic subjects to vascular dysfunction, atherosclerosis, and acute vascular events.[38,73,85] In an earlier study, we demonstrated that drug-induced hyperglycemia results in the altered production of platelet and vessel wall-derived metabolites of AA via Cox pathway.[38,73] Similar alterations have been observed the production of NO and endothelin 1. Ouvina et al. have demonstrated increased levels of endothelin, von Willebrand factor, and soluble selectin in the plasma of diabetic subjects.[86] The authors concluded that presence of increased endothelial damage markers and low nitric oxide bioavailability in diabetic subjects could lead to a higher risk for development of thrombotic events. To demonstrate a similar alteration in the vasodilators and vasoconstrictors, Tretjakovs et al. studied AA incorporation into phospholipids and nitric oxide end products in diabetic subjects.[87] Their study demonstrated that development of diabetes in CAD patients decreased the ability to produce platelet-derived NO and enhanced AA incorporation into phospholipids. Whereas, Huszka et al. demonstrated in their study that endothelial-derived NO is reduced in diabetes suggesting vascular damage.[88] They concluded that decreased NO production may lead to increased platelet activation in these individuals.

Alterations in the balance between various bioactive metabolites generated by platelets and vessel wall lead to either hyper- or hypofunction of platelets. Level of cytosolic calcium and degree of actin assembly and phosphorylation of contractile proteins dictate the degree of platelet activation.[9,21,22-26] Pellegatta et al. studied both resting calcium levels and agonist-mediated rise in the levels and concluded that poor metabolic control (HbA_{1c} >8) altered calcium homeostasis as well as stimulation–response coupling.[89] Schaeffer et al. based on their results concluded that platelets of diabetic subjects have enhanced calcium signaling due to excessive superoxide production.[90] Fukuda et al. have studied the phosphorylation of myosin light chain (MLC) in platelets of diabetic subjects as well as age- and sex-matched controls.[91] They found that MLC phosphorylation was significantly higher in platelets of diabetic subjects irrespective of their age. Results of these studies and the earlier observations demonstrate that hypoglycemia oxidative stress, platelet activation, and vascular dysfunction contribute significantly to the pathogenesis of diabetes mellitus, a chronic metabolic disorder.

BLOOD CELLS AND BLOOD COMPONENTS

There is increasing evidence suggesting that the inflammatory mediators play a pathogenic role in the atherogenesis as well as in acute coronary syndromes.[92] Several recent studies suggest that inflammatory cytokines such as TNF-α, IL-1, and various chemokines (IL-8) may activate matrix metalloproteinases and induce degradation of connective tissue and promote apoptosis of cells in the atherosclerotic lesion, promoting plaque destabilization and rupture. There is considerable evidence to show that platelets contribute significantly to the pathogenesis of acute coronary events by other mechanisms including stimulation of an inflammatory response within the atherosclerotic plaque. They secrete a wide range of growth factors and inflammatory mediators.[92] In addition, they activate other cells such as monocytes and macrophages and promote expression of tissue necrosis factor and tissue factor. They also modulate the function of leukocytes and promote the expression of chemotactic and adhesive properties of endothelial cells as well as IL-1 production in smooth muscle cells. Increased leukocyte-platelet aggregation has been demonstrated in acute MI and cerebral infarction. Similar platelet interaction with other blood cells has been studied in diabetics.[93-95] Telejko et al. found increased leukocyte-platelet aggregation formation in CAD patients.[93] They also found positive correlation with monocyte-platelet aggregation and fasting insulin levels.[93] In a separate study, Hilberg et al. found increased number of platelet-granulocyte and platelet-lymphocyte aggregates in diabetic subjects.[94] High levels of the soluble fragment of CD40 ligand (sCD40L) has been implicated with adverse vascular outcomes. Lim et al. found that the plasma levels of sCD40L, soluble P-selectin, and IL-6 are higher in diabetic subjects.[95] In the same study, highest amounts of tissue factor were found in those patients with overt CAD. A recent study in South Indians have shown increased levels of sP-selectin and sCD40L in subjects with impaired glucose tolerance and type 2 diabetes compared to those with normal glucose tolerance.[96] It is clear from the available evidence that several platelet-derived factors, both membrane bound (P-selectin, pCD40L) and soluble (S-selectin, sCD40L), are involved in the inflammatory response mediated by the activation of platelets, leukocyte, monocytes, macrophages, and endothelial cells. Some studies have demonstrated the presence of platelets in MI and CD40L expression.[97] Levels of circulating markers of inflammation, CRP have been found to be higher in patients with unstable coronary syndromes.[92] Furthermore, according to the Harvard researchers, persistent elevation of CRP in patients with unstable angina seems to be a good predictor of future coronary events such as ischemia and MI.[97-99] In a recent study, Mohan and associates demonstrated an association of elevated CRP with body fat, diabetes, and CAD in Indian subjects.[100]

ROLE OF PLATELETS IN VASCULAR PATHOLOGY

Platelet activation in vivo seems to play a role in diabetes-related micro- and macro-angiopathies. To investigate the role of platelets in macroangiopathy,

Diamantopoulos et al. monitored platelet levels of β-thromboglobulin (β-TG), a protein secreted by platelets in diabetic subjects with peripheral arterial disease.[101] Plasma levels of β-TG were higher in those with well-characterized peripheral occlusive arterial disease. Based on the results of platelet aggregation tests, Chitre and Velaskar concluded that platelet hyperfunction plays a significant role in the development of diabetic microangiopathies.[102] In a separate study, fibrinogen binding to platelets and AA metabolism was used to monitor the platelet function in diabetic subjects. Authors of this study concluded that increased fibrinogen binding and hyperaggregability of platelets from non-retinopathic diabetics to be related to their capacity to form more prostaglandin, endoperoxides, and thromboxanes.[104] In addition to platelet activation, some studies have demonstrated generalized hypercoagulation in diabetic retinopathy.[105] On the other hand, Lysenko et al. studied 407 diabetic patients and found relapsing hemorrhage syndrome in 40% of these subjects.[106]

Available evidence suggests a critical role for platelet activation as well as hypercoagulation in diabetic vascular complications including diabetic nephropathy.[107] A study from Mayo clinic, Rochester, Minnesota, using a combination of dipyridamole and aspirin suggests a role for thromboxane in the pathogenesis of human glomerular disease.[108] Japanese researchers monitored platelet-derived microparticles and activation markers CD62/CD63 and concluded that increased platelet activity and its related procoagulant activity may play a role in the development of diabetic nephropathy.[109] Toth et al. monitored plasma thromboxane and β-TG levels as well as urinary β-TG levels in diabetic subjects.[110] They found that these platelet activation markers were higher in diabetic group compared to normal control subjects. Further large-scale clinical trials are needed to critically assess the role of platelet hyperfunction and hypercoagulation in the pathogenesis of vascular complications such as retinopathy, neuropathy, nephropathy, and vasculopathy.

MANAGEMENT OF HEMATOLOGICAL PARAMETERS

Patients with diabetes have an approximately threefold risk for all cardiovascular diseases. There seems to be a strong association between hyperfunction and hypercoagulability and diabetes-related vascular complications. Therefore, there is a great need to evaluate the role of antiplatelet and antithrombotic drugs in reducing risk for the development of end-organ failure. Results from several hundred clinical trials have demonstrated that aspirin is as effective as any other drug in reducing the development of acute vascular events. Aspirin at low (80 mg) to medium (160 mg) doses seems to offer significant benefits to patients suffering from various vascular diseases, including diabetes mellitus.[111] In recent years, there is some degree of concern that patients on antiplatelet drugs such as aspirin and clopidogrel develop resistance to the action of these drugs.[112] Limited number of studies have demonstrated poor outcome in those who are considered nonresponders to the action of antiplatelet drugs.[112]

A recent study has suggested that increased protein glycation in diabetes mellitus is associated with decreased aspirin-mediated protein acetylation and reduced sensitivity of platelets to aspirin.[113] In a separate study, Angiolillo et al. assessed platelet function profile in diabetic and nondiabetic subjects on aspirin and clopidogrel therapy.[114]

They found that diabetic subjects had increased platelet reactivity and decreased sensitivity to antiplatelet drugs. They also found that in diabetic group, there were more nonresponders to the action of clopidogrel. Aspirin in low doses inhibits platelet production of thromboxane and reduces in vivo activation of platelets. Physicians recommend clopidogrel if aspirin is found to be ineffective in some patients. Therefore, if this phenomenon of drug resistance is found to be true, there is a real need for alternate therapy. In a meta-analysis of six clinical trials in diabetic subjects with acute coronary syndromes, intravenous GPIIb-IIIa inhibitors reduced 30-day mortality.[115]

Eibl et al. studied the effect of improved metabolic control on platelet activation markers. They monitored platelet activation markers such as CD36, CD49, CD62, and CD63 and found that all were elevated in diabetic subjects. After 3 months of improved metabolic control, all the markers except CD36 were reduced in diabetic subjects.[116] Studies by Watala and associates also demonstrated a relationship between metabolic control and platelet sensitivity to aspirin.[117] They found a correlation between reduced response of platelets to the action of aspirin and increased level of HbA_{1c} in diabetic subjects. In a recent study, the role of $P2Y_{12}$ receptors in the development of platelet microaggregation was demonstrated in diabetic patients.[118] In the same study they showed that aspirin as well as ticlopidine reduced microaggregate formation induced by ADP or shear stress. Shouzu et al. showed that platelet-derived microparticles and activated platelets stimulate the activation of monocytes and promote the production of monocyte-derived microparticles and also that ticlopidine may be useful in reducing the hypercoagulability in these diabetic subjects.[119] Several studies have demonstrated a beneficial role for antiplatelet drugs in reducing the vascular complications associated with diabetes. However, there is a great need for large-scale clinical trials to evaluate the role of antiplatelet drugs as well as antithrombotic drugs in reducing the diabetes-related vascular complications.

CONCLUSION

Global prevalence and the burden of diabetes mellitus are increasing rapidly due to aging populations, life style changes, reduced physical activity, stress, and obesity.[120] India used to be the capital of type 2 diabetes for quite some time, but China has taken over the lead. According to the Institute for Health Matrices and Evaluation (IHME), currently, 2.1 billion people—nearly 30% of the global population are either obese or overweight—a new, first-of-a-kind analysis of trend data from 188 countries. Obesity increased two-fold since 1980, whereas type 2 diabetes by fourfold. Overweight, obesity, as well as noncommunicable diseases are largely preventable. Hyperglycemia, oxidative stress, obesity, endothelial dysfunction, platelet hyperfunction, and prothrombotic coagulation pathways contribute significantly to the pathogenesis of this complex chronic metabolic disease. Approximately 80% of patients with diabetes mellitus die of cardiovascular disease.[121] A comprehensive management of all the risks associated with this disease is the only choice available for subjects with this disease. Early diagnosis of people at risk for developing these metabolic abnormalities will contribute significantly to the success of primary prevention efforts. Large clinical trials investigating the role of antiplatelet drugs and antithrombotic compounds in the prevention of CAD in diabetic subjects are needed.[122]

REFERENCES

1. Rao GHR, White JG. Coronary artery disease: an overview of risk factors. Indian Heart J. 1993;45:143-53.
2. Rao GHR, Mohanty D, Rao ASC. Coronary artery disease: risk factors for Indian men and women. Indian J Hematol Blood Transf. 1997;15:3-8.
3. Rao GHR, Kakkar VV. Coronary Artery Disease in South Asians: Epidemiology, Risk Factors and Prevention. New Delhi: Jaypee Brothers Medical Publishers; 2001.
4. Rao GHR, Thanikachalam S. Coronary Artery Disease: Risk Promoters, Pathophysiology, and Prevention. New Delhi: Jaypee Brothers Medical Publishers; 2005.
5. King H, Auberti RE, Herman HH. Global burden of diabetes 1995-2025. Numerical estimate and projection. Diabetes Care. 1998;2:1414-31.
6. Ramachandran A, Snehalatha C, Latha E, Vijay V, Viswanathan M. Rising prevalence of NIDDM in an urban population in India. Diabetologia. 1997;40:232-7.
7. Rao GHR. Platelet hyperfunction as a risk promoter for acute coronary events. In: Rao GHR, Thanikachalam S (Eds). Coronary Artery Disease: Risk Promoters, Pathophysiology and Prevention. New Delhi: Jaypee Brothers Medical Publishers; 2005. pp. 192-201.
8. Zeiher A, Drexler H, Wollschlagen H, Just H. Modulation of coronary vasomotor tone in humans Progressive endothelial dysfunction with different early stages of coronary atherosclerosis. Circulation. 1990;83: 391-401.
9. Rao GHR. Physiology of blood platelet activation. Indian J Physiol Pharmacol. 1993;37: 263-75.
10. Ross R. Atherosclerosis—an inflammatory disease. N Engl J Med. 1999;340:115-26.
11. Libby P, Ridker PM, Maseri A. Inflammation and atherosclerosis. Circulation. 2002;105: 1135-43.
12. Libby P. Current concepts of the pathogenesis of the acute coronary syndromes. Circulation. 2001;104:365-72.
13. Stern MP. Diabetes and cardiovascular disease. The "common soil" hypothesis. Diabetes. 1995;44;369-74.
14. Das UN. Metabolic syndrome X. Type-2 diabetes mellitus and disorders are common in Indians: but why and how? In: Rao GHR, Thanikachalam S (Eds). Coronary Artery Disease: Risk Promoters, Pathophysiology and Prevention. New Delhi: Jaypee Brothers Medical Publishers; 2005. pp. 73-84.
15. Celermajer DS, Sorensen KE, Gooch VM, Spiegelhalter DJ, Miller OI, Sullivan ID, et al. Non-invasive detection of endothelial dysfunction in children and adults at risk for atherosclerosis. Lancet. 1992;340:1111-5.
16. Ravikumar R, Deepa R, Shanthirani CS, Mohan V. Comparison of carotid-medial thickening, arterial stiffness ad brachial artery dilation in diabetic and non-diabetic subjects. Am J Cardiol. 2002;90:702-7.
17. Sobol AB, Watala C. The role of platelets in diabetes-related vascular complications. Diabetes Res Clin Pract. 2000;50:1-16.
18. Keaney JF, Loscalzo J. Diabetes, oxidative stress and platelet activation. Circulation. 199;99:189-91.
19. Ruoslahti E. Integrins. J Clin Invest. 1991; 87:1-4.
20. Ruoslahti E, Peerchbacher MD. New Perspective in cell adhesion. RGD and integrins. Science. 1987;238:491-7.
21. Rao GHR. Signal transduction second messengers and platelet function. J Lab Clin Med. 1993;121:18-20.
22. Rao GHR. Signal transduction second messengers and platelet pharmacology. Pharmacol. 1994;13:39-44.
23. Hallam TJ, Sanchej A, Rink TJ. Stimulus response coupling in human platelets. Biochem J. 1984;218:819-27.
24. Seiss W. Molecular mechanisms of platelet activation. Physiol Rev. 1989;69:59-78.
25. Rana RS, Hokin LE. Role of phosphoinositides in transmembrane signaling. Physiol Rev. 1990;70:115-64.
26. Hokin LE. Receptors and phosphoinositide generated second messengers. Annu Rev Biochem. 1985;54:205-35.
27. Marcus AJ. The role of lipids in platelet function: with particular reference to arachidonic acid pathway. J. Lipid Res. 1978;19: 793-826.
28. Aukurst P, Waehre T, Damas JK, Gullestad L, Solum NO. Inflammatory role of platelets in

acute coronary syndromes. Heart. 2001;86: 605-6.
29. Roth GJ, Stanford N, Majerus PW. Acetylation of prostaglandin synthetase by aspirin. Proc Natl Acad Sci U S A. 1975;72:3073-6.
30. Needleman P, Raz A, Minkes, Ferrendelli JA, Sprecher H. Triene prostaglandins: prostacyclin and thromboxane biosynthesis and unique biological properties. Proc Natl Acad Sci U S A. 19179;76:944-8.
31. Hamberg M, Svensson J, Samuelsson B. Mechanisms of anti-aggregating effect of aspirin on human platelets. Lancet. 1974;2:223-4.
32. Hamberg M, Svensson J, Samuelsson B. Thromboxanes: a new group of biologically active compounds derived from prostaglandin endoperoxides. Proc Natl Acad Sci U S A. 1975;72:2994-8.
33. Rao GHR, Rao AT. Pharmacology of platelet activation—inhibitory drugs. Indian J Physiol Pharmacol. 1994;38:69-84.
34. Stampler J, Vaccaro O, Neaton JD, Wentworth D. Diabetes, other risk factors, and 12-yr cardiovascular mortality for men screened in multiple risk factor interventions trial. Diabetes Care. 1993;16:434-44.
35. Kannel WB, McGee DL. Diabetes and cardiovascular risk factors: the Framingham study. Circulation. 1979;59:8-13.
36. Bridges JM, Dalby AM, Millar JHD, Weaver JA An effect of D-glucose on platelet stickiness. Lancet. 1965;1:75-7.
37. Kwaan HC, Colwell JA, Cruz S, Suwanwela N, Dobbie JG. Increase platelet aggregation in diabetes mellitus. J Lab Clin Med. 1972;80:236-46.
38. Gerrard JM, Stuart MJ, Rao GHR, Steffes MW, Mauer SM, Brown DM, et al. Alteration in balance of prostaglandin and thromboxane synthesis in diabetic rats. J Lab Clin Med. 1980;95:950-7.
39. Mandal S, Sarode R, Dash S, Dash RJ. Hyperaggregation of platelets detected by whole aggregometry in newly diagnosed non-insulin dependent diabetes mellitus. Am J Clin Pathol. 1993;100:103-7.
40. Nomura S, Suzuki M, Kastura K, Xie GL, Miyazaki Y, Miyake T, et al. Platelet-derived micro-particles may influence the development of atherosclerosis in diabetes mellitus. Atherosclerosis. 1995;116:235-40.
41. Tschoepe D, Roesen P, Eser J, Schwippert B, Nieuwenhuis HK, Kehrel B, et al. Large platelets circulate in an activated state in diabetes mellitus. Semin Thromb Hemost. 1991;17:433-8.
42. Tshoepe D, Roesen P, Schiwppert B, Gries FA. Platelets in diabetes: the role in the hemostatic regulation in atherosclerosis. Semin Thromb Hemost. 1993;19:122-8.
43. Fattah MA, Shaheen MH, Mafouz B. Disturbances of hemostasis in diabetes mellitus. Dis Markers. 2003-2004;19:251-8.
44. Deepa R, Mohan C. Tissue plasminogen activator inhibitor and coronary artery disease in Indians. In: Rao GHR, Thanikachalam S (Eds). Coronary Artery Disease: Risk Promoters, Pathophysiology and Prevention. New Delhi: Jaypee Medical Publishers; 2005. pp. 133-41.
45. Wincour PD. Platelet abnormalities in diabetes mellitus. Diabetes. 1992;41:26-31.
46. Kawamori R, Imano E Watarai T, Nishizawa H, Matsushima H, Kodama M, et al. Platelet activation in diabetic patients with asymptomatic atherosclerosis. Diabetes Res Clin Pract. 1994;24:89-95.
47. Nakajima S, Noguchi T, Taka T, Ueda T, Kaizu K, Fukamizu M, et al. A global platelet test of thrombosis and thrombolysis detects a prothrombotic state in some patients with non-insulin-dependent diabetes in some patients with stroke. Platelet. 2000;11:459-66.
48. Carr ME, Krishnaswami A, Martin EJ. Platelet contractile force (PCF) and clot elastic modulus (CEM) are elevated in diabetic patients with chest pain. Diabet Med. 2000;19:862-6.
49. Gresele P, Guglimini G, De Angelis M, Ciferri S, Ciofetta M, Falcinelli E, et al. Acute, short-term hyperglycemia enhances shear stress-induced platelet activation in patients with type-2 diabetes mellitus. J Am Coll Cardiol. 2003;19:1013-20.
50. Witztum JL, Steinberg D. Role of oxidized low density lipoprotein in atherosclerosis. J Clin Invest. 1991;88:1785-92.
51. Nomura S, Shouzu A, Omoto S, Nishikawa M, Iwasaka T, Fukuhara S. Activated platelet and oxidized LDL induce endothelial

membrane vesiculation: clinical significance of endothelial cell-derived micro-particles in patients with type-2 diabetes. Clin Appl Thromb Hemost. 2004;10:205-15.

52. Dalle-Donne I, Scsaloni A, Glustarini D, Cavarra E, Tell G, Lungarella G, et al. Proteins as biomarkers of oxidative stress in diseases: the contribution of redox proteomics. Mass Spectrom Rev. 2005;24:55-99.
53. Roberts LJ, Morrow JD. The generation and actions of isoprostanes. Biochim Biophys Acta. 1997;1345:121-35.
54. Gopaul NK, Anggard EE, Mallet AL, Betteridge DJ, Wolff SP, Nourooz-Zadeh J. Plasma 8-epi-PGF$_1$alpha levels are elevated in individuals with non-insulin dependent diabetes mellitus. FEBS Lett. 1995;3668:225-39.
55. Nenci CG, Pilani U. Diabetes, coagulation and vascular events. Recenti Prog Med. 2000;91:86-90.
56. De Cristofaro R, Rocca B, Vitacolonna E, Falco A, Marchesani P, Ciabattoni G, et al. Lipid and protein oxidation contribute to a prothrombotic state in patients with ype-2 diabetes mellitus. J Thromb Hemost. 2003;1:25-56.
57. Yamagashi SI, Edelstein D, Du XL, Brownlee M. Hyperglycemia potentiates collagen-induced platelet activation through mitochondrial superoxide production. Diabetes. 2001;50:1491-4.
58. Vericel E, Januel C, Carreras M, Moulin P, Lagarde M. Diabetic patients without vascular complications display enhanced platelet activation and decreased antioxidant status. Diabetes. 2004;53:1046-51.
59. Rao GHR, Parthasarathy S. Antioxidants, atherosclerosis, and thrombosis. Prostaglandins Leukot Essent Fatty Acids. 1996;54:155-66.
60. Radha E, Hill TD, Rao GHR, White JG. Glutathione levels in human platelets play a circadian rhythm *in vitro*. Thromb Res. 1985;40:823-31.
61. Hill TD, White JG, Rao GHR. The influence glutathione depleting agents on human platelet function. Thromb Res. 1989;53: 457-65.
62. Hill TD, White JG Rao GHR. Role of glutathione and glutathione peroxidase inhuman platelet arachidonic acid metabolism. Prostaglandins. 1989;38:21-32.
63. Hill TD, White JG, Rao GHR. Platelet hypersensitivity induced by 1-chloro-2, d-dinitrobenzene, hydroperoxides and inhibition of lipoxygenase. Thromb Res. 1989; 53:447-55.
64. Franconi F, Bennardini F, Mattana A, Miceli M, Ciuti M, Milan M, et al. Taurine levels in plasma and platelets in insulin-dependent and non-insulin dependent diabetes mellitus. Correlation with platelet aggregation. In: Huxtable R, Michalk DV (Eds). Taurine in Health and Disease. New York: Plenum Press; 1994;419-23.
65. Di Simplicio P, De Giorgion A, Caradaioli E. Glutathione, glutathione utilizing enzymes and thioltransferase in platelets of insulin-dependent diabetic patients: relation with platelet aggregation and with macro-angiopathic complications. Eur J Clin Invest. 1995;25:665-9.
66. Franconi F, Bennardinin F Mattana A, Miceli M, Ciuti M, Mian M, et al. Plasma and platelet taurine are reduced in subjects with insulin-dependent diabetes mellitus: effects of taurine supplementation. Am J Clin Nutr. 1995;61:1116-59.
67. Seghieri G, Martinoli L, di Fellice M, Anichini R, Fazzini A, Ciuti M, et al. Plasma and Platelet ascorbate pools and lipid peroxidation in insulin-dependent diabetes mellitus. Eur J Clin Invest. 1998;28:659-63.
68. Seghieri G, Di Simplicion P, De Giorgio A, Anichini R, Alberti L, Franconi F. Relationship between metabolic control and platelet content of glutathione and its related enzymes, in insulin-dependent diabetes mellitus. Clin Chim Acta. 2000;299:109-17.
69. Seghieri G, Di Simplicio P, Anichini R, Alviggi L, De Bellis A, Bennardini F, et al. Platelet antioxidant enzymes in insulin-dependent diabetes mellitus. Clin Chim Acta. 2001;309:19-23.
70. Sinclair AJ, Girling AJ, Gary L, Le Guen C, Lunec J, Barnett AH. Disturbed handling of ascorbic acid in diabetic patients with and without micro-angiopathy during high dose ascorbate supplementation. Diabetologia. 1991;34:171-5.
71. Davi G, Giabottoni G, Consoli A, Mezzetti A, Falco A, Santarone S, et al. In vivo formation

of 8-iso-prostaglandinF_2 alpha and platelet activation in diabetes mellitus: effects of improved metabolic control. Circulation. 1999;99:224-9.

72. Pieper GM, Jordan M, Dollinger LA, Adams MB, Roza AM. Peroxidative stress in diabetic blood vessels: reversal by pancreatic islet transplantation. Diabetes. 1995;44: 884-9.
73. Gerrard JM, Rao GHR, Stuart MJ. Alterations in the balance of thromboxane and prostacyclin synthesis in platelet and the vessel wall in a diabetic animal model. In: Hirsch J, Steele PP, Vernier RL (Eds). The Effects of Platelet Active Drugs on Cardiovascular System. Denver: University of Colorado Press; 1981. pp. 207-23.
74. Cohn J, Finkelstein JN. Abnormalities of vascular compliance in hypertension, aging and heart failure. J Hypertens Suppl. 1992;10: S61-4.
75. Vane JK Anggard EE, Botting RM. Regulatory function of the vascular endothelium. N Engl J Med 1990;323:27-36.
76. Marcus AJ. The eicosanoids in biology and medicine. J Lipid Res. 1984;25:1511-6.
77. Ferro CJ, Webb DJ. Endothelial dysfunction and hypertension. Drugs. 1997;53:30-41.
78. De Meyer GRY, Herman AG. Vascular endothelial dysfunction. Prog Cardiovasc Dis. 1997;34:325-42.
79. Bank AJ. Physiologic aspects of drug therapy. Vasc Med. 1997;2:44-50.
80. McVeigh GE, Allen PB, Morgan DR. Evaluation of mechanical properties: clinical experimental and therapeutic aspects. Clin Sci (Lond). 2001;100:387-93.
81. McVeigh GE, Hamilton PK, Morgan DR, Hanratty CG, Silke B. Nitric oxide modulation of blood vessels identified by arterial wave form analysis. Clin Sci (Lond). 2001;100:387-93.
82. Cohn JN. New approaches to screening for vascular and cardiac risk. Am J Hypertens. 2001;14:2185-205.
83. Naidu MUR, Reddy BM, Yashmaina S, Patnaik N, Usha Rani P. Validity and reproducibility of arterial pulse wave velocity measurements using a new device with oscillometric technique: a pilot study. Biomed Eng On line. 2005;4:49.
84. Rema M, Mohan V, Deepa R. Association of carotid intima-media thickness and arterial stiffness with diabetic retinopathy. The Chennai Urban Epidemiology Study (CURES-2). Diabetes Care. 2004;27:1962-7.
85. Marinopoulos S, Berkenbilt S, Rami G, Brancati FL, Powe NR, Golden SH, et al. Meta-analysis: glycosylated hemoglobin and cardiovascular disease in diabetes mellitus. Ann Intern Med. 2004;21:421-31.
86. Ouvina SM, La Grecca RD, Zanaro NL, Palmer L, Sassetti B. Endothelial dysfunction, nitric oxide and platelet activation in hypersensitive and diabetic type-2 patients. Thromb Res. 2001;102:107-17.
87. Tretjakovs P, Kalnins U, Dabina I, Erglis A, Dinne I, Jurka A, et al. Nitric oxide production and arachidonic acid metabolism in platelet membranes of coronary heart disease patients with and without diabetes. Med Prin Pract. 2003;12:10-6.
88. Huszka M, Kaplar M, Rejto L. The association of reduce endothelium derived relaxing factor-NO production with endothelial damage and increased in vivo platelet activation in patients with diabetes mellitus. Thromb Res. 1997;86:173-80.
89. Pellegatta F, Folli F, Ronchi P, Caspani L, Galli L, Vicari AM. Deranged platelet calcium homeostasis in poorly controlled IDDM patients. Diabetes Care. 1993;16:178-83.
90. Schaeffer G, Wascher TC, Kostner GM, Graier WF. Alterations in platelet Ca^{2+} signaling in diabetic patients is due to increased formation of superoxide and reduced nitric oxide production. Diabetologia. 1999;42:167-76.
91. Fukuda K, Ozaki Y, Satoh K, Kume S, Tawata M, Onaya T, et al. Phosphorylation of myosin light chain in resting and platelets from NIDDM patients is enhanced: correlation with spontaneous aggregation. Diabetes. 1997;46:488-93.
92. Entman ML, Ballantyne CM. Inflammation and acute coronary syndromes. Circulation. 1993;88:800-3.
93. Telejko B, Zak J, Bachorzewska-Gajewska H, Nowak K, Nikołajuk A, Dobrzycki S, et al. Platelet-monocyte aggregate formation in patients with coronary artery disease and disorders of carbohydrate metabolism. Pol Arch Wewn. 2004;112:1067-73.

94. Hilberg T, Eicher E, Glaser D, Schmidt V, Gabriel HH. Platelet activity, reactivity and platelet-leucocyte conjugate formation before and after exhaustive or moderate exercise in patients with IDDM. Platelets. 2004;15:101-8.
95. Lim HS, Blann AD, Lip GY. Soluble CD40 ligand, soluble P-selectin interleukin-6, and tissue factor in diabetes mellitus: relationship to cardiovascular disease and risk factor intervention. Circulation. 2004;109:2524-8.
96. Gokulakrishnan K, Deepa R, Mohan V, Gross MD. Soluble P-selectin and CD40L levels in subjects with prediabetes, diabetes mellitus and metabolic syndrome—the Chennai Urban Epidemiology Study. Metabolism. 2006;55:237-42.
97. Ridker PM, Glynn RJ, Hennekens CH. C-reactive protein adds to the predictive value of total cholesterol in determining risk for first myocardial infraction. Circulation. 1998;97:2007-11.
98. Ridker PM. High sensitivity C-reactive protein potential adjunct for global risk assessment in the primary prevention of cardiovascular disease. Circulation. 2001;103:1813.
99. Rifai N, Ridker PM. High sensitivity C-reactive protein: a novel and promising marker of coronary artery disease. Clin Chem. 2001;47:403-11.
100. Mohan V, Deepa R, Vemurugan K. Association of C-reactive protein with body fat, diabetes and coronary artery disease in South Asians. The Chennai Urban Epidemiology Study (CURES-6). Diabetes Med. 2005;22:863-70.
101. Diamantopoulos EJ, Raptis SA, Moulopulous SD. Increased platelet activity in diabetic macroangiopathy. Horm Metab Res Suppl. 1992;26:95-102.
102. Chitre AP, Velaskar DS. Role of platelets in diabetic microangiopathy—an additional factor. Angiology. 1988;39:458-65.
103. Di Mino G, Cerbone AM, Irde C. The binding of fibrinogen to platelets in diabetes mellitus. Wien Klin Wochenschr. 1986;4:217-21.
104. Olson JA, Whitelaw CM, McHardy KS. Soluble leukocyte adhesion molecules in diabetic retinopathy stimulate retinal capillary endothelial migration. Diabetology. 1997;40:1166-71.
105. Evagrafov Vlu, Markova OA, Grishin VL. Changes in general hemostasis in patients with diabetic retinopathy. Vestn Oftalmol. 2004;120:29-31.
106. Lysenko VS, Mukha AL, Bunnin Ala, Fedorova NV. Thrombo-cytopathies and their role in the development of hemorrhagic syndrome in vascular diseases of the fundus oculi. Vestn Oftalmol. 2001;117:24-6
107. Malyszko J, Malyszko J, Musliwiee M. Blood platelet function, plasma serotonin and lipid metabolism in patients with diabetic nephropathy. Pol Arch Med Wewn. 1995;94:26-31.
108. Donaldson JV Jr, Listrup DM, Holley KE, Romero JC. Platelet-inhibitor treatment of diabetic nephropathy: a year prospective study. Mayo Clin Proc. 1988;81:3-15.
109. Omoto S, Nomura S, Shouzu A, Hayakawa T, Shimizu H, Miyake Y, et al. Significance of platelet-derived micro-particles and activated platelets in diabetic nephropathy. Nephron. 1999;81:271-7.
110. Toth L, Szenasi P, Varasanyi MN, Szilvási I, Lehoczky E, Kammerer L, et al. Elevated levels of plasma and urine beta thromboglobulin or thromboxane-B2 as markers of real platelet hyper-activation in diabetic nephropathy. Haemostasis. 1992;22:334-9.
111. Antiplatelet Trialists' Collaboration. Collaborative overview of randomized trials of antiplatelet therapy. 1: Prevention of death, myocardial infarction and stroke by prolonged antiplatelet therapy in various categories of patients. BMJ. 1994;308:81-106.
112. Rao GHR. Aspirin resistance: a fact or myth? Exp Clin Cardiol. 2005;10:17-20.
113. Watala C, Pluta J, Golanski H, Rozalski M, Czyz M, Trojanowski Z, et al. Increased glycation in diabetes mellitus associated with decreased aspirin-mediated protein acetylation and reduced sensitivity of blood platelets to aspirin. J Mol Med (Berl). 2005;83:148-58.
114. Angiolillo DJ, Fernandes-Ortiz A, Bernardo E, Ramírez C, Sabaté M, Jimenez-Quevedo P, et al. Platelet function profiles in patients with type-2 diabetes and coronary artery disease on combined aspirin and clopidogrel treatment. Diabetes. 2005;54:2430-5.

115. Colwell JA, Nesto RW. The platelet in diabetes: focus of ischemic events. Diabetes Care. 2003;26:2181-8.
116. Eibl N, Krugluger W, Strett G, Schrattbauer K, Hopmeier P, Schernthaner G. Improved metabolic control decreases platelet activation markers in patients with type-2 diabetes. Eur J Clin Invest. 2004;34:205-9.
117. Watala C, Golanki J, Plutta J, Boncler M, Rozalski M, Luzak B, et al. Reduced sensitivity of platelets from type-2 diabetes patients to acetylsalicylic acid (aspirin): its relation to metabolic control. Thromb Res. 2004;113:101-13.
118. Matsuno H, Tokuda H, Ishisaki A, Zhou Y, Kitajima Y, Kozawa O. P2Y12 receptors play a significant role in the development of platelet micro aggregation in patients with diabetes. J Clin Endocrinol Metab. 2005;90:920-7.
119. Shouzu A, Nomura S, Omoto S, Hayakawa T, Nishikawa M, Iwasaka T. Effect of ticlopidine on monocyte-derived micro particles and activated platelet markers in diabetes mellitus. Clin Appl Thromb Hemsot. 2004;10;167-73.
120. Wild S, Roglic G, Green A, Sicree R, King H. Global prevalence of Diabetes. Estimates for the year 2000 and projections for 2030. Diabetes Care. 2004;27:1047-53.
121. O'Keefe JH, Miles JM, Harris WH. Improving the adverse cardiovascular progress of type-2 diabetes. Mayo Clin Proc. 1999;74:171-80.
122. Pellegrini SM, Roncaglioni MC, Avanzini F. Primary prevention of cardiovascular event with low-dose aspirin and vitamin E in type-2 diabetic patients: results of the Primary Prevention Project (PPP) trial. Diabetes Care. 2003;26:3264-72.

Reprinted with permission from Jaypee Brothers Medical Publishers. Article published In: V Mohan, Rao GHR (Eds). Type-2 Diabetes in South Asians: Epidemiology, Risk Factors and Prevention. 2007. pp. 264-80.

Platelet Hyperfunction as a Risk Promoter for Acute Coronary Events

CHAPTER 13

INTRODUCTION

Rupture of the "vulnerable" atherosclerotic plaque seems to be the pivotal event in the development of acute coronary syndromes. However, the primary sequence of events responsible for sudden onset of intracoronary thrombosis causing acute coronary syndromes is at best speculative. Inflammations within the vulnerable coronary plaques seem to cause unstable angina by promoting rupture and erosion. Global risk assessment with cardiovascular risk factors has changed considerably over the years. Coronary artery disease (CAD) can be effectively predicted, by and large, using the evidence developed by the Framingham Heart Study. However, in the two large cohort studies done in Germany, the actual risk of CAD was overestimated by 100% when Framingham-based risk charts were used for risk prediction, suggesting the limitations of such applications. Risk factors commonly used in the predictions are age, sex, cholesterol, high-density lipoprotein (HDL), diabetes mellitus, and cigarette smoking. Although a beneficial effect of antiplatelet therapy has been demonstrated in over 400 clinical trials, hematological parameters have not been considered as major classical risk factors for CAD.

Studies from the Harvard Epidemiology group showed that significant deaths due to myocardial infarction (MI) occurred in early hours of the day. Furthermore, they also showed that circulating adrenaline levels and platelet activity were higher in the early hours of the day in patients with MI. In a separate study, beneficial effect of daily dose 160 mg of aspirin was demonstrated. In one of the major studies on the hormone replacement therapy (HRT), postmenopausal women were administered hormone therapy and various CAD risk were monitored for over 5 years. Although HRT significantly lowered all the risk factors studied, the end results were no different for HRT group compared to the control group, as far as the overall cardiovascular events were concerned. These studies did not evaluate any hematological parameters. Finally, the patients who receive mechanical heart valves are advised to take anticoagulant medications every day. However, significant numbers of these patients develop thromboembolic events, suggesting a critical role for platelets in precipitating these complications. Platelets play a critical role in the pathogenesis of thrombus formation, thromboembolic events, and may even serve as a source of circulating immune-reactive tissue factor. Summary of over 400 clinical trials have demonstrated that any antiplatelet drugs offers some degree of protection against cardiovascular events. It is therefore essential to thoroughly evaluate the risk associated with platelet hyperfunction in precipitating acute coronary events.

Risks of Platelet Hyperfunction

Atherosclerosis is a multifactorial disease, which leads to the narrowing and hardening of the arteries.[1-6] Thrombosis, another associated multifactorial disease, causes reduction and blockage of the flow of blood to the tissues causing ischemia and tissue injury.[7,8] Together these diseases of the cardiovascular system are the leading causes of morbidity and mortality in the industrialized nations.[9] A variety of risk factors contribute to the pathogenesis of these diseases. Some of the well-known risk factors include smoking, hypertension, diabetes, repeated injury of the vascular tissues, elevated levels of low-density lipoproteins (LDLs), low levels of HDLs, central abdominal obesity, and sedentary lifestyle.[10] Some of the newer emerging risk factors include increased levels of fibrinogen, elevation of circulating platelet-activating factor, increased stress, decreased levels of vitamin B_{12}, elevated blood phosphorous, C-reactive protein (CRP), increased transfatty acids in red blood cells (RBCs), platelet microparticles, tissue factor, platelet hyperfunction, and hypercoagulability. In spite of decades of research in this field, role of platelets in the initiation of infection, inflammation, vascular dysfunction, and atherosclerosis is not very well defined. In this chapter, an attempt is made to provide some evidence to support the hypothesis that platelets play a very significant role in the promotion of events leading to acute coronary events. Additional evidence is presented to show a correlation between platelet activation, stimulation of other circulating blood cells, and the process of inflammation.

PLATELET PHYSIOLOGY

Blood platelets interact with a variety of soluble agonists, such as epinephrine and adenosine diphosphate, many insoluble cell matrix components, including collagen, laminin, and biomaterials used for the construction of invasive medical devices.[11] These interactions stimulate specific receptors and glycoprotein-rich domains (integrins and nonintegrins) on the plasma membrane of platelets and lead to the activation of intracellular effector enzymes.[12] Majority of the regulatory events appear to require free calcium. Ionized calcium is the primary bioregulator, and a variety of biochemical mechanisms modulate the level and availability of free cytosolic calcium. Major enzymes that regulate the free cytosolic calcium levels via second messengers include phospholipase C, phospholipase A_2, and phospholipase D together with adenylyl and guanylyl cyclases. Activation of phospholipase C results in the hydrolysis of phosphatidyl inositol 4,5-bisphosphate and formation of second messengers 1,2-diacylglycerol and inositol 1,4,5-trisphosphate (IP_3). Diglyceride induces activation of protein kinase C, whereas IP_3 mobilizes cytosolic calcium from internal membrane stores.[13] Elevation of cytosolic calcium stimulates phospholipase A_2 and liberates arachidonic acid. Free arachidonic acid is transformed to a novel metabolite, thromboxane A_2 by fatty acid synthetase (Cox-1, cyclooxygenase). Thromboxane A_2 is the major metabolite of this pathway and plays a critical role in platelet recruitment, granule mobilization, and secretion. Secretory granules contain a variety of growth factors, mitogens, and inflammatory mediators. Secretion of granules promote P-selectin and CD40 expression on the platelet membrane. Furthermore, activation also promotes the expression of acidic lipids on the membrane and tissue factor expression, thus making these cells procoagulant. Fully activated platelets can modulate the function of other circulating blood cells, such as leukocytes, monocytes, macrophages, as well as vascular endothelial cells (ECs).[14] Agonist-mediated stimulation of platelets promotes the expression of an epitope on glycoprotein IIb/IIIa receptors. Activation of this receptor is essential for the binding of circulating fibrinogen. Fibrinogen forms a bridge between individual platelets and facilitates the thrombus formation. von Willebrand factor (vWF) binds platelet GPIbIX complex only at high shear rate unlike fibrinogen, which can bind platelets at low shear. Upregulation in signaling pathways will increase the risk for clinical complications associated with acute coronary events. Downregulation of signal transduction mechanisms may precipitate bleeding diathesis or stroke.

ACTIVATION OF CIRCULATING BLOOD CELLS AND INFLAMMATION

There is increasing evidence suggesting that the inflammatory mediators play a pathogenic role in the atherogenesis as well as in acute coronary syndromes.[14-16] Several recent studies suggest that inflammatory cytokines, such as tumor necrosis factor-α (TNF-α), interleukin (IL-1), and various chemokines (IL-8) may activate matrix metalloproteinases and induce degradation of connective tissue and promote apoptosis of cells in the atherosclerotic lesion, thus promoting plaques destabilization and rupture. There is considerable evidence to show that platelets contribute significantly to the pathogenesis of acute coronary syndromes by facilitating thrombus formation. They may also trigger acute coronary events by other mechanisms, including stimulation of an inflammatory response within the atherosclerotic plaque. They secrete a wide range of growth factors and inflammatory mediators.[17-19] In addition, they activate other cells, such as monocytes and macrophages and promote the expression of tissue necrosis factor and tissue factor. They also modulate the function of leucocytes and promote the expression of chemotactic and adhesive properties of ECs as well as IL-1 production in smooth muscle cells. Increased leucocyte–platelet aggregation has been demonstrated in acute MI and cerebral infarction. It has been shown that release of CC-chemokines RANTES by platelets triggers the arrest of monocytes on inflamed atherosclerotic endothelium.[20] Furthermore, in vulnerable plaque, significant amounts of tissue factor expression also have been demonstrated. It is clear from the available evidence that several platelet-derived factors both membrane bound (P-selectin, pCD40L) as wells soluble (S-selectin, sCD40L) are involved in the inflammatory response mediated by the activation of platelets, leucocytes, monocytes, macrophages, and ECs. Some studies have demonstrated the presence of platelet activation markers, such as P-selectin and CD40 in patients with MI. There is some evidence to suggest that overexpression of CD40L on platelets is correlated with the need for reangioplasty. Expression of this protein promotes the expression of adhesion molecules, chemokines and inflammatory cytokines, and recruitment of leucocyte within the vulnerable plaque. Levels of circulating markers of inflammation, CRP have been found to be higher in patients with unstable coronary syndromes.[21,22] Furthermore, according to Harvard researchers, persistent elevation of CRP in patients with unstable angina seems to be a good predictor of future coronary events, such as ischemia and MI.[22]

VASCULAR DYSFUNCTION

Functional and structural changes in the arterial wall precede the development of atherosclerosis, obstructive coronary artery disease, and may even serve as an early marker for the hypertensive disease.[23,24] Functional and structural changes of vascular ECs are modulated by a variety of thrombogenic factors as well as antithrombogenic factors.[24] Some of the vasoactive compounds released by the ECs include vasodilatory compounds, such as adenosine, prostacyclin and nitric oxide and vasoconstrictory molecules like cyclooxygenase-derived endothelium-dependent constriction factor (EDCF), hypoxia-induced endothelium-dependent constriction factor, and endothelin. Lipid peroxides, oxidized lipids, and lipoproteins promote the formation of vasoconstrictors by platelets. These lipid mediators inhibit enzymes that promote the formation of vasodilators by the healthy endothelium and lower endogenous production of vasodilators. Alterations in the balance between platelet-associated vasoconstrictors and EC-derived vasodilators result in the vascular dysfunction.[25-27] This is probably the earliest stage at which one can detect the manifestation of the arterial dysfunctions, hypertension, and atherosclerosis. Indeed, one can classify the risk according to the level of EC dysfunction and presence of additional CAD risk factors. One can use acetylcholine, L-arginine, nitric oxide synthetase inhibitor, LNNMA, and monitor the flow response in the forearm to determine the degree of EC dysfunction.[28-34] Alternatively, one can use CV Profilor (DO-2020, Hypertension Diagnostics, Eagan, MN) or Periscope (Genesis Medical Systems, Hyderabad, India) and monitor the pulse waveform of the small arteries.[24]

HORMONES, STRESS, AND ACUTE CORONARY EVENTS

Studies from our laboratory demonstrated the existence of such an imbalance in the production of these vasoactive compounds in cigarette smokers as well as users of oral contraceptives. In a separate study, in an animal model, we also demonstrated such an imbalance in the production of platelet-derived thromboxane and vascular prostacyclin in drug-induced diabetes.[35]

It is of interest to note that a variety of factors can initiate, promote, and precipitate acute coronary events. Harvard researchers have reported that heart attacks, stroke, angina, and sudden death occur close to 9 AM in the morning. The period from 6 AM to noon is also the time when various physiological processes that contribute to the sudden onset of coronary events also manifest.[36-39] Blood levels of adrenaline, platelet stickiness, levels of circulating vasoconstrictory compounds, arterial pressure contribute to plaque rupture, and coagulable state increases in the morning hours. Unstable angina and MI are precipitated by thrombus formation over a disrupted plaque. β-block and aspirin, which can diminish these physiological processes, have been shown to reduce or abolish the morning peak onset of MI. Physical and mental stress also seems to play a role in the onset of MI, stroke, and sudden death.

Classical example for stress-induced onset of cardiac death is the effect a major earthquake had on the citizens of Los Angeles (LA). Major earthquake occurred in this city on January 17, 1994. The data from State coroner's office shows that death due to cardiac events went up by 150% for that one single day compared to number of deaths that occurred on that date in previous years.[39,40] Over half of the deaths related to atherosclerosis on the day of the earthquake occurred between midnight and 6 AM, whereas, only 3 out of 32 of the deaths during the 7 days before the earthquake occurred at that time of the day. Similar increase in cardiac deaths due to fear and trauma has been recorded during LA riots and Gulf war. On a separate note, it is worthwhile to study the effect of stress on the development of CVD risk factors. In view of the fact due to the recent information technology revolution in India, more and more young individuals are exposed to highly demanding jobs as well as altered lifestyle.

Framingham study, initiated some 50 years ago, established for the first time significant risk associated with the elevated levels of blood cholesterol to the development of CAD.[41,42] Since that time many studies have demonstrated the increased risk for CAD with the increase in total blood cholesterol. In view of these findings over the years many lipid-lowering drugs have been developed and tested. National Cholesterol Education Program has been developed by the National Institutes of Health, United States, and appropriate guidelines have been established for the better management of risks associated with abnormal lipid metabolism. Indeed, Framingham risk assessment protocol as well as PROCOM risk assessment calculator uses the common risk factors for CAD for assessing the risk for coronary events. Although lipid abnormalities have been shown to increase the risk for CAD, their exact role in precipitating acute coronary events has not been demonstrated. Therefore, it is not clear as to whether or not lipid-lowering drugs offer full protection against CVD events.

Results of one of the clinical trials with high-risk patients provide partial answer to this question. Postmenopausal women have increased risk for developing heart disease and often results are fatal. Several studies are in progress to evaluate the beneficial effects or otherwise of HRT. Outcome of one of the multicenter placebo control studies [Heart and Estrogen/Progestin Replacement Therapy (HERS)] sheds some light on the importance of hematological parameters in the precipitation of acute coronary events.[43] HERS study was a randomized trial of estrogen and progestin for the secondary prevention of CAD in postmenopausal women (2,700, 4.1 years). Antihypertensive agents and lipid-lowering drugs were used as concomitant therapy. HRT significantly lowered serum lipids and associated CAD risk promoters. However, HRT did not lower the cardiovascular events associated with postmenopausal conditions. No studies were done on the hemostatic variables in this clinical study. The results of this study clearly suggest the importance of hemostatic variables in precipitating coronary events. In a randomized placebo-controlled 12-week study, it was found that there was a shift in the procoagulant–anticoagulant balance toward a procoagulant state following HRT.[44]

A separate study evaluating the beneficial effect of HRT on arterial compliance and endothelial dysfunction failed to demonstrate any such benefit in postmenopausal women.[45] Short-term HRT also has been shown to increase circulating activated platelets as measured by flow cytometry.[46] It is well known that activated platelets are procoagulant and promote the expression of tissue factor on other circulating blood cells. Another short-term study on HRT demonstrated increased CRP levels following short-term therapy. There is considerable evidence to suggest a role for activated platelets in mediating inflammatory response. Such inflammatory response can lead to the elevation of CRP in the circulation.[47] These observations suggest that just the management of the known classical risk promoters for CAD may not be sufficient to protect the postmenopausal women from the risk for future coronary events. It is important to look at the role of platelets, coagulation factors, and degree of inflammation in precipitating coronary events in these high-risk individuals.

THERAPEUTIC IMPLICATIONS

It is clear from the available evidence that platelets play a very important role in promoting the pathogenesis of inflammation, atherosclerosis, and acute coronary events.[14-16] The potential role played by the platelets in the initiation and propagation of this multifactorial disease process has several therapeutic implications. Platelet function inhibitors, such as aspirin, glycoprotein IIb/IIIa antagonists, and ADP receptor blockers (clopidogrel) are already in use in the treatment of acute coronary syndrome.[48]

ReoPro (abciximab) is a high-affinity binding antibody for the GP IIb/IIIa receptor. Binding is rapid and completed in minutes. It binds both nonactivated platelets and activated platelets. It does not activate platelets. It prevents binding of fibrinogen and vWF. EPIC trial, a multicenter (56 sites) randomized, double-blind placebo-controlled study evaluated the efficacy of infusion of this inhibitor in 2,099 patients undergoing high-risk balloon angioplasty or directional atherectomy.[49] Results demonstrated relative reduction in death or MI of 40% at 48 hours postprocedure, 37% after 30 days, and 31% after 6 months. Phase III trials of ReoPro, looking at the primary end point, death or MI at 30 days, showed 33% (EPIC), 50% (EPILOG), 29% (CAPTURE), and 51% (EPILSTENT) reduction in the occurrence of acute events in the treated group.[50-52] EPILOG trial evaluated the benefit of combined therapy with GPIIb/IIIa and low-dose heparin during percutaneous transluminal coronary angioplasty (PTCA). Combined therapy markedly reduced the risk of acute ischemic complications in patients undergoing PTCA without increasing the risk of hemorrhage. The results of the 4P Acute Coronary Syndrome Trials [PARAGOR (2,282), PRISM (5,231), PRISM Plus (1,570), PURSUIT (10,948)] demonstrated overall reduction in death or nonfatal MI in the treated group compared to the placebo control.[53-55] EPISTENT, a multicenter (63 sites) study evaluated the efficacy of abciximab, heparin, and ticlopidine in patients (2,399) undergoing coronary stent implantation.[52] Observations up to 6 months' postprocedure demonstrated a significant benefit with the use of abciximab during the PTCA. Use of a stent and the inhibitor further improved the benefit in patients undergoing PTCA. These results held good even at a 1-year follow-up period post PTCA. These observations clearly demonstrate the overall beneficial effect of GPIIb/IIIa inhibitors in a variety of high-risk interventional procedures.

Aspirin (acetyl salicylic acid) selectively acetylates the hydroxyl groups of a single serine residue (position 529) in the prostaglandin (PG) synthetase and causes irreversible inhibition of the activity of this enzyme. Single oral dose of 100 mg of aspirin can significantly inhibit the PG synthetase activity in circulating platelets. Since these cells lack DNA and the ability to resynthesize the enzyme, the dysfunction caused by aspirin cannot be overcome. Therefore, platelets exposed to aspirin lose the ability to make prostanoids completely. However, one should keep in mind that once the aspirin is hydrolyzed to salicylic acid, ability to inhibit PG synthesis is lost. Hence, the newly produced platelets from the bone marrow after the aspirin is hydrolyzed will have the active enzyme. Approximately 10% of fresh platelets are added on to the circulating blood every day. Furthermore, studies from our laboratory have demonstrated that aspirin-treated platelets respond to the agonists in a normal fashion after prior exposure to epinephrine.[48] Therefore, one should keep in mind that though aspirin is a potent antiplatelet drug, it does not offer full protection against platelet activation by multiple agonists.

There is considerable evidence to support the use of aspirin in the prevention of risk associated with unstable angina. However, in spite of the observed beneficial effects, the patients seem to develop MI. Therefore, there is considerable concern that the patients with CVD may have variable response to the action of aspirin. Of all the aspirin clinical trials, most convincing evidence on the beneficial effects of this drug comes from ISIS-2 trial.[56] In this study, 17,187 patients received streptokinase or oral aspirin (160 mg/day). Patients on aspirin alone had a highly significant reduction (23%) in mortality. The risk reduction for nonfatal MI was 49% and nonfatal stroke was 46%.

Antithrombotic Trialists' Collaboration (ATC) Group of the clinical service unit, Radcliffe Infirmary, Oxford, UK, reviewed over 400 randomized clinical trials assessing the benefit of antiplatelet treatment.[57] This large overview of clinical trials confirms that antiplatelet treatment reduces vascular events by about a quarter in high-risk patients. Nonfatal MI and stroke were reduced by one-third. Vascular deaths (from fatal MI and stroke) fell by one-sixth. In this heterogeneous group of patient's benefits were apparent irrespective of age, sex, blood pressure, or the presence of diabetes. Aspirin alone, at doses ranging from 75 to 325 mg, seems as effective as any other antiplatelet regimen, with little risk of adverse effects. ATC group reached the following conclusion based on their extensive review of the subject: antiplatelet therapy protects a wider range of patients at high risk for occlusive vascular disease than is currently treated routinely. It should be considered for almost all with suspected MI, unstable angina, or history of MI, angina, stroke, transient ischemic attack, arterial bypass surgery, or angioplasty. Medium dose of aspirin (75–325 mg/day) is the most widely tested antiplatelet regimen, and no other regimen appeared significantly effective at preventing MI, stroke, or death. We would like to mention that aspirin or clopidogrel may not offer the same beneficial effect in all the patients, as the response of platelets may vary considerably. Aspirin or clopidogrel inhibit only one of the many platelet activation pathways. Therefore, these drugs can only offer limited beneficial effect.

Potential beneficial effect of antiplatelet therapy in reducing cardiovascular events is well documented.[57] However, little is known about their effect on inflammation. Although, few reports suggest anti-inflammatory role for antithrombotic drugs as well as for statins, our knowledge in this area is considerably poor. It will be of importance to explore if antiplatelet drugs also have the potential to inhibit platelet-mediated inflammation, and if not, new and effective drugs should be developed. Recent studies have shown that a variety of bioactive molecules and inflammatory mediators play a key role in the platelet-mediated inflammation (P-selectin, S-selectin, CD4OL, sCD40L, and other chemokines).[14-16] Targeted treatment for the prevention of expression of these molecules such as tissue factor, CRP, and tissue necrosis factor may represent a novel approach in downregulation of inflammation mediated by activated blood cells and in the treatment of acute coronary events.

NEED FOR A POINT-OF-CARE ASSAY FOR MONITORING ANTIPLATELET AND ANTITHROMBOTIC THERAPIES

The Framingham studies instituted by National Institutes of Health in the 50s identified the major risk factors for the development of

CVD. Specific lipid-lowering drugs and a variety of blood pressure-lowering drugs were developed to better manage these CVD risk factors. Along with the use of these therapeutic modalities, the means to monitor risk factors after medical intervention was also developed. However, in spite of the fact that antiplatelet therapies are in use for longer than the statin therapy, no simple, specific, cost-effective assays are available for monitoring antiplatelet therapy.

The need for such an assay for monitoring antithrombotic therapies is greater in stroke patients. According to American Heart Association (AHA) update,[58] on an average every 45 seconds someone in the United States has a stroke. Of all strokes, 88% are ischemic and 9% are intracerebral hemorrhagic. Therefore, majority of stroke patients are on antiplatelet therapy. Drugs of choice for antiplatelet therapy are, aspirin, Plavix, or a combination of both. Since there is some concern that patients with CVD may have variable response to the action of aspirin, there is a tendency to recommend Plavix, combination of aspirin and Plavix, or Aggrenox (combination of aspirin and extended-release dipyridamole). In view of this, there is a great need to monitor the antiplatelet therapy in these patients, so that the therapy could be optimized to suit the individual requirement.

Several methods are available for monitoring platelet function. Hurlen et al. have used the method of Wu and Hoak to determine the platelet aggregate ratio as a marker of assessing platelet function.[59,60] Gum et al. have used aggregometry to evaluate aspirin sensitivity by monitoring platelet response to ADP and arachidonic acid.[61] They also used Platelet Function Analyzer (PFA-100 Dade International Inc, Miami), a method that measures platelet function to study their patient population. Malinin et al. used Ultegra RPFA-ASA (VerifyNow, Accumetrics, Inc San Diego, CA) to monitor the effect of single-dose aspirin (325 mg) in subjects with multiple risk factors.[62] In spite of the fact researchers are monitoring platelet function over five decades, there are no simple, specific, cost-effective assays available for monitoring antiplatelet therapies. However, we strongly feel that platelet aggregation studies will still provide valuable information to the clinicians on the status of platelet reactivity.

Studies in our laboratory over several decades using both optical and impedance aggregometry have failed to show any aspirin or clopidogrel resistance in normal healthy subjects.[63-65] Performing whole blood aggregometry is simple and results are reproducible. Whole blood is drawn into sterile plastic syringes using a butterfly needle (20 x G) and mixed with 3.2% sodium citrate (anticoagulant, 9:1 ratio). Platelet aggregation studies are performed with whole blood diluted 1:1 ratio with 0.9% saline. As in optical aggregometry with platelet-rich plasma, during whole blood aggregometry ATP secretion from the dense granules of platelets could be monitored by using firefly luciferin and luciferase reaction. Using arachidonic acid or ADP as agonists, one can monitor aspirin or clopidogrel resistance in patient populations, using whole blood aggregometry. Studies from our laboratory as well as that of others have demonstrated that whole blood aggregometry by impedance method is superior to optical method.[66,67]

According to AHA, every 3 minutes someone in the United States dies of a stroke. It is noteworthy that 8–12% of ischemic stroke and 37–38% of hemorrhagic stroke result in death of stroke patients within 30 days. It is therefore essential to monitor activation profiles of both platelet and coagulation pathways, so that better therapeutic protection could be provided to those with high risk for acute vascular events. In the absence of a point-of-care assay capable of monitoring both the mechanisms that promote thrombosis, whole blood aggregometry is a good choice for monitoring antiplatelet therapies.

CONCLUSION

In conclusion, South Asians have a very high incidence of CAD compared to any other ethnic group in the world. Elevated risk factors classically associated with CAD do not adequately explain the increased risk for CAD in patients with syndrome X or in South Asians. Although, there is heavy emphasis on the benefits of lipid-lowering drugs, evidence from some studies suggests that this approach may not provide the full protection to the high-risk populations. At present, no group has been identified and followed prospectively to establish a causal relationship between abnormalities of coagulation tests, levels of coagulation factors, or activity of platelets, infection, inflammation, and the presence of hyperthrombotic state.

Platelets play a very important role in hemostasis and thrombosis. Their role in the maintenance of hemostasis and their contribution to the promotion of thrombotic events is well documented. However, least is known about their modulating role in the initiation and promotion of a variety of events associated with vascular dysfunction, arterial stiffness, inflammation, atherosclerosis, and acute coronary events. Interventional procedures are costly and do not provide complete protection from future acute cardiovascular events. Prevention of the development of CAD risk is the only cure and is very cost-effective. In the South Asian countries, there is a great need for the development of cost-effective early diagnostic procedures capable of detecting the disease itself, better management of the identified risks for CVD and prevention. It is also important to develop new guidelines for CAD risk factors for this population, so that people with high risk can be identified and treated aggressively. We also should keep in mind that even a low-dose aspirin (75 mg/day) is as effective as any other antiplatelet treatment in significantly reducing the risk for acute coronary events.

REFERENCES

1. Harker LA, Ross R, Schlicter SJ, Scott CR. Homocystine induced atherosclerosis. The role of endothelial cell injury and platelet response in its genesis. J Clin Invest. 1976; 58:731–41.
2. McGill HC Jr. George Lyman Duff memorial lecture. Persistent problems in the pathogenesis of atherosclerosis. Arteriosclerosis. 1984;4:443-51.
3. Niewiarowski S, Rao AK. Contribution of thrombogenic factors to the pathogenesis of atherosclerosis. Prog Cardiovasc Dis. 1983;26:197-221.
4. Ross R, Glomset JA. The pathogenesis of atherosclerosis (first of two parts). N Engl J Med. 1976;295:369-77.
5. Ross R. The pathogenesis of atherosclerosis—an update. N Engl J Med. 1986;314:488-500.
6. Scharf RE, Harker LA. Thrombosis and atherosclerosis: regulatory role of interactions among blood components and endothelium. Blut. 1987;55:131-44.
7. Marcus AJ. Stratton lecture 1989. Thrombosis and inflammation as multicellular processes: pathophysiologic significance of transcellular metabolism. Blood. 1990;76:1903-7.
8. Nachman RL. Review: Stratton Lecture. Thrombosis and atherogenesis: molecular connections. Blood. 1992;79:1897-1906.
9. Rao GHR, White JG. Coronary artery disease: an overview of risk factors. Indian Heart J. 1993;45:143-53.
10. Rao GHR, Mohanty D, Rao ASC. Coronary artery disease: risk factors for Indian men and women. Indian J Hematol. 1997;15:3-7.

11. Rao GHR. Physiology of blood platelet activation. Indian J Physiol Pharmacol. 1993;37: 263-73.
12. Siess W. Molecular mechanisms of platelet activation. Physiol Rev. 1989;69:58-177.
13. Rana RS, Hokin LE. Role of phosphoinositides in transmembrane signaling. Physiol Rev. 1990;70:115-64.
14. Aukrust RJ, Waehre T, Damas JK, Gullestad L, Solum NO. Inflammatory role of platelets in acute coronary syndromes. Heart. 2001;86:605-7.
15. Robbie L, Libby P. Inflammation and atherothrombosis. Ann N Y Acad Sci. 2001;947: 167-79.
16. Shebuski RJ, Kilgore KS. Role of inflammatory mediators in thrombogenesis. J Pharmacol Exp Ther. 2002;300:729-35.
17. Brandt E, Ludwig A, Petersen F, Flad HD. Platelet-derived CXC chemokines: old players in new games. Immunol Rev. 2000;177: 204-16.
18. Clemetson KJ, Clemetson JM, Proudfoot AE, Power CA, Baggiolini M, Wells TN. Functional expression of CCR1, CCR3, CCR4, and CXCR4 chemokine receptors on human platelets. Blood. 2000;96:4046-54.
19. Garlichs CD Eskafi S, Raaz D, Schmidt A, Ludwig J, Herrmann M, et al. Patients with acute coronary syndromes express enhanced CD40 ligand/CD154 on platelets. Heart. 2001;86:649-55.
20. van Hunbdelshausen P, Weber KSC, Huo Y, Proudfoot AE, Nelson PJ, Ley K, et al. RANTES deposition by platelets triggers monocyte arrest on inflamed and atherosclerotic endothelium. Circulation. 2001;103:1772-7.
21. Zebrack JS, Mulhestein JH, Horne BD, Anderson JL; Intermountain Heart Collaboration Study Group. C-reactive protein and angiographic coronary artery disease: independent and additive predictors of risk in subjects with angina. J Am Coll Cardiol. 2002;39:632-7.
22. Rifai N, Ridker PM. High-sensitivity C-reactive protein: a novel and promising marker of coronary heart disease. Clin Chem. 2001;47: 403-11.
23. Ware JA, Heistad DD. Seminars in medicine of the Beth Israel Hospital, Boston. Platelet-endothelium interactions. N Engl J Med. 1993;328:628-35.
24. Cohn JN, Finkelstein J, McVeigh G, Morgan D, LeMay L, Robinson J, et al. Noninvasive pulse wave analysis for the early detection of vascular disease. Hypertension. 1995;26: 503-8.
25. Fitzerlad GA, Smith B, Pedersen AK, Brash AR. Increased prostacyclin biosynthesis in patients with severe atherosclerosis and platelet activation. N Engl J Med. 1984;310: 1065-8.
26. Panza JA, Quyyum AA, Brush JE, Epstein SE. Abnormal endothelium-dependent vascular relaxation in patients with essential hypertension. N Engl J Med. 1990;323:22-7.
27. Tesfamcrian B, Brown ML, Cohen RA. Elevated glucose impairs endothelium-dependent relaxation by activating protein kinase C. J Clin Invest. 1991;87:1643-8.
28. Freiman PC, Mitchell GG, Heistad DD, Armstrong ML, Harrison DG. Atherosclerosis impairs endothelium-dependent vascular relaxation to acetylcholine and thrombin in primates. Circ Res. 1986;58:783-9.
29. Kugiyama K, Kerns SA, Mowisett JD, Roberts R, Henry PD.. Impairment of endothelium-dependent arterial relaxation by lysolecithin in modified low-density lipoproteins. Nature. 1990;344:160-2.
30. Ludmer PL, Selwyn AP, Schook TL, Wayne RR, Mudge GH, Alexander RW, et al. Paradoxical vasoconstriction induced by acetylcholine in atherosclerotic coronary arteries. N Engl J Med. 1986;315:1046-51.
31. Golino P, Piscione F, Willerson JJ, Cappelli-Bigazzi M, Focaccio A, Villari B, et al. Divergent effects of serotonin on coronary-artery dimensions and blood flow in patients with coronary atherosclerosis and control patients. N Engl J Med. 1991;324:641-8.
32. Williams JK, Adam MR, Klopenstein HS. Estrogen modulates responses of atherosclerotic coronary arteries. Circulation. 1990;81:1680-7.
33. Drexler H, Zeiher AM, Meinzeer K, Just H. Correction of endothelial dysfunction in coronary microcirculation of hypercholesterolaemic patients by L-arginine. Lancet. 1991;338:1546-50.

34. Petros A, Bennet D, Vallance P. Effect of nitric oxide synthase inhibitors on hypotension in patients with septic shock. Lancet. 1991;338:1557-8.
35. Gerrard JM, Stuart MJ, Rao GHR, Steffes MW, Mauer SM, Brown DM, et al. Alteration in the balance of prostaglandin and thromboxane synthesis in diabetic rats. J Lab Clin Med. 1980;95:950-8.
36. Willich SN, MaClure M, Mittleman M, Arntz HR, Muller JE. Sudden cardiac death. Support for a role of triggering in causation. Circulation. 1993;87:1442-50.
37. Willich SN. Epidemiologic studies demonstrating increased morning incidence of sudden cardiac death. Am J Cardiol. 1990;66:15G-17G.
38. Willich SN, Klatt S, Arntz HR. Circadian variation and triggers of acute coronary syndromes. Eur Heart J. 1998;19:12-23.
39. Kloner RA, Leor J, Poole WK, Perritt R. Population-based analysis of the effect of the Northridge Earthquake on cardiac death in Los Angeles County, California. J Am Coll Cardiol. 1997;30:1174-80.
40. Leor J, Poole WK, Kloner RA. Sudden cardiac death triggered by an earthquake. N Engl J Med. 1996;334:413-9.
41. Anderson KM, Castchi WP, Levy D. Cholesterol and mortality. 30 years of follow-up from the Framingham study. JAMA. 1987;257:176-80.
42. McManus RJ, Mant S, Menlendijks CF, Salter RA, Pattison HM, Roalfe AK, et al. Comparison of estimates and calculations of risk of coronary heart disease by doctors and nurses using different calculation tools in general practice: cross sectional study. BMJ. 2002;324:459-64.
43. Hulley S, Grady D, Bush J, Furberg C, Herrington D, Riggs B, et al. Randomized trial of estrogen plus progestin for secondary prevention of coronary heart disease in postmenopausal women. Heart and Estrogen/progestin Replacement Study (HERS) Research Group. JAMA. 1998;280:605-13.
44. van Baal WM, Emeris JJ, van deer Mooren MJ. Impaired procoagulant-anticoagulant balance during hormone replacement therapy? A randomised, placebo-controlled 12-week study. Thromb Haemost. 2000;83:29-34.
45. Teede HJ, Liang YL, Kotsopailos D. placebo-controlled trial of long-term oral combined continuous hormone replacement therapy in postmenopausal women: effects on arterial compliance and endothelial function. Clin Endocrinol. 2001;55:673-82.
46. Thijs A, van Baal WM, vander Mooren MJ, Kenemans P, Dräger AM, Huijgens PC, et al. Effects of hormone replacement therapy on blood platelets. Eur J Clin Invest. 2002;32:613-8.
47. van Baal WM, Kenemans P, van der Mooren MJ, Kessel H, Emeis JJ, Stehouwer CD. Increased C-reactive protein levels during short-term hormone replacement therapy in healthy postmenopausal women. Thromb Haemost. 1999;81:925-8.
48. Rao GHR, Rao AT. Pharmacology of platelet activation-inhibitory drugs. Indian J. Physiol Pharmacol. 1994;38:69-84.
49. Lefkovits J, Blankenship JC, Anderson K, Stoner GL, Talley JD, Worley SJ, et al. Increased risk of non-Q wave myocardial infarction after directional atherectomy is platelet dependent: evidence from the EPIC trial. Evaluation of c7E3 for the Prevention of Ischemic Complications. J Am Coll Cardiol. 1996;28:849-55.
50. The EPILOG investigators. Platelet glycoprotein IIb/IIIa receptor blockade and low-dose heparin during percutaneous coronary revascularization. N Engl J Med. 1997;336: 1689-96.
51. The CAPTURE investigators. Randomised placebo-controlled trial of abciximab before and during coronary intervention in refractory unstable angina: the CAPTURE Study. Lancet. 1997;349:1429-35.
52. The EPISTENT investigators. Randomised placebo-controlled and balloon-angioplasty-controlled trial to assess safety of coronary stenting with use of platelet glycoprotein-IIb/IIIa blockade. Lancet. 1998;352:87-92.
53. The PRISM investigators. A comparison of aspirin plus tirofiban with aspirin plus heparin for unstable angina. N Engl J Med. 1998;338:1498-505.
54. The PRISM-Plus investigators. Inhibition of the platelet glycoprotein IIb/IIIa receptor with tirofiban in unstable angina and non-Q-wave myocardial infarction. N Engl J Med. 1998;338:1488-97.

55. Schulman SP, Goldschmidt-Clemont PJ, Topol EJ, Califf RM, Navetta FI, Willerson JT, et al. Effects of integrelin, a platelet glycoprotein IIb/IIIa receptor antagonist, in unstable angina. A randomized multicenter trial. Circulation. 1996;94:2083-9.
56. ISIS-2 (Second International Study of Infarct Survival) Collaborative Group. Lancet. 1988; 2(8607):349-60.
57. Antiplatelet Trialists' Collaboration. Secondary prevention of vascular disease by prolonged antiplatelet treatment. Antiplatelet Trialists' Collaboration. BMJ. 1998;296:320-31.
58. Heart Disease and Stroke Statistics-2006 Update. A report from the American Heart Association Statistics committee and Stroke Statistics Subcommittee. Circulation. 2006;113e85-e151. https://doi.org/10.1161/CIRCULATION.105.171600.
59. Hurlen M, Seijeflot I, Arnesen H. The effect of different antithrombotic regimens on platelet aggregation after myocardial infarction. Scand Cardiovasc J. 1998;32:233-7.
60. Wu KK, Hoak JC. A new method for the quantitative detection of platelet aggregates in patients with arterial insufficiency. Lancet. 1974;11:924-6.
61. Gum PA, Kottke-Marchnat K, Poggio ED, Gurm H, Welsh PA, Brooks L, et al. Profile and prevalence of aspirin resistance in patients with cardiovascular disease. Am J Cardiol. 2001;88:230-5.
62. Malinin A, Spergling M, Muhlestein B, Steinhubl S, Serebruany V. Assessing aspirin responsiveness in subjects with multiple risk factors for vascular disease with a rapid platelet function analyzer. Blood Coagul Fibrinolysis. 2004;1:295-301.
63. Rao GHR. Aspirin resistance: a fact or a myth? Exp Clin Cardiol. 2005;10:17-20.
64. Rao GHR. Need for a noninvasive diagnostic platform for early detection and management of cardiometabolic disorders. World Heart J. 2006;1:63-78.
65. Rao GHR, Michiels JJ. Aspirin resistance: does it exist? Semin Thromb Hemost. 2007;33:210-4.
66. Dyszkiewicz-Korpanty AM, Frenkel EP, Sarode R. Approach to the assessment of platelet function: comparison between optical-based platelet-rich plasma and impedance-based whole blood platelet aggregation methods. Clin Appl Thromb Hemost. 2005;11:25-35.
67. Ivandic BT, Schilick P, Saritz P, Kurz K, Katus HA, Giannitsis E. Determination of clopidogrel resistance by whole blood platelet aggregometry and inhibitors of the P2Y12 receptor. Clin Chem. 2006;52:383-8.

Reprinted with permission from Jaypee Brothers Medical Publishers. Article published In: Rao GHR, Thanikachalam S. Coronary Artery Disease: Risk Promoters, Pathophysiology, and Prevention. 2005. pp. 192-201.

CHAPTER 14

Epinephrine-induced Platelet Membrane Modulation

INTRODUCTION

Studies at the University of Minnesota in the early 70s discovered a phenomenon called "platelet membrane modulation" that demonstrated the ability of epinephrine to restore the sensitivity of refractory platelets to the action of agonists.[1-79] These studies became a part of the National Institutes of Health (NIH)-funded investigation in the 80s. In this chapter, we will describe how this mechanism of membrane modulation was discovered and its role and significance in the pathophysiology of platelet function.

MECHANISM OF MEMBRANE MODULATION

In this paragraph, we have described the studies we proposed to the National Institutes of Health, USA, to obtain funds for our ongoing studies on the mechanisms of platelet membrane modulation. Recent investigations in this laboratory have established existence of a novel mechanism capable of securing irreversible platelet aggregation independent of adenosine diphosphate (ADP) secretion, prostaglandin synthesis, or the generation of platelet-activating factor (PAF). The new mechanism, termed membrane modulation, is associated with the platelet surface, mediated through α-adrenergic receptors and stimulated by exposure to epinephrine. Platelets rendered refractory to a variety of aggregating agents can be restored to a normal state of sensitivity through activation of the mechanism of membrane modulation. This includes platelets treated with aspirin in vivo or in vitro, and the aspirin-treated platelet will serve as a principal model for the studies to be carried out during this investigation. The purpose of this proposal is to explore and define the mechanism of platelet membrane modulation in detail. It is possible that generation of products of the lipoxygenase pathway in aspirin-treated platelets, elevation of endogenous levels of cyclic guanosine monophosphate (cGMP), exposure of fibrinogen receptors, mobilization of calcium, phosphorylation of membrane-associated proteins, or reduction of heme proteins may underlie the epinephrine-induced activation of membrane modulation and correction of membrane sensitivity in aspirin-treated cells. Appropriate biochemical, physiological, and morphological methods will be used to study each of these possibilities in detail. Accomplishment of these specific aims will reveal the fundamental mechanisms underlying the platelet modulation. The ability to gain pharmacological control of this newly discovered mechanism regulating platelet membrane activation and capable of securing irreversible aggregation of refractory cells in the absence of prostaglandin synthesis or ADP secretion may provide a new approach to the management and prevention of thrombotic disease (1985–1987).

In our Thrombosis Research Laboratory at the University of Minnesota, during the early 70s, we were evaluating platelet function using a variety of animal models.[5,7-10] The reason why we were interested in testing the function of animal platelets was because of the extensive use of animal models in the device development industry. At the Hershey laboratories in Pennsylvania, cows are used as model for the development of implantable medical devices. Whereas, at the Utah Heart Research Institute, preferred animal model was horses. Several other laboratories use sheep and goats as preferred animal models. In our own experimental surgery laboratories, dogs, pigs, piglets, and primates are used for experimental surgery. Canadian researchers extensively use rabbit platelets for studies. Studies at our laboratory for the first time demonstrated that there was considerable difference in the response of animal platelets to common platelet agonists.

Since dogs were preferred animal models for various studies at the nationally and internationally recognized division of experimental surgery, at the University of Minnesota, we decided to study the function of dog platelets first. To our surprise, we found that whenever we tried to obtain the platelets from the whole blood obtained from the animals at the "Dog Labs," blood had very low number of platelets or none at all. To understand the significance of this finding, we explored how our colleague Prof Gerhard Johnson and associates were doing their studies on dog platelets at the Veterans Administration Hospital, Minneapolis, Minnesota.[7-10] We found out that the dogs used in their laboratory were conditioned to the laboratory environment and were not excited too much when the blood was drawn from them. On the other hand, at the University of Minnesota, where dozens of dogs are kept in individual cages under one roof, all dogs get excited when any one enters the facility and start barking like crazy. In view of this behavior, we assumed that due to the increased in vivo adrenaline rush generated by excitation, the platelets in circulation become sticky and get sequestered. This observation demonstrated the role of (excitation related) adrenaline for the first time in initiating platelet stickiness.

We also found out during these early attempts in our studies on dog platelets that not all dogs respond the same way to the action of various agonists.[7] The platelet-rich plasma (PRP) from most dogs aggregates in response to ADP, collagen, and thrombin. Dog PRP generally does not aggregate in response to epinephrine, and previous studies found that dog PRP uniformly failed to aggregate when exposed to arachidonic acid (AA) prepared (as arachidonate) in an ethanol–sodium carbonate medium. Our studies demonstrated that 30% of randomly selected mongrel dogs have PRP, which aggregates when exposed to sodium arachidonate dissolved in modified Tyrode buffer, PRP from these dogs also aggregates with lower concentrations of ADP and collagen than PRP, which is unresponsive to arachidonate. Dog PRP, which aggregates with arachidonate releases ^{14}C-serotonin, while nonaggregating PRP does not. However, arachidonate stimulates malondialdehyde production in both aggregating and nonaggregating PRP, suggesting that cyclooxygenase pathway is intact in both the types of dog platelets. In view of the fact that our earlier studies on dog platelets led us to believe that somehow epinephrine was responsible for the sequestration of platelets in dogs that were excited or agitated, we tried the influence of epinephrine on arachidonate-nonresponsive dog platelets.

We found that preincubation of PRP from AA-nonresponsive dogs with epinephrine

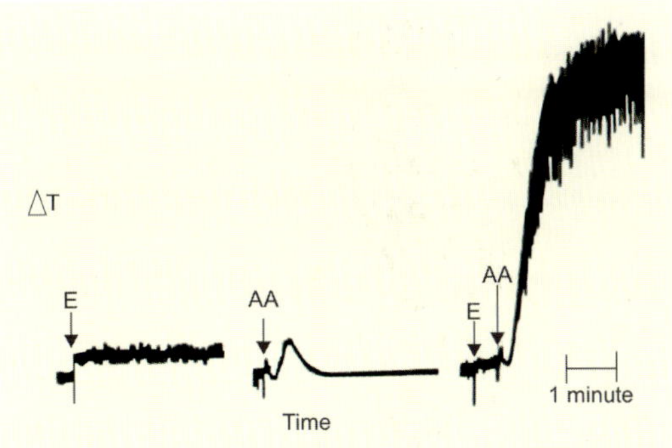

Fig. 14.1: Response of arachidonic acid (AA)—nonresponsive dog platelets to epinephrine and arachidonate. Restoration of response to arachidonate by epinephrine (ΔT: Change in light transmission; E: Epinephrine).

uniformly transformed PRP, which does not aggregate on exposure to arachidonate alone into arachidonate-aggregating PRP (Fig. 14.1). Whereas AA-responsive dog PRP, which aggregates with arachidonate, releases ^{14}C-serotonin while nonaggregating PRP does not.

The results of these studies indicate that dog platelets are heterogeneous in regard to their aggregation response to arachidonate. The mechanism of this heterogeneity is unknown; however, since prostaglandin metabolism is intact and the platelets of some dogs respond to arachidonate alone, it appears to be the result of variable sensitivity to endoperoxides and thromboxane A_2 (TXA_2). Most dogs, mongrel, or purpose-bred have platelets that form TXA_2, but fail to aggregate irreversibly or to secrete granule contents in response to the TXA_2 formed.[80-85] These TXA_2 insensitive platelets also fail to aggregate irreversibly or to secrete in response to TXA_2 analogs such as U46619 or I-BOP. However, some mongrel dogs have TXA_2-sensitive platelets that aggregate and secrete in response to the endogenous TXA_2 formed as do human platelets. Each dog's response to TXA_2 is consistent and genetically defined.[80] Although dog platelets that aggregate with arachidonate alone are generally more responsive to other aggregating agents, normal aggregation with ADP and collagen has been observed in dog platelets that are unresponsive to arachidonate. This unresponsiveness is not due to any detectable defect in the arachidonate pathway of platelet prostaglandin metabolism, since both aggregating and nonaggregating platelets of dogs synthesize TXA_2 in normal quantities.[80] Micromolar quantities of epinephrine uniformly convert arachidonate-insensitive platelets (AIP) into arachidonate-sensitive platelets (ASP), despite the fact that epinephrine at that concentration failed to induce aggregation in the dog platelets. These studies on dog platelets, serendipitously, introduced us to a newly discovered phenomenon, which for the lack of a better term, we called "membrane modulation."

One of the principal mechanisms regulating platelet signal transduction mechanisms is linked to cyclic nucleotide metabolism [cyclic adenosine monophosphate (cAMP)/cGMP), and the endogenous level of adenosine 3′-5′-monophosphate (cAMP), which plays an important role in cytosolic calcium modulation and regulation of the platelet response to aggregating agents. Substances that elevate cAMP by and large inhibit platelet aggregation, and agents that lower cAMP enhance platelet aggregation. Since epinephrine lowers previously elevated platelet cAMP and uniformly converts AIP to ASP, we postulated that AIP might differ from ASP in regard to the mechanisms that control or modulate cAMP levels. However, AIP appear to have cAMP-dependent mechanisms that modulate their responsiveness to products of prostaglandin metabolism. Prostacyclin (PGI_2), the most potent naturally occurring inhibitor of human and dog platelet aggregation, may play an important role in inhibiting platelet aggregation in vivo by elevating platelet cAMP. We observed that low concentrations of PGI_2 in vitro converted ASP to AIP. We also observed that the effects of PGI_2 on dog platelets are relatively longlasting and that ASP recovered from PGI_2 inhibition of ADP induced aggregation more rapidly than AIP.

Prostacyclin is the major metabolite formed from the AA metabolism following stimulation of prostaglandin synthesis in blood vessels. Despite its lability, it is a powerful vasodilator and potent inhibitor of blood platelet function. It stimulates adenylyl cyclase, elevates endogenous levels of cAMP, and blocks the response of platelets to aggregating agents. In view of our earlier observations on the role of cyclic nucleotides in modulating platelet function in dog platelets, we explored further the role of prostacyclin on dissociation of human platelet aggregates and the ability of epinephrine to restore the function of drug-induced refractory platelets. Dissociation of ADP aggregates was concentration dependent, caused complete disappearance of platelet clumps, and restored platelet discoid form.[12] The dispersed platelets were refractory to further stimulation by ADP, thrombin, arachidonate, or the calcium ionophore A23187. Measurement of cAMP revealed no detectable change in the levels after ADP-mediated aggregation, but showed a rapid increase in the levels following addition of PGI_2. Reduction of high levels of cAMP by addition of epinephrine did not result in aggregation of platelets. However, epinephrine addition to refractory platelets restored in large measure their sensitivity to aggregation by arachidonate, thrombin, ADP, and A23187.

The shape changes and aggregation of washed platelets induced by AA can be reversed by prostacyclin, but these platelets can be reactivated by treatment with epinephrine and arachidonate. These events may be modulated by cAMP since 2 mM dibutyryl cAMP also reversed activation without reactivation by epinephrine and AA. We examined protein phosphorylation and formation of cytoskeletal cores resistant to 1% triton X-100 extraction of these platelets and correlated these processes with aggregation, fibrinogen binding, and changes in ultrastructure.[30] Unactivated platelet cores contained 15% of total actin and no detectable myosin or actin-binding proteins. AA-induced cytoskeletal cores, which contained 60–80% of the total actin myosin and actin-binding protein as the major components were disassembled back to unactivated levels by PGI_2 and then fully assembled by epinephrine and AA. Phosphorylation of myosin light chain (MLC) and a 40,000 Da protein triggered by AA (two- to five-fold) was reversed to basal levels by PGI_2 but was completely reversed to peak levels upon addition of the epinephrine and AA mixture. The reversibility of actin-binding protein phosphorylation could not be established. With this possible exception, cytoskeletal assembly with associated protein phosphorylation, aggregation, fibrinogen binding, and changes in ultrastructure triggered by activation are readily and concertedly recyclable (Fig. 14.2).

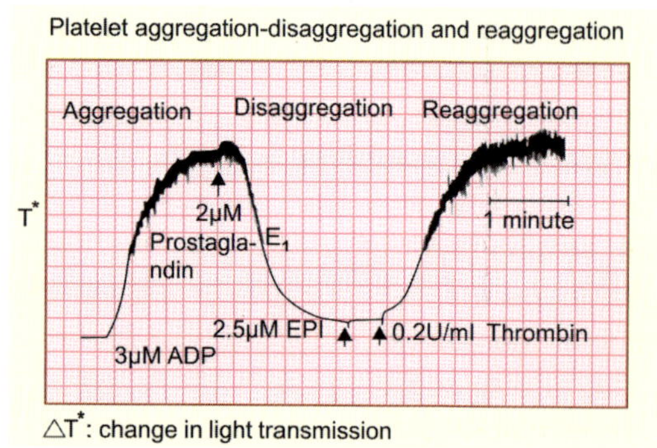

Fig. 14.2: Dissociation of adenosine diphosphate (ADP)-induced aggregates of platelets by PGE_1. Restoration of aggregation response to thrombin by epinephrine exposure of refractory platelets.

Now that we had discovered a way to disassociate aggregated platelets and reaggregate them by exposing to epinephrine and challenging them with addition of other agonists, we used this in vitro assay system to further evaluate and characterize the inhibitory effects of potentially effective antiplatelet drugs. Agents that elevate intracellular levels of cAMP were potent inducers of platelet dissociation in aggregates caused by ADP. On the other hand, antimalarials, calmodulin complexing agents, and phospholipase inhibitors caused dissociation of platelet aggregates irrespective of agonist used to cause aggregation.[12,16,32,52] By and large, the dissociated cells were refractory to the action of agonists. Restoration of the sensitivity of disaggregated platelets by treatment with epinephrine demonstrated the ability of inhibitor-treated refractory platelets to recover fully functional capacity almost immediately. A major finding of these studies is the fact that epinephrine-induced membrane modulation could restore the functional state of the platelet membrane in the majority of antiplatelet drug-induced refractory situations (Fig. 14.3). By and large, exposure of platelets to antagonists caused the refractory state. However, depending on the dosage inhibitory effect of some of the antagonists could be reversed. For instance, the inhibitory effect of adenylate cyclase stimulators such as PGE_1, PGI_2, PGD_2, and forskolin could be reversed by epinephrine. In this series of studies, we demonstrated that epinephrine-induced membrane modulation restored the functional state of the platelet membrane, irrespective of the drug used for disassociating agonist-induced preformed platelet aggregates.

Now that we had demonstrated the ability of epinephrine-induced membrane modulation, it was time to test whether it would also work in platelets of patients who are on aspirin

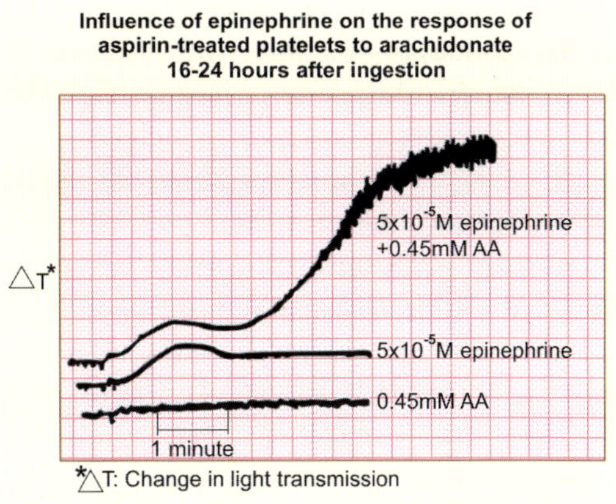

Fig. 14.3: Response of in vivo aspirin-exposed platelets to in vitro action by epinephrine and arachidonic acid (AA). Restoration of platelet response to AA by epinephrine.

prophylaxis. In order to mimic this condition, we used volunteers who took 600 mg of aspirin. We used three groups of volunteers in these studies. All volunteers took 600 mg of aspirin for these studies.[11] The blood was drawn for these studies from the first group, 2 hours after they took aspirin. In the second group, the blood was drawn 24 hours after they took aspirin. In the third group (representing individuals under aspirin prophylaxis), the blood was drawn after they had taken a daily dose of 600 mg aspirin for several weeks. In these studies, addition of epinephrine did not restore the sensitivity of platelets to the action of arachidonate in samples that were exposed to in vitro aspirin or the platelets obtained from volunteers who had taken aspirin 2 hours before the experiment. However, sample of PRP from donors 10–16 hours after aspirin ingestion as well as those whose platelets were exposed for longer periods developed irreversible aggregation when exposed to epinephrine followed by sodium arachidonate. Platelets from individuals who had taken aspirin 10–16 hours before were unable to metabolize ^{14}C-AA and exposure to epinephrine did not improve their ability to synthesize endoperoxides or thromboxanes, suggesting that epinephrine-induced restoration of platelet response to arachidonate did not need the mediation of newly synthesized endoperoxides or thromboxanes.

Several individuals, families, and under different clinical symptoms of hemorrhage and thrombotic conditions seem to have altered in vivo eicosanoid metabolism or impaired in vivo prostaglandin synthesis.[23] During our routine studies, we discovered an individual who had no history of bleeding, whose platelets lacked cyclooxygenase activity. Since we had demonstrated the ability of epinephrine-induced membrane modulation to restore the sensitivity of aspirin-treated platelets to the action of arachidonate, we evaluated the influence of epinephrine on the response of her platelets to sodium arachidonate-induced aggregation and secretion (Fig. 14.4). The results of our studies demonstrated that even though her platelets were unable to convert AA into endoperoxides and thromboxanes, they were able to undergo irreversible aggregation in response to AA and other agents when pretreated with epinephrine.

The fact that adrenaline can override the effect of aspirin and restore the response of platelets to the action of arachidonate prompted us to do some additional studies on aspirin and its effect both in human platelets and in animal models. At the time we were doing these studies, one of the groups published an article indicating that aspirin has no inhibitory effect on bovine platelets. After some preliminary investigations, we demonstrated that in ruminants the oral aspirin had no inhibitory effect as it was hydrolyzed to its inactive form (salicylic acid) in the stomach before it reached the circulation. We showed if aspirin was administered

Influence of epinephrine on the response of cyclo-oxygenase deficient platelets to arachidonate

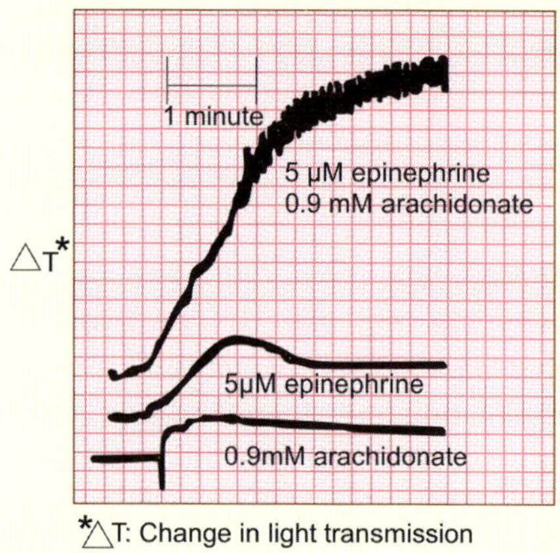

Fig. 14.4: Platelets of patient with cyclooxygenase deficiency did not respond with aggregation when stirred with arachidonate. Similarly, they did not respond to the action of epinephrine. However, when they were pretreated with epinephrine, they responded with irreversible aggregation to the action of arachidonate.

as suppository through anal route, it was equally effective in inhibiting cyclooxygenase in bovine platelets.[57] We also followed in vivo aspirin metabolism in both dogs and in human volunteers.[13,14,24]

A single oral dose of aspirin in human subjects inhibits the aggregation response of platelets to arachidonate and other weak agonists for approximately 1 week after ingestion. In a series of studies in our laboratory, we evaluated the rate at which cyclooxygenase active platelets return to the circulation in humans and dogs and compared the response curves obtained to arachidonate stimulation of aspirin-exposed platelets to assess the recovery of cyclooxygenase activity.[24] Studies on dogs were done as collaborative studies, at the VA Hospital, Minneapolis, Minnesota, with Prof Gerhard Johnson's research group. After a single dose of aspirin, dog platelet function was compromised for several days. Normal responses to AA and other agonists were normal by 6 days. However, cyclooxygenase active platelets returned to the circulation in the dogs more rapidly than in humans. More rapid return of competent cells in the dogs probably relates to the more rapid turnover and shorter half-life span of canine platelets. It was of interest to note that even though sufficient number of cyclooxygenase active platelets had returned to the circulation, they were refractory to the action of agonists. In vitro studies showed that addition of 10% of normal platelets to aspirin-treated platelets was sufficient to restore the response of aspirin-exposed platelets to the action of arachidonate.

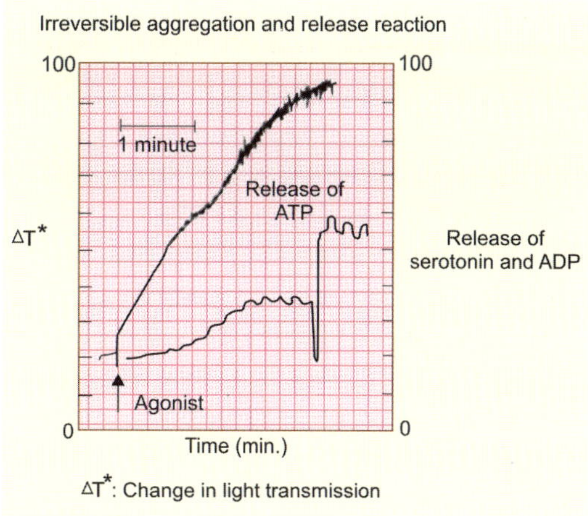

Fig. 14.5: Irreversible aggregation with primary and secondary waves and release of ATP. (ADP: Adenosine diphosphate; ATP: adenosine triphosphate).

Weak agonists or threshold concentrations of potent agonists cause two distinct phases of aggregation when added to stirred samples of citrated platelet-rich plasma. The second wave is irreversible and develops before the primary reversible wave dissipates completely.

Second wave of aggregation is temporally related to onset of the platelet release reaction and has been considered to be dependent on the action of secreted products such as ADP, serotonin, and other storage granule contents (Fig. 14.5). Aspirin treatment, for example, acetylates cyclooxygenase, prevents endoperoxide and thromboxane synthesis and blocks the release of granule contents and abolishes second wave aggregation response. Also, platelets of patients with storage pool deficiency fail to develop second waves of aggregation when stimulated by threshold concentrations of aggregating agents. We also demonstrated that the products of prostaglandin synthesis formed by storage pool-deficient platelets could cause the release of granule contents from aspirin-treated platelets resulting complete normal second waves of irreversible aggregation in mixtures of two cell populations stirred with epinephrine or collagen, even though neither population of cells alone will develop a second wave aggregation with the same concentrations of agonists.

Human platelets do not demonstrate the variation in sensitivity to arachidonate as revealed by dog platelets. However, exposure to small quantities of agonists that stimulate adenylyl cyclase at concentrations that were too low to elevate cAMP converted human platelets to AA-insensitive platelets (similar to AA-insensitive dog platelets). Exposure of these AA-refractory platelets to concentrations of epinephrine too low to cause aggregation restored the ability of these refractory platelets to aggregate irreversibly when stirred with arachidonate. Thus, the mechanism of membrane modulation detected first time in canine platelets was present in human platelets also.[12,19] This mechanism was further demonstrated in studies with aspirin-treated platelets. By using α-adrenergic receptor blockers, we demonstrated that epinephrine-mediated membrane modulation was dependent on α-adrenergic receptor stimulation. Studies with storage pool-deficient platelets, cyclooxygenase-deficient platelets, and aspirin-treated platelets demonstrated that the intrinsic mechanism of membrane modulation appears capable of promoting irreversible aggregation in the absence of secretion and prostaglandin synthesis.[20,31]

In view of the fact that our studies demonstrated that the mechanism of platelet membrane modulation was dependent on α-adrenergic receptor function, we explored the significance and nature of this dependency. Since this mechanism seems to be critical for the restoration of the sensitivity of refractory platelets to the action of a variety of agonists, any impairment of α-adrenergic function will, therefore, interfere with the mechanism of membrane modulation. Phospholipase A_2 has been shown to modulate α-adrenergic receptor function in rat cortical membranes and in human platelet membranes.[45] We followed the effect of commercially available phospholipases (PLAs) on ligand binding to platelet and on regulation and coupling of physiological functions via membrane modulation. Platelets exposed to the PLAs responded with normal aggregation when stimulated by common agonists. However, the treatment abolished the second wave aggregation response in response to epinephrine. Proteases and PLAs have been shown to inactivate yohimbine binding sites (adrenergic receptors) on human platelet membranes suggesting that these enzymes specifically attack α_2-adrenergic receptor domains.

There are conflicting reports as to the number of α-adrenergic receptors on platelet membranes and their functional status. For instance, platelets from patients with Hermansky–Pudlak syndrome, and myeloproliferative disorders respond poorly to epinephrine stimulation. However, these epinephrine refractory platelets still maintain their α-adrenergic receptor function as evidenced by our studies on epinephrine-mediated restoration of function in these platelets. Although PLA-treated platelets did not develop second wave response to the action of epinephrine, the potentiating influence of adrenaline could be demonstrated in these platelets, suggesting that the mechanism involved in restoration of membrane sensitivity to the action of agonists in refractory platelets was conserved in PLA-treated platelets. This is a very significant finding because adrenalin-induced membrane modulation may be the only salvage mechanism available for restoration of membrane sensitivity to the action of agonists in platelets with compromised function.

To explore further the mechanism of membrane modulation, we used Quni-2, a calcium fluorophores to probe calcium-dependent and calcium-independent events that underlie the mechanism of membrane modulation. Quin-2 causes a significant compromise in the calcium-dependent signal transduction mechanisms including phospholipase C–mediated turnover of phosphoinositides, increases in cytosolic calcium levels, MLC phosphorylation, PLA_2 activation and release of AA, endoperoxide and thromboxane formation, contraction, and secretion of granule contents.[36,52] However, Quin-2 failed to inhibit epinephrine-induced membrane modulation. Platelets made refractory by Quin-2 loading upon exposure to epinephrine and arachidonate aggregated irreversibly, suggesting that these biochemical events requiring cytosolic calcium are not required for the development of stickiness and irreversible aggregation.

What is the real clinical significance of this finding? Studies from our laboratory using both animal models and human subjects demonstrated the existence of an intrinsic mechanism, termed membrane modulation, capable of securing irreversible aggregation of platelets that were made refractory by exposing them to antiplatelet drugs. The newly discovered mechanism was α-adrenergic receptor–mediated membrane calcium-dependent and not dependent on cytosolic calcium. In view of these observations, we felt that individuals on antiplatelet therapy may not be well protected in situations where circulating levels of catecholamines are increased. Several studies have demonstrated that noradrenaline levels are increased manyfold higher than adrenaline during stress, exercise, age hypertension, congestive heart failure, angina, and trauma. Therefore, we evaluated the ability of noradrenaline (NA) to mediate membrane modulation and restore function of drug-induced refractory platelets.[52]

Aspirin-exposed platelets were obtained for these studies from volunteers who had ingested 80 mg of aspirin. PGE_1-exposed platelets were obtained after dissociation of ADP aggregates by PGE_1. Low calcium platelets were obtained by using Quni-2 to buffer cytosolic calcium.[52] Drug-exposed platelets did not aggregate irreversibly when stirred with arachidonate or noradrenaline (NA) alone. However, when treated with NA first, drug-exposed refractory platelets regained their sensitivity to the action of arachidonate and aggregated irreversibly. The ability of NA to restore the sensitivity of drug-induced refractory platelets was effectively blocked by yohimbine, an α-adrenergic antagonist.

Despite the universal use of aspirin as a potent antiplatelet drug, it has not been shown to be a universally effective antithrombotic agent. Investigations in our laboratory have shown that some effects of aspirin on platelet function can be reversed in vitro as well as in vivo through a mechanism, which we have described in our earlier studies as membrane modulation. Platelets made refractory to aggregating agents by exposure to aspirin in vitro or in vivo regain their sensitivity and ability to undergo irreversible aggregation on exposure to epinephrine. Various studies in our laboratory have shown that this salvage mechanism does not depend on reversing the effects of aspirin on cyclooxygenase. Restoration of the sensitivity to agonists does not depend on secreted components of granule contents or prostaglandin synthesis. In other words, restoration of function of refractory platelets is independent of inositol phosphatide metabolism, second messenger generation, increase in phospholipase activity, elevation of cytosolic calcium, release of arachidonic acid, prostaglandin synthesis, contraction, and secretion of granule contents. These observations prompted us to examine whether a similar mechanism exists in vivo, which might reverse the effects of aspirin on platelet vessel wall interactions.

We used a well-established method called Baumgartner techniques for testing aspirin effect on vessel wall interactions. Freshly obtained human blood was used for these studies. The effect of aspirin on the interaction of platelets with exposed subendothelium of perfused segments of rabbit aorta has been evaluated in many laboratories. Aspirin does not interfere with contact or subsequent spreading of platelets on the denuded vascular surface. In fact, as others have shown, aspirin pretreatment appears to increase the amount of vascular surface covered by platelets. Aspirin does, however, interfere with platelet–platelet interaction as manifested by the reduction in the number of thrombi present compared to controls.[37] The effect of epinephrine was striking. Pretreatment of platelets with epinephrine before combining with washed red cells to make reconstituted blood reversed the effect of aspirin. The number of platelet thrombi observed on denuded vessel surface was essentially identical to controls. Under various situations due to trauma or emotional strain, endogenous epinephrine or non-epinephrine may increase in the circulating blood. In such situations, newly introduced hormones may be able to reverse the influence of aspirin and neutralize the beneficial or prophylactic effect of antiplatelet therapies.

Based on our observations, we reported in the Lancet (1988) that aspirin ingestion does not totally inhibit platelet function, and inhibition can be reversed by adrenaline-induced α-adrenergic receptor modulation.[44] Using animal models, we also demonstrated that acute platelet thrombi form periodically in stenosed dog and pig coronary arteries and in stenosed rabbit carotid arteries, and the periodic thrombus formation could be abolished with aspirin 5 mg/kg given intravenously.[44,86-90] However, in 75% of the animals, infusion of epinephrine 0.4 µg/kg/min after the aspirin caused renewal of thrombus formation temporarily until adrenaline had been metabolized. We further demonstrated using similar animal model that this mechanism was α-adrenergic receptor mediated and calcium dependent. In these studies, we used verapamil, a known calcium channel blocker and α-adrenergic receptor antagonist to demonstrate that the in vivo membrane modulation by adrenaline indeed was via adrenergic receptor modulation and was membrane calcium dependent.[44]

Toffler et al. from Harvard University have suggested that certain "triggers" are responsible for the onset of sudden death.[91] These investigators found a significantly higher incidence of myocardial infarction (MI), ventricular tachyarrhythmia, and sudden death due to cardiac causes in the morning hours than at other times of the day, and they have suggested that these events may be triggered by increase in the adrenergic activity, heart rate, systemic arterial pressure, and blood coagulability that occur in the morning. Toffler et al. in their seminal article in the N Engl J Med (1987) reported that the frequencies of MI and sudden cardiac death are highest during the period from 6 a.m. to noon. Since platelet stickiness or increased aggregability may have a role in triggering these acute cardiac events, they measured platelet activity at 3-hour intervals for 24 hours in 15 healthy individuals. The period from 6 to 9 a. m. was the only interval in the 24-hour period during which platelet aggregability increased significantly. They also observed that morning increase in platelet aggregability was not observed when the subjects remained supine and inactive. Based on their observation, they speculated that there was a temporal association between increased platelet aggregability in the morning hours and an increased frequency of MI and sudden cardiac death.[91-93]

In our article in *Coronary Artery Disease* (1991) based on the results of our studies using several animal models, we too speculated how certain risk factors could promote prothrombotic conditions by elevating circulating hormones.[86] For instance, cigarette smoking is a major risk factor for cardiovascular morbidity and mortality. It has been shown that cigarette smoking acutely enhances platelet aggregation, which suggests that increased platelet function might be the mechanism by which cigarette smoking is linked to arterial thrombotic disease. Cigarette smoking elevates catecholamines and aspirin alone does not block the enhanced platelet function in men with coronary artery disease.[94] In early studies, a circadian function of cardiac function has been noted in the early morning hours.[92,93] In addition, studies by Toffler et al. have demonstrated that there is increased aggregability during the early morning hours. Based on several in vitro and in vivo studies from our laboratory at the University of Minnesota, we too speculated that a combination of low-dose aspirin and an α or β blocker might be an effective strategy for prevention of this observed acute cardiac events in the morning hours.[21,53,95]

Another factor that may contribute to this observed morning increase in platelet aggregation may be altered prostaglandin metabolism as well as increase in blood pressure. Several earlier studies have demonstrated a circadian variation in blood pressure.[96,97] Based on some of these observations, several suggestions were made as to what time of the day prophylactic drugs should be taken. We and other researchers suggested that taking a low-dose aspirin in the evening is better than taking after one wakes up.[54,73] Both the Harvard's Physicians' Health Study (1989) and a Spanish study in 2005 found that taking aspirin at bedtime would provide the maximum platelet inhibition and protection during this vulnerable period (early morning hours). Based on the results of a small randomized clinical study, Dr Tobias Bonnet and associates from Leiden University Medical Center, the Netherlands, reported that taking an aspirin at night might boost its benefits better than taking it in the morning. These researchers also found that morning platelet activity was reduced to a much greater degree when the aspirin was taken at night. The timing of the aspirin, however, had no impact on morning blood pressure levels (New York Times; November 19, 2103; Clinical Trial Registration-http://clinicaltrials.gov/: NCT01379079).

On January 17, 1994, at 4.31 a.m. Los Angeles County was jolted by an earthquake. One of the strongest earthquakes reported in a major city in North America (NEJM, 1994). Leor et al. reviewed the mortality figures and determined the underlying causes of death, the age, and the sex of all persons whose deaths were investigated by the Los Angeles County coroner's office for the 7-day period before the earthquake and the 6 days after the earthquake.[98] Fifty percent of the deaths that occurred were found to be associated to underlying atherosclerotic cardiovascular disease. Not surprisingly, trauma was the second most frequent cause of death assigned by the coroner. The authors concluded that the average daily number of deaths determined by the Coroner's office to be due to atherosclerotic cardiovascular disease from the 7 days before the earthquake to the 6 days after the earthquake was 15.6–9.6. A sharp increase in the number of deaths during the earthquake followed by a decrease suggests that the earthquake precipitated death among people who were "at risk" for developing acute vascular events. Because of this trigger, they died a few days earlier.

Authors in their concluding paragraphs discuss the works of Muller, Toffler, and their associates, who in their earlier article on this subject, had suggested that the act of waking up and emotional and physical stress can trigger the onset of cardiac events by perhaps stimulating the release of catecholamines and inducing hypercoagulability factors that may contribute to the vulnerable atherosclerotic plaque and subsequent coronary artery thrombosis.[91] They further state that the hypothesis related to the triggering effect of acute events is supported by the observation that 35% increase in 72 coronary care units in southern California in the week after the earthquake. When considering practical and future implications, they suggest that administration of drugs such as β-adrenergic-blocking agents and aspirin to patients who are at high risk because of atherosclerotic cardiovascular disease might be beneficial.[21,53,95]

Are there other such examples in which stress-related excess risk of cardiovascular events was observed? Authors of a report in NEJM found a significant increase in the incidence of cardiovascular events (consisting of both the acute coronary syndrome and symptomatic cardiac arrhythmia) in a defined population of Germans in association with soccer matches involving the German team during the FIFA World Cup held in Germany in 2006.[99] According to Chi and Kloner of The Heart Institute, USC, Los Angeles, the seriousness of the coronary artery disease is heightened by the fact that approximately a third of the patients present with sudden death as their first manifestation and efforts to prevent infarctions before they occur have fueled an area of research, which investigates inciting events or "triggers" of MI, arrhythmias, and sudden death.[100] These authors, for instance, speculate that mechanisms by which watching sporting events (soccer, cricket, etc.) could contribute to cardiac events are increased in the sympathetic nervous system stimulation and circulating catecholamines induced by emotional involvement in the game.

From the time, we discovered an intrinsic mechanism of membrane modulation in the early 70s, in the dogs that their platelets sequester when they are excited or agitated to the present time, numerous studies have demonstrated possible role of stress, emotion, and trauma-related occurrence of acute cardiac events. Yet, we have not been able to come up with appropriate strategies to prevent these triggering events for "at-risk" patients. One of the reasons being, it is hard to monitor "at-risk" population. Since taking an aspirin and a β blocker could prevent such an event, it is possible this strategy may be a part of the educational programs by the professional societies and public health policy makers. It could be used as a warning or a reminder to those avid watchers of sports, or those engaged in professional activities, which put them at such risk (participants of competitive sports, law enforcement officers, or military personnel on active duties).

Studies from our laboratory demonstrated that circulating levels of catecholamines could induce stickiness in blood platelets. If the levels are not high enough, the minimally activated platelets could reverse back into their normal inactivated state. This intrinsic mechanism of catecholamine-induced membrane modulation is capable of restoring the sensitivity of drug-induced refractory platelets to the action of agonists. The restoration of sensitivity to various agonists is not dependent on the potentiation of various activating and signaling mechanism such as phosphatide inositol metabolism, formation of second messengers: diglyceride, inositol trisphosphate, elevation of cytosolic calcium, activation of phospholipases, release of arachidonic acid, formation of endoperoxides, thromboxanes, assembly of cytosolic actin, contraction of cytoskeletal proteins, or release of granule contents. The mechanism of membrane modulation is mediated by α-adrenergic receptor stimulation and is dependent on the availability of membrane-associated calcium.

Professional societies and organizations such as American Heart Association, National Health Services of the United Kingdom, and South Asian Society on Atherosclerosis and Thrombosis, United States, advocated taking aspirin before bedtime than in the morning based on a large body of evidence that suggested that majority of heart attacks occur in the morning. We would like to suggest on the basis of our work on the mechanism of membrane modulation that an α-adrenergic receptor antagonist or a β blocker may be added to this prophylactic measure in those cases, where an emotional or stress-related release of endogenous catecholamines are anticipated, as a temporary measure to block adrenergic response on platelet receptors and thus prevent sudden death or acute cardiac event.

REFERENCES

1. White JG, Rao GHR, Estensen RD. Investigation of the release reaction in platelets exposed to phorbol myristate acetate. Am J Pathol. 1974;75:301-14.
2. White JG, Rao GHR, Gerrard JM. Effects of ionophore, A23187, on blood platelets. 1. Influence on Aggregation and secretion. Am J Pathol. 1974;7(2):135-50.
3. Gerrard JM, White JG, Rao GHR. Effects of ionophore, A23187 on blood platelets. 11. Influence on ultrastructure. Am J Pathol. 1974;77(2):151-66.
4. Clawson CC, Rao GHR, White JG. Platelet interaction with bacteria. 1V. Stimulation of the release reaction. Am J Pathol. 1975;81:411-20.
5. White KJG, Matlack C, Mundschenk D, Rao GHR. Platelet disorders in normal and bleeder horse. First International Symposium on Equine Hematology. Colorado: American Association of Equine Practitioners; 1976. pp. 209-21.
6. Gerrard JM, Stoddard SF, Shapiro RS, Coccia PF, Ramsay NKC, Nesbit ME, et al. Platelet storage pool deficiency and prostaglandin synthesis in chronic myelogenous leukemia. Br J Haematol. 1978;40:597-607.
7. Johnson GJ, Rao GHR, White JG. Platelet dysfunction induced by parenteral carbenicillin and ticarcillin: Studies of the dose response relationship and mechanism of action. Am J Pathol. 1978;91:85-106.
8. Johnson GJ, Leis LA, Rao GHR, White JG. Arachidonate-induced platelet aggregation in the dog. Thromb Res. 1979;15:147-54.
9. Johnson GJ, Rao GHR, Leis LA, White JG. Effects of agents, which alter cyclic AMP on arachidonic acid-induced platelet aggregation in the dog. Blood. 1980;55:222-79.
10. Gerrard JM, Stuart MJ, Rao GHR, Steffes MM, Mauer SM, Brown DM, et al. Alteration in the balance of prostaglandin and thromboxane synthesis in diabetes. J Lab Clin Med. 1980;95:950-7.
11. Rao GHR, Johnson GJ, White JG. Influence of epinephrine on the aggregation response of aspirin-treated platelets. Prostaglandin Med. 1980;5:45-58.
12. Rao GHR, Reddy KR, White JG. The influence of epinephrine on prostacyclin- induced dissociation of ADP aggregated platelets. Prostaglandins Med. 1980;5:385-97.
13. Einzig S, Rao GHR, White JG. Differential sensitivity of regional vascular beds in the dog to low dose prostacyclin infusion. Can J Pharmacol. 1980;58:940-6.
14. Einzig S, Sotomora R, Rao GHR, Gerrard JM, Folker JE, White JG. Prostacyclin does not increase blood flow in acute ischemic canine myocardium. Prostaglandins Med. 1980;5:209-21.
15. White JG, Hagert K, Nipper JHJ, Rao GHR. Functional platelets after storage in vitro for fifteen to twenty days. Am J Pathol. 1980;101:613-34.
16. Rao GHR, Reddy KR, White JG. Influence of trifluoperazine on platelet aggregation and disaggregation. Prostaglandins Med. 1980;5:221-34.
17. Gerrard JM, Phillips DR, Rao GHR, Plow EF, Walz DA, Ross R, et al. Biochemical studies of two patients with the gray platelet syndrome: selective deficiency of alpha granules. J Clin Invest. 1980;66:102-9.
18. Peterson DA, Rao GHR, Gerrard JM, White JM. Epinephrine and other activators of prostaglandin endoperoxide synthetase can reduce Fe^{3+} to Fe^{2+} heme. Prostaglandins Med. 1980;5:357-65.
19. Rao GHR, Reddy KR, White JG. Modification of human platelet response to sodium arachidonate by membrane modulation. Prostaglandins Med. 1981;6:75-90.
20. Rao GHR, Gerrard JM, Witkop CJ, White JG. Platelet aggregation independent of ADP release or prostaglandin synthesis in patients with Hermansky-Pudlak syndrome. Prostaglandins Med. 1981;6:459-72.
21. Rao GHR, Reddy KR, White JG. Low dose aspirin, platelet function and prostaglandin

synthesis: influence of epinephrine and alpha-adrenergic blockade. Prostaglandins Med. 1981;6:485-94.
22. Gerrard JM, Rao GHR, Stuart MJ, White JG. Alterations in the balance of thromboxane and prostacyclin synthesis in platelet and the vessel wall in a diabetic model. In: Hirsch J, Steele PP, Vernier RL (Eds). The Effects of Platelet Active Drugs on the Cardiovascular System. University of Colorado Press; 1981. pp. 207-23.
23. Rao GHR, White JG. Epinephrine potentiation of arachidonate-induced aggregation of cyclooxygenase deficient platelets. Am J Pathol. 1981;11:355-66.
24. Rao GHR, Johnson GJ, Reddy KR, White JG. Rapid return of cyclooxygenase active platelets in dogs after a single oral dose of aspirin. Prostaglandins. 1981;22:761-72.
25. Peterson DA, Gerrard JM, Glover SM, Rao GHR, White JG. Epinephrine reduction of heme: Implications for understanding the transmission of agonist stimulus. Science. 1982;215:71-3.
26. Rao GHR, Schmidt HHO, Pierpont ME, White JG. Human platelet activation by an alkyl-acetyl analogue of phosphatidylcholine. Biochim Biophys Acta. 1982;715:205-14.
27. Rao GHR, White JG. Platelet activating factor (PAF) causes human platelet aggregation through the mechanism of membrane modulation. Prostaglandins Med. 1982;9:459-72.
28. White JG, Reddy KR, White JG. Penicillin induced human platelet dysfunction and its reversal by epinephrine. Prostaglandins Leukot Med. 1983;11:199-211.
29. Rao GHR, Radha E, White JG. Effect of docosahexaenoic acid (DHA) on arachidonic acid metabolism and platelet function. Biochem Biophys. Res Commun. 1983;117:540-56.
30. Cox AC, Carrol RC, White JG, Rao GHR. Recycling of platelet phosphorylation and cytoskeletal assembly. J Cell Biol. 1984;98:8-15.
31. Rao GHR, White JG. Role of arachidonic acid metabolism in human platelet activation and irreversible aggregation. Am J Hematol. 1985;19:339-47.
32. Rao GHR, White JG. Disaggregation and reaggregation of irreversibly aggregated platelets: a method for more complete evaluation of antiplatelet drugs. Agents Actions. 1985;16:425-34.
33. Rao GHR White JG. Comparative pharmacology of cyclooxygenase inhibitors. Prostaglandins Med. 1985;18:119-31.
34. Rao GHR, Radha E, White JG. Irreversible platelet aggregation does not depend upon lipoxygenase metabolites. Biochem Biophys Res Commun. 1985;131:50-7.
35. Radha E, Hill TD, Rao GHR, White JG. Glutathione levels in human platelets displays a circadian rhythm in vitro. Thromb Res. 1985;40:823-31.
36. Rao GHR, Peller JD, Semba CP, White JG. Influence of the calcium sensitive fluorophore Quin 2 on platelet function. Blood. 1986;67:354-61.
37. Rao GHR, Escolar G, White JG. Epinephrine reverses the inhibitory influence of aspirin on platelet-vessel wall interactions. Thromb Res. 1986;44:65-74.
38. Rao GHR, White JG, Cox CA. Influence of a calcium-dependent protease inhibitor on platelet activation and secretion. Thromb Res. 1987;47:625-37.
39. Burris SM, Smith CM, Rao GHR, White JG. Aspirin treatment reduces platelet resistance to deformation. Arteriosclerosis. 1987;7:385-8.
40. Rao GHR. Influence of antiplatelet drugs on platelet-vessel wall interactions. Prostaglandins Leukot Med. 1987;30:133-45.
41. Rao GHR. Influence of a calmodulin antagonists (Stelazine) on agonist-induced calcium mobilization and platelet activation. Biochem Biophys Res Commun. 1987;149:768-75.
42. Smith CM, Burris SM, Rao GHR, White JG. Epinephrine reversal of aspirin effects on platelet deformability. Thromb Res. 1988;51:35-44.
43. Rao GHR. Measurement of ionized calcium in normal human platelets. Anal Biochem. 1988;169:400-8.
44. Folts JD, Rowe CG, Rao GHR. Problem with aspirin as anti-thrombotic agent in coronary artery disease. Lancet. 1988;1:937.
45. Rao GHR, White JG. Influence of phospholipase A2 on human platelet alpha-adrenergic receptor function. Thromb Res. 1989;53:427-34.

46. Rao GHR, White JG. Epinephrine-induced platelet membrane modulation. In: Myers KM, Barnes CD (Eds). Platelet Storage Granules. Boca Raton: CRC Press; 1992. pp. 117-49.
47. Grouse LH, Rao GHR, Weiss DJ, Perman V, White JG. Surface activated bovine platelets do not spread, they unfold. Am J Pathol. 1990;136:399-408.
48. Rao GHR, Raij L, Lester B, White JG. Inhibition of agonist-induced human platelet activation by nitric oxide. In: Moncada S, Higgs EA (Eds). Proceeding Roy Social Symposium. New York: Elsevier; 1990. pp. 355-67.
49. Krishnamurthi S, Wheeler-Jones CPD, Patel Y, Sadowska K, Kakkar, Rao GHR. Nitroprusside inhibits platelet function primarily by inhibiting calcium mobilization. Biochem Soc Transact. 1990;18:460-70.
50. Rao GHR, Krishnamurthi S, Raij L, White JG. Influence of nitric oxide on agonist-mediated calcium mobilization in platelets. Biochem Med Metab Biol. 1990;43:271-5.
51. Weiss DJ, McClay CB, Smith CM, Rao GHR, White JG. Platelet function in the racing thorough bred. Implications for exercise-induced hemorrhage. Vet Clin Pathol. 1990;19:35-9.
52. Rao GHR, White JG. Aspirin, PGE1, and Quin-2 AM induced platelet dysfunction. Restoration of function by norepinephrine. Prostaglandins Leukot Essent Fatty Acids. 1990;39:141-6.
53. Rao GHR, Escolar G, Zavoral J, White JG. Influence of adrenergic receptor blockade on aspirin-induced inhibition of platelet function. Platelets. 1990;1:145-50.
54. Prikyl P, Siegelova J, Rao GHR. Chronotherapeutic treatment daily of low-dose aspirin. University of Minnesota Medtronic Chronobiology Seminar Series. 1991;3:1-8.
55. Rao GHR. The role of membrane lipids in the platelet storage lesion commentary. Blood Cells. 1992;18:498-500.
56. Rao GHR, Smith 11, white JG. Influence of calcium antagonists on thrombin-induced calcium mobilization and platelet-vessel wall interactions. Biochem Med. Metab Biol. 1992;47:226-31.
57. Rao GHR, Ericson DG, Weiss DJ, Parks PG, White JG. Influence of aspirin and carbacyclin on bovine platelet function. ASAIO J. 1992;38:830-4.
58. Rao GHR. Influence of storage on signal transduction pathways and platelet function. Blood Cells. 1992;18:383-96.
59. Rao GHR, Rao ASC, White JG. Influence of low-dose enteric coated aspirin on platelet function. Indian Heart J. 1992;44:365-71.
60. Herzberg MC, Krishnan LK, MacFarlane GD. Involvement of α2-adrenoreceptors and G-proteins in the modulation of platelet secretion in response to Streptococcus sanguis. Crit Rev Oral Biol Med. 1993;4:435-42.
61. Smith CM, Burris SM, Rao GHR, White JG. Detergent-resistant cytoskeleton of the surface activated platelets differ from the suspension-activated cytoskeleton. Blood. 1992;80:2774-80.
62. Rao GHR. Signal transduction, second messengers and platelet function. J Lab Clin Med. 1993;121:18-22.
63. Rao GHR, Escolar G, White JG. Biochemistry, physiology and function of platelets stored as concentrates. Transfusion. 1993;33:766-78.
64. Rao GHR, Escolar G, Smith CM, White JG. Influence of heat on platelet biochemistry, physiology and function. J Lab Clin Med. 1993;122:455-65.
65. Rao GHR, Gerrard JM, Murthy M, White JG. Possible mechanisms of epinephrine actions in human platelets that are refractory to arachidonic acid. Biochem Med Metab Biol. 1993;50:322-37.
66. Rao GHR, Tate M, Hebbel R, White JG. Influence of antioxidants on arachidonic acid metabolism and platelet function. Biochem Med Metab Biol. 1994;51:74-9.
67. Rao GHR, Escolar G, White JG. Monitoring signal transduction and cytoskeletal alterations by fluorescent imaging and confocal microscopy. Ann NY Acad Sci. 1994;714:297-300.
68. Rao GHR, White JG. Influence of various doses of aspirin *(in vivo)* on platelet arachidonic acid metabolism (ex vivo) and function. Prostaglandins Leukot Essent Fatty Acids. 1994;51:63-9.
69. Rao GHR, Smith CM 11, Doni MG, White JG. Intracellular calcium imaging in adherent human platelets. Arterioscler Thromb. 1994;5:95-105.

70. Rao GHR, Fields CM, White JG, Fields G. Promotion of human platelet adhesion and aggregation by a synthetic, triple-helical mini-collagen. J Biol Chem. 1994;269:13899-903.
71. Rao GHR. Signal transduction second messengers and platelet pharmacology. Pharmacol (Life Sci). 1994;13:39-44.
72. Rao GHR, Peller JD, Prakash YS, Doni MG, White JG. Monitoring signal transduction and cytoskeletal alterations in adherent platelets. Arterioscler Thromb. 1994;5:155-65.
73. Rao GHR. Circadian variations and coronary artery disease. Chronobiologia. 1994; 21:63-4.
74. White JG, Rao GHR. Aggregated-disaggregated, refractory platelets retain sensitivity to ristocetin. Thromb Res. 1996;84:253-6.
75. Rao GHR, White JG. Epinephrine and platelet function. J Lab Clin Med. 1997;130:238-9.
76. Rao GHR. Role of platelet adhesion and aggregation on thrombus formation. Thromb Haemost. 1998;79:454-5.
77. Chandy T, Mooradian DL, Rao GHR. Platelet adhesion and spreading on protein coated surfaces. Variations in behavior in washed cells, PRP, and whole blood. J Biomater Appl. 1998;13:46-65.
78. Rao GHR, Fareed J. Aspirin prophylaxis for the prevention of thrombosis: expectations and limitations. Thrombosis. 2012;2012: 104707.
79. Rao GHR. Aspirin resistance: clinical significance. J Clin Prevent Cardiol. 2012;1(3): 118-29.
80. Johnson GJ. Platelet thromboxane receptors: biology and function. In: Rao GHR (Ed). Handbook of Platelet Physiology and Pharmacology. Boston: Kluwer Academic Publishers; 1999. pp. 38-79.
81. Johnson GJ, Leis LA, Dunlop PC. Thromboxane-insensitive dog platelets have impaired activation of phospholipase C due to receptor-linked G protein dysfunction. J Clin Invest. 1993;92:2469-79.
82. Johnson GJ, Leis LA, King RA. Thromboxane responsiveness of dog platelets is inherited as an autosomal trait. Thromb Haemost. 1991;65:578-80.
83. Dunlop PC, Leis LA, Johnson GJ. Epinephrine correction of impaired platelet thromboxane receptors signaling. Am J Cell Physiol. 2000;279:C1760-71.
84. Dudley A, Thompson S, Fritz J, Grady J, Stokes J, Wills R, et al. Cyclooxygenase and platelet function in healthy dogs receiving low-dose aspirin. J Vet Intern Med. 2013;27: 141-9.
85. Thomason J, Archer T, Wills S, Press, Mackin A. The effect of cyclosporine and aspirin on platelet function in normal dogs. J Vet Intern Med. 2017;30:1022-30.
86. Bonebrake FC, Bertha B, Folts JD, Rao GHR. Verapamil combined with aspirin for inhibiting epinephrine-stimulated platelet thrombus formation in stenosed canine arteries. Coron Artery Dis. 1991;2:487-92.
87. Folts JD, Gallapher K, Rowe CG. Cyclical flow reductions in stenosed canine coronary arteries: vasospasm or platelet aggregation? Circulation. 1982;65:248-55.
88. Folts JD. Experimental arterial thrombosis, platelet inhibitors and their possible clinical relevance. J Cardiovasc Rep. 1982;3: 370-82.
89. Folts JD, Rowe CG. Epinephrine potentiation of in vivo stimuli reverses aspirin inhibition of platelet thrombus formation in stenosed canine coronary arteries Thromb Res. 1988;50:507-16.
90. Karlsberg RP, Cryer PE, Roberts R. Serial plasma catecholamines response early in the course of clinical acute myocardial infarction: relationship to infarct extent and mortality. Am Heart J. 1981;102:24-9.
91. Toffler GH, Bredzinski D, Schafer AI, Czeisler CA, Rutherford JD, Willich SN, et al. Concurrent morning increase in platelet aggregability and the risk for myocardial infarction and sudden death. N Engl J Med. 1987; 316:1514-8.
92. Willich SN, Levy D, Rocco MB, Toffler GH, Stone PH, Muller JE. Circadian variation in the incidence of sudden cardiac death in the Framingham Heart Study Population. Am J Cardiol. 1987;60:801-6.
93. Muller JE, Ludmer PL, Willich SN, Toffler GH, Aylmer G, Klangos I, et al. Circadian variation in the frequency of sudden cardiac death. Circulation. 1987;75:131-8.
94. Davis JW, Hassanein KM, Hignite CE, Ruttnger HA. Cigarette smoking-induced

enhancement of platelet function: lack of prevention by aspirin in men with coronary artery disease. J Lab Clin Med. 1985;105:479-83.

95. Frishman WH, Laifer LI, Furberg CD. Beta-adrenergic blockers in the prevention of sudden death. In: ME Josephson (Ed.) Sudden Cardiac Death. FA Davis, Philadelphia; 1985:249-64.
96. Hermida RC, Ayala DE, Portaluppi F. Circadian variations of blood pressure: the basis for the chronotherapy of hypertension. Adv Drug Deliv Rev. 2007;59:904-22.
97. Cough AR, Loughran JH, Slaughter MS. Circadian variations in health and disease. Implications for patient management. Chronophysiol Therapy. 2011;1:17-31.
98. Leor J, Poole K, Kloner RA. Sudden cardiac death by an earthquake. N Engl J Med. 1996;334:413-9.
99. Wilbert-Lampen U, Leistner D, Greven MS, Pohl T, Sper S, Völker C, et al. Cardiovascular events during world cup soccer. N Engl J Med. 2008;358:475-83.
100. Chi JS, Kloner RA. Stress and myocardial infarction. Heart. 2003;89:475-6.

Platelet–Vessel Wall Interactions

CHAPTER 15

INTRODUCTION

The circulating system performs a variety of vital functions, such as carrying oxygen and nutrients to the cells and tissues as well as removal of the waste from the body. The heart is a four-chambered muscular organ that beats approximately 70 times a minute for over half a billion times in its lifetime. The circulatory system is a complex network of tubes of varying sizes and textures. It is estimated that the system is approximately equivalent to 60,000 miles of vessels carrying about 5 L of blood throughout the body every minute. The entire length of these vessels is lined with a monolayer of endothelial cells (it is believed that endothelial cells of a normal human body can cover about six tennis courts).

Major players in the platelet vessel wall interactions are circulating platelets, red cells and endothelial cells covering the vascular wall. Scanning electron micrographs of inactivated platelets, red cells and endothelial cells are shown in Figures 15.1 to 15.3.

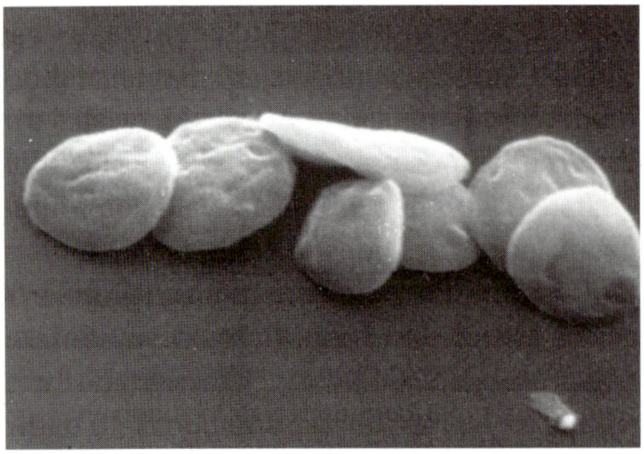

Fig. 15.1: Scanning electron micrograph of discoid platelets.

BLOOD VESSEL COVERED BY A MONOLAYER OF ENDOTHELIAL CELLS

Vascular system has three types of arteries: arterioles, muscular arteries, and elastic arteries. Morphology of these vessels varies according to the functional needs. Arterioles are the smallest with narrow lumen and

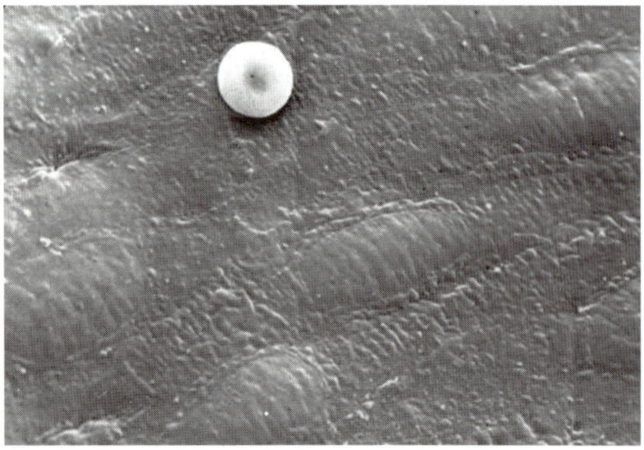

Fig. 15.2: Red cell on vascular surface.

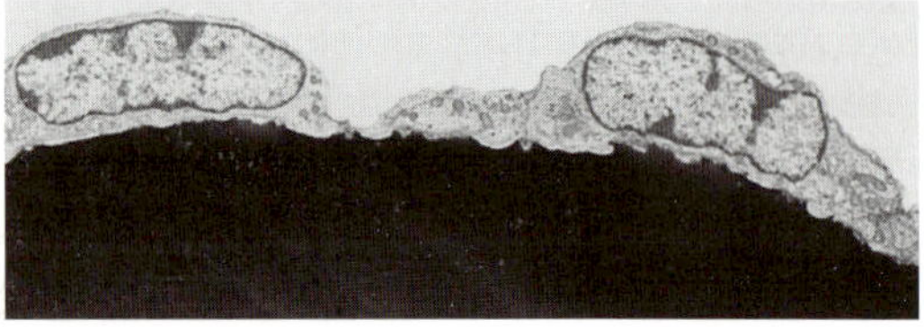

Fig. 15.3: Endothelial cells.

muscular walls. Muscular arteries are responsible for distribution of oxygenated blood throughout the body. Elastic arteries are larger vessels and their walls contain elastin. Presence of these specialized cells as well as the composition of the cellular matrix plays a very important role in the modulation of the flow velocity, fluid dynamics, vascular physiology, platelet–vessel wall interactions, and various functions of the circulatory system. The human cardiovascular system is an internal closed loop with multiple branches circulating complex fluid with variable speed and pressure. Important features of blood flow in arteries are pulsatile in nature with numerous branches, which cause vessel wall shear stress (VWSS) to be cyclical and nonuniform. Walls of all the blood vessels except in the smallest consist of three layers, namely the tunica intima, tunica media, and tunica externa. The tunica intima reduces friction between vessel walls and blood; the tunica media controls vasoconstriction and vasodilation of the vessels; and the tunica externa reinforces and anchors the vessel to surrounding tissues.

When we look at the blood vessel anatomy, average lumen diameter (D) and vessel wall thickness (T) varies considerably. According to published literature, the vessel wall anatomy is as follows: elastic artery (D: 1.5 cm, T: 1 mm); muscular artery (D: 6 mm, T: 1 mm); arteriole (D: 37 µm, T: 6 µm); capillary (D: 9 µm, T: 0.5 µm); venule (D: 20 µm, T: 1 µm); vein (D: 5 mm, T: 0.5 mm).

PLATELET PHYSIOLOGY

Blood platelets interact with a variety of soluble agonists, such as epinephrine and adenosine diphosphate (ADP), many insoluble cell matrix components, including collagen, laminin, and biomaterials used for the construction of invasive medical devices.[1] These interactions stimulate specific receptors and glycoprotein-rich domains (integrins and nonintegrins) on the plasma membrane of platelets and lead to the activation of intracellular effector enzymes.[2] Majority of the regulatory events appear to require free calcium. Ionized calcium is the primary bioregulator, and a variety of biochemical mechanisms modulate the level and availability of free cytosolic calcium. Major enzymes that regulate the free cytosolic calcium levels via second messengers include phospholipase C, phospholipase A_2, and phospholipase D, together with adenylyl and guanylyl cyclases. Activation of phospholipase C results in the hydrolysis of phosphatidyl inositol 4, 5-bisphosphate and formation of second messengers 1, 2-diacylglycerol and inositol 1, 4, 5-trisphosphate (IP_3). Diglyceride induces activation of protein kinase C, whereas IP_3 mobilizes cytosolic calcium from internal membrane stores.[3] Elevation of cytosolic calcium stimulates phospholipase A_2 and liberates arachidonic acid (AA). Free AA is transformed to a novel metabolite, thromboxane A_2 by fatty acid synthetase (Cox-1, cyclooxygenase). Thromboxane A_2 is the major metabolite of this pathway and plays a critical role in platelet recruitment, granule mobilization, and secretion. Secretory granules contain a variety of growth factors, mitogens, and inflammatory mediators. Secretion of granules promote P-selectin and CD40 expression on the platelet membrane. Furthermore, activation also promotes the expression of acidic lipids on the membrane and tissue factor expression, thus making these cells procoagulant. Fully activated platelets can modulate the function of other circulating blood cells, such as leukocytes, monocytes, macrophages, as well as vascular endothelial cells.[4,5] Agonist-mediated stimulation of platelets promotes the expression of an epitope on glycoprotein IIb/IIIa receptors.

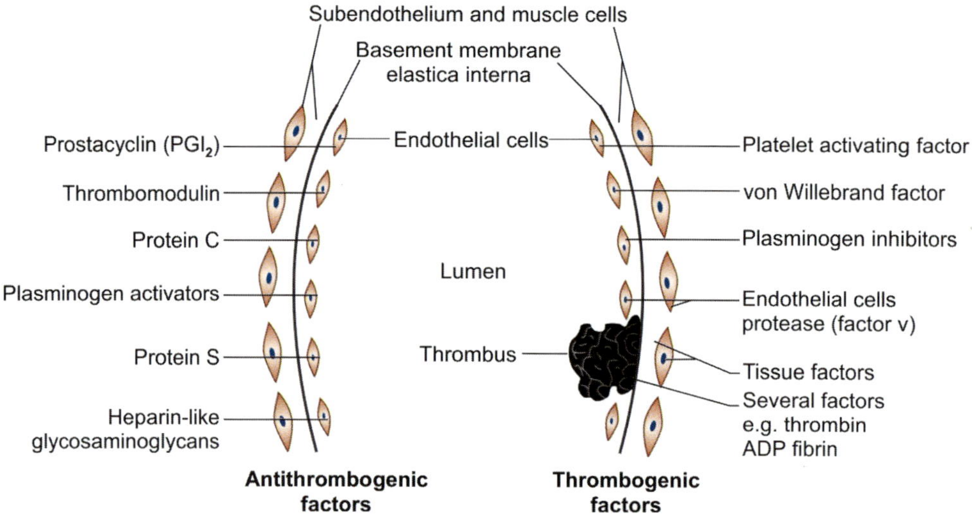

Fig. 15.4: Factors modulating thrombogenesis. In this figure, some of the vasoactive compounds generated by endothelium are represented. Listed on the right side, platelet activating factor, von Willebrand factor, plasminogen inhibitors, endothelial cell proteases, tissue factors, thrombin, ADP, and fibrin are prothrombotic compounds; whereas, those listed on the left side, prostacyclin, thrombomodulin, protein C, plasminogen activators, protein S, heparin and heparin-like compounds are antithrombotic components.

Activation of this receptor is essential for the binding of circulating fibrinogen. Fibrinogen forms a bridge between individual platelets and facilitates the thrombus formation. von Willebrand factor (vWF) binds to platelet GPIbIX complex only at high shear rate unlike fibrinogen, which can bind platelets at low shear. Upregulation in signaling pathways will increase the risk for clinical complications associated with acute coronary events. Downregulation of signal transduction mechanisms may precipitate bleeding diathesis or stroke.

VASCULAR DYSFUNCTION

Functional and structural changes in the arterial wall precede the development of atherosclerosis, obstructive coronary artery disease, and may even serve as an early marker for the hypertensive disease.[6-10] Functional and structural changes of vascular endothelial cells (ECs) are modulated by a variety of thrombogenic factors as well as antithrombogenic factors (Fig. 15.4).[11-13] Some of the vasoactive compounds released by the ECs include vasodilatory compounds, such as adenosine, prostacyclin and nitric oxide, and vasoconstrictory molecules like cyclooxygenase-derived endothelium-dependent constriction factor (EDCF), hypoxia-induced endothelium-dependent constriction factor, and endothelin. Lipid peroxides, oxidized lipids, and lipoproteins promote the formation of vasoconstrictors by platelets.[8] These lipid mediators inhibit enzymes that promote the formation of vasodilators by the healthy endothelium and lower endogenous production of vasodilators. Alterations in the balance between platelet-associated vasoconstrictors and EC-derived vasodilators result in the vascular dysfunction.[9] This is probably the earliest stage at which one can detect the manifestation of the arterial dysfunctions, hypertension, and atherosclerosis. Indeed, one can classify the risk according to the level of EC dysfunction and additional coronary artery disease (CAD) risk factors present. One can use acetylcholine, L-arginine, and nitric oxide synthetase inhibitor, LNNMA and monitor the flow response in the forearm to determine the degree of EC dysfunction.[13,14] Alternatively, one can use CV Profilor (DO-2020, Hypertension Diagnostics, Eagan, MN) or Periscope (Genesis Medical Systems, Hyderabad, India) and monitor the pulse waveform of the small arteries.[15,16] Platelet interaction with collagen fibrils and exposed subendothelium of rabbit aorta are shown in Figures 15.5A and B.

Signaling mechanisms involved in platelet–vessel wall interaction is not well characterized. However, large body of literature suggests that the mechanisms are similar, underlying adhesion, shape change, spreading, calcium mobilization, second messenger generation, contraction, secretion, and thrombus formation. The major difference being in cell–cell interaction leading to aggregation, fibrinogen binding to GPIIb/IIIa receptor plays the primary role. In platelet–vessel wall interactions, a variety of interactive membrane glycoprotein domains play an important role. The membrane glycoproteins of human platelets act as receptors or interactive domains that mediate adhesion to the subendothelial matrix and platelet aggregation and growth of these aggregates. These glycoprotein domains exist as noncovalently linked heterodimers belonging to the supergene family of adhesion receptors called the integrins.[18,19] Platelets contain at least five members of this supergene family, including a collagen receptor (GPIa-IIa: α_2, β_1), a fibronectin receptor (GPIc-IIa; αv, β_3). Majority of the integrin receptors bind a tripeptide sequence, arginine–glycine, aspartic acid (RGD) on the adhesive proteins. In addition to the integrins referred above, platelets contain other membrane glycoproteins, such as GPIb-IX complex, a receptor that binds vWF, thought to be the primary receptor responsible for platelet adhesion to the subendothelial matrix under flow conditions. A less-known domain called GPV and GPIV function as receptors for thrombospondin and collagen. It is noteworthy that a form of GPIIb/IIIa is

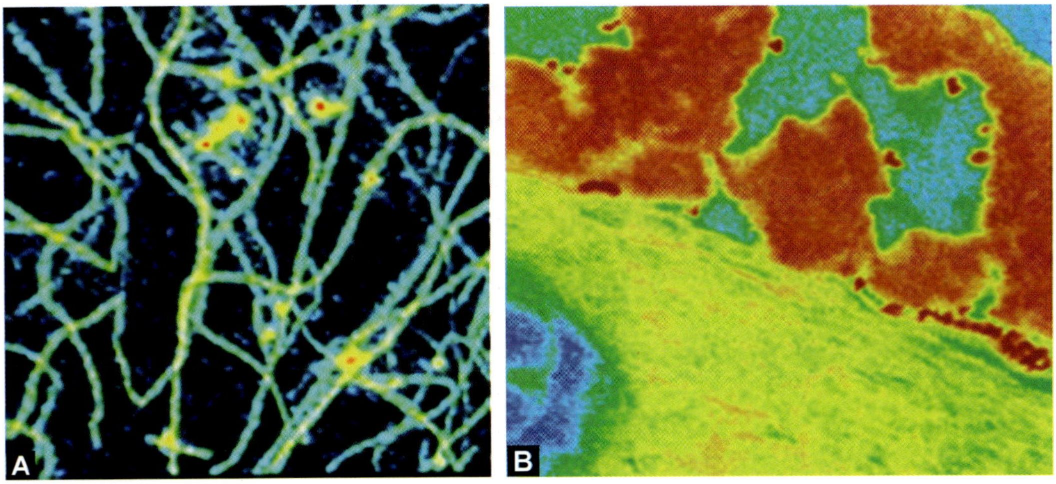

Figs.15.5A and B: Platelet microthrombi on collagen surface. Platelet thrombi on subendothelium. Fluorescent imaging of platelet thrombi on collagen microfibrils and rabbit subendothelium.

expressed on unactivated platelets and acts as functional receptor that mediates irreversible aggregation to immobilized (surface bound) fibrinogen. This reaction can occur in the presence of elevated cAMP unlike the activation of platelets in suspension, which is inhibited by rise in cAMP. On the other hand, platelet-binding to vWF through GPIb is inhibited by elevated levels of cAMP. Therefore, GPIb and GPIIb/IIIa induce platelet activation by binding with vWF and fibrinogen on vessel wall surface in the absence of exogenous agonists.[19] Studies on platelet and vessel wall interactions (with components, such as glycoprotein-rich domains) have shown that such interactions cannot be inhibited by aspirin and clopidogrel.[20,21]

In the previous section on epinephrine-induced membrane modulation, we described how the studies on irreversibly aggregated platelets could be used as a "model" to understand the modulation of platelet function by agonists and antagonists. Since platelet–vessel wall interactions leading to platelet adhesion, aggregation and thrombus formation provide a better model for testing the effectiveness or otherwise of antiplatelet and antithrombotic drugs, we will describe the methodology used for these studies in detail.

Blood for these studies were obtained from adult volunteers, who had not taken any medications for at least 2 weeks prior to venesection and mixed immediately with citrate–citric acid–dextrose (CCD) anticoagulant (citrate 0.1 M, citric acid 7 mM, dextrose 0.14 M, pH 6.5) in a ratio of 9 parts blood to 1 part anticoagulant. Platelet-rich plasma (PRP) was obtained by centrifuging the whole blood at room temperature for 20 minutes at 100 g for 20 minutes. Platelet-poor plasma (PPP) was obtained by spinning the remaining blood at 200 g for 20 minutes. PPP was stored frozen at –35°C during the platelet washing period. Freshly thawed PPP was used for reconstituting platelet concentrates. Platelets from PRP were washed twice with equal volumes of CCD containing 5 mM adenosine and 3 mM theophylline. Washed platelets were resuspended in PPP obtained from the same donor and tested on the aggregometer for their response to the action of agonists before evaluating by the Baumgartner method.[22-27]

Concentration of platelets was adjusted to 4–5 × 10^5 platelets/μL with PPP. This reconstituted PRP was incubated for 30 minutes at 37°C, divided into four aliquots, and incubated with aspirin (100 μM), epinephrine (10 μM), aspirin + epinephrine (100 + 10 μM), and buffer (control group). Perfusates consisted of treated PRP combined with a 40% volume of washed red cells. The final concentrations of platelets in these perfusates were always between 1.5 × 10^5 and 2.5 × 10^5 cells/μL. Perfusions were carried out at 37°C in perfusion chambers developed by Prof Baumgartner with an effective annular width of 2.2 mm and rod length of 7.2 cm[22] (Fig. 15.6).

Flow of blood was obtained by pumping the reconstituted blood through a Cole Parmer Masterflex pump with autoclude head. Blood was perfused at 140 mL/min (wall shear rate 800 sec^{-1}) Denuded rabbit abdominal aorta segments were used in all the experiments in this series of studies (Fig. 15.7).

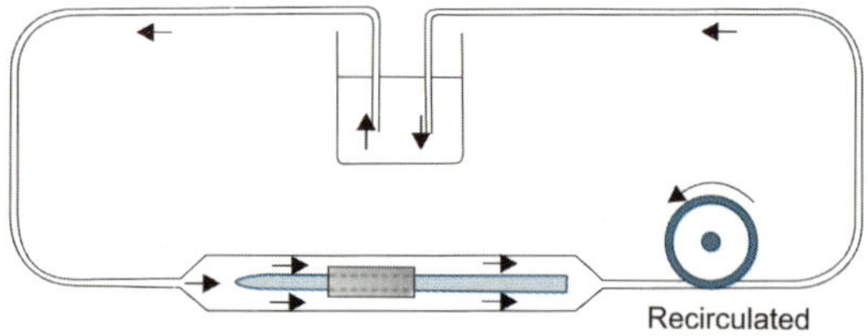

Fig. 15.6: Baumgartner perfusion chamber: a closed loop circulation of reconstituted human blood over denuded rabbit aorta.
Courtesy: Prof Gienes Escolar, Barcelona, Spain.

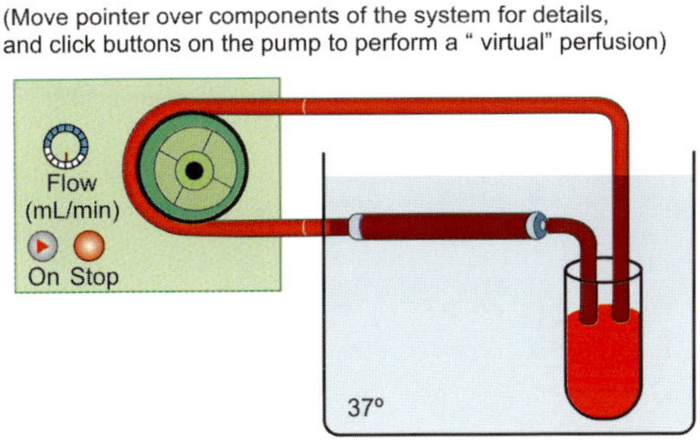

Fig. 15.7: Schematics of an annular perfusion chamber.
Source: Published with permission from Prof Gines Escolar and Dr Jordi Bozzo (02-02-2017).

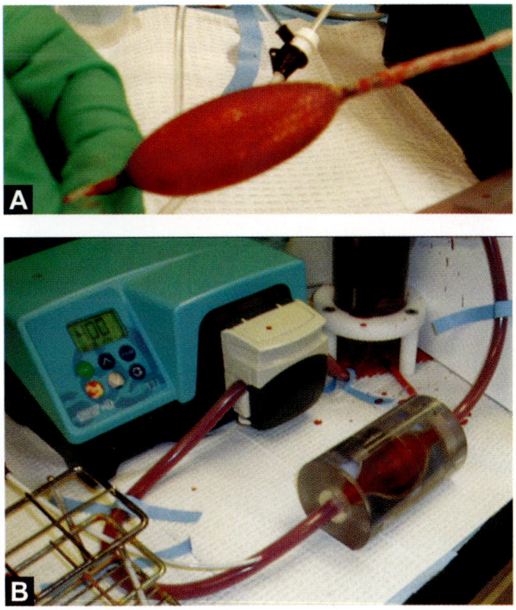

Figs. 15.8A and B: Screening of a balloon catheter for blood compatibility.

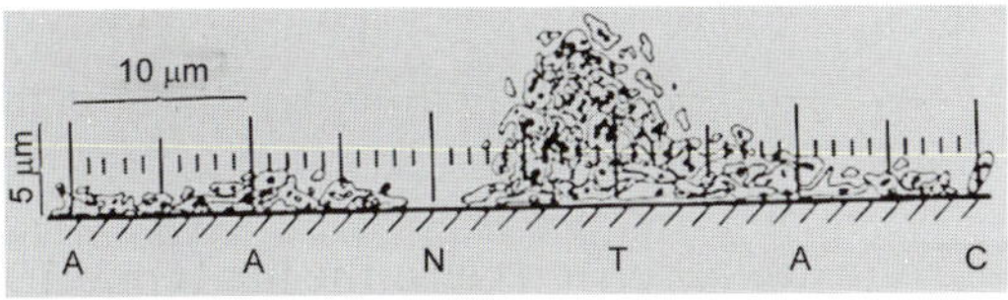

Fig. 15.9: Diagram of a micrometer.
Courtesy: Prof Gienes Escolar, Barcelona, Spain.

Aortic segments were mounted on the plastic rods and rinsed with phosphate buffer for 10 minutes. After 5 minutes of perfusion with reconstituted blood, the segments were fixed with 3% glutaraldehyde in White saline buffer (Figs. 15.8A and B). The fixed samples were separated and processed for electron microscopy. Platelet interaction was evaluated in JB-4 sections of 3-µm thickness. Two series of axial slices, each 0.5 mm, were cut from the block. A microscope with an eyepiece micrometer divided into 100 parts was used for these evaluations (Fig. 15.9).

Platelets or groups of platelets were classified as contact (C), platelets that were attached but not spread on the subendothelium (spread), platelets that were spread on the subendothelium surface, and aggregates (Agg). A further stage in which adherent platelets had formed with multiple layers but did not exceed 5 µm in height (Figs. 15.10A and B); thrombi (T) platelet aggregates of more than 5 µm in height. All of these basic parameters were expressed as percentages of the total surface examined.

The results of this study presented as percentage of area covered in Table 15.1. Photomicrographs as shown in Figures 15.10 to 15.14 represent various stages of platelet interaction on rabbit subendothelium.

Under the conditions of this study, aspirin did not prevent platelet interaction with subendothelium. The total number of platelets covered on the vascular surface in the aspirin group (56%) was as high as in that of untreated normal control group (55%). However, the percentage of thrombi formed were significantly less in the aspirin group (4%) compared to 21% in the untreated group. This dramatic decrease in the thrombogenicity was offset by the

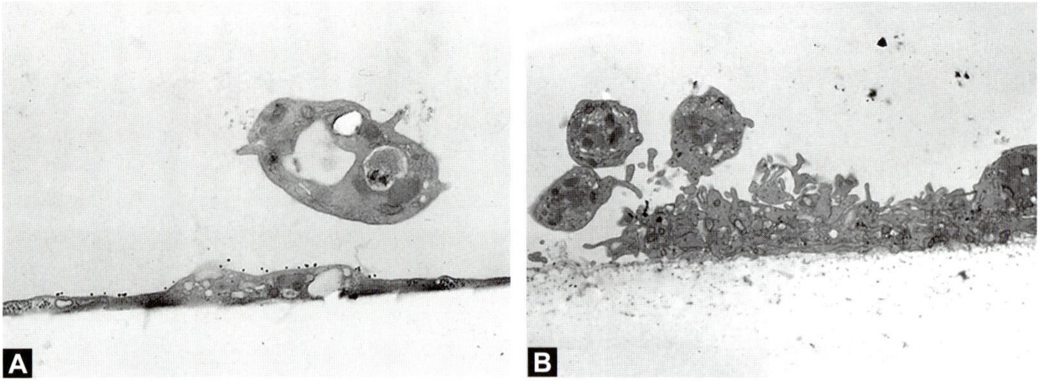

Figs. 15.10A and B: Platelet approaching a spread platelet. Platelet aggregates on surface.

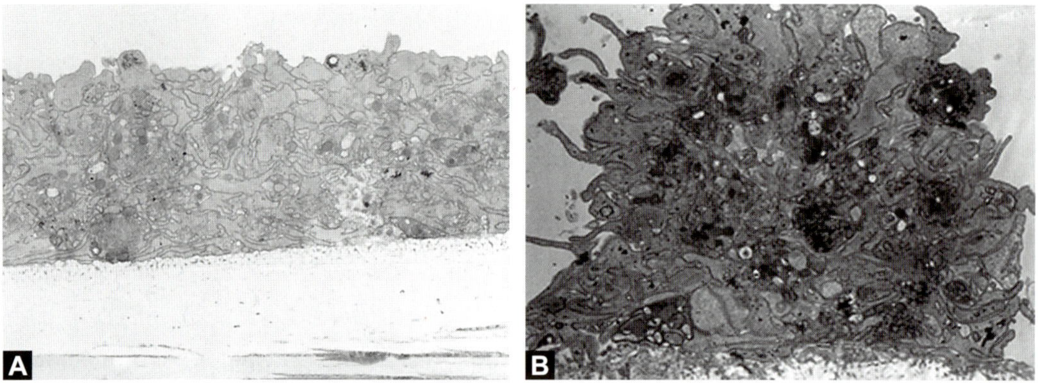

Figs. 15.11A and B: Platelet aggregates on vessel surface. Platelet thrombus on vessel surface.

Table 15.1: Platelet vessel-wall Interactions: Using denuded rabbit aorta platelet interaction with the exposed subendothelial surface was followed using a flow model developed in our laboratory. Data presented show percentage of area covered by reactive platelets following various drug treatments, such as aspirin (ASA), epinephrine (Epi), ASA+Epi.

Platelet interaction with subendothelium				
	Spread	Aggregates	Thrombus	Surface covered
Control	7.6 ± 0.6	24.3 ± 0.9	21.5 ± 0.1	55.5 ± 1.2
ASA (100 uM)	33.0 ± 1.2	17.6 ± 0.9	4.1 ± 0.3	56.7 ± 1.4
Epi (10 uM)	10.0 ± 0.8	20.6 ± 0.4	17.3 ± 0.8	50.3 ± 1.7
Epi + ASA	12.0 ± 1.0	22.5 ± 0.9	20.8 ± 2.0	56.8 ± 1.2

increase in spread platelets in aspirin-treated group (33%) compared to that of only 8% in the control group. Results of these studies showed that epinephrine could reverse the inhibitory influence of aspirin on platelet-vessel wall interaction (Figs. 15.11A and B). The existence of this salvage pathway was first demonstrated in our laboratory at the University of Minnesota with studies on dog platelets, as reported in the Chapter 14: Epinephrine-induced platelet Membrane Modulation.

Platelets initiate hemostasis by using their glycoprotein receptors to form attachments to the damaged tissue, which arrests them from

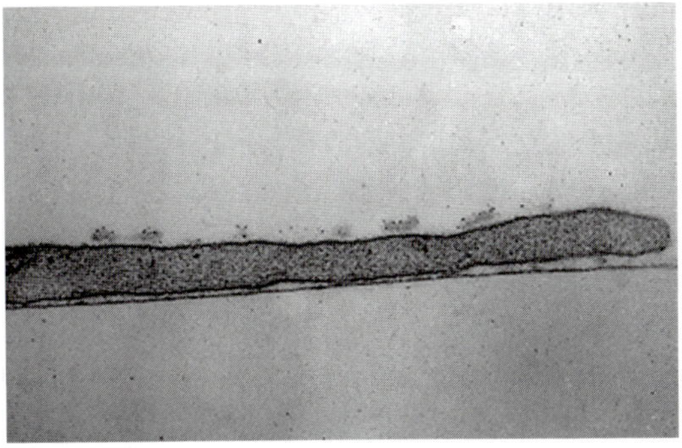

Fig. 15.12: Platelet spreading on a surface.

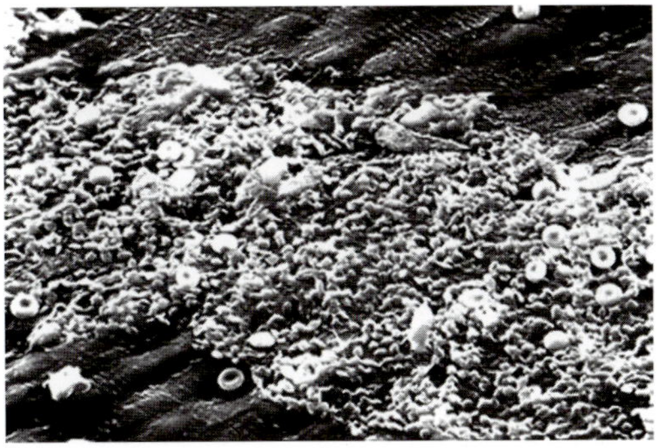

Fig. 15.13: Platelet interaction on rabbit aorta.

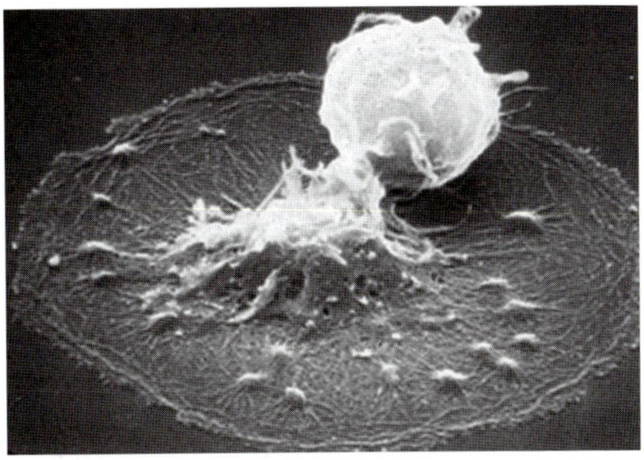

Fig. 15.14: 16.0 cytoskeleton of a spread platelet.

circulating in the blood. Once attached on the surface, depending on the cell matrix components that they interact, they adhere, change their shape, spread or form aggregates. For instance, if the substrate is fibronectin, then they spread on the surface as shown in the Figure 15.12.

On the other hand, if it is a denuded surface or an injured vessel, they will adhere, spread, aggregate, release a variety of soluble agonists and adhesive proteins from their granules to activate and recruit more platelets to the injured site (Fig. 15.13).

Fully activated platelets promote thrombin generation, initiate clot formation, and participate in the formation of a hemostatic plug. Cytoskeletal changes following activation promotes more physical contact of the wounded surface and the actin–myosin interactions help pull the clot into a more compact structure that stabilizes it against the wounded vessel wall.

As we have discussed earlier, glycoprotein domains or receptors on platelet membranes bind to ligands on the injured vessel wall within the extracellular matrix. Extracellular matrix (ECM) of the blood vessel wall not only consists predominantly collagen and laminin, but also adhesive proteins like vWF, fibrinogen, and fibronectin. According to researchers, initial arrest of a platelet from the circulating blood involves the glycoprotein receptor GPIb-IX-V and subsequent engagement with GPIV to collagen. In addition, P-selectin receptors on the surface of activated endothelial cells can mediate platelet adhesion through interactions with P-selectin glycoprotein ligand 1 (PSGL-1) on a platelet membrane after degranulation.

Receptors GPIb-IX-V and $\alpha IIb\beta_3$ also play an important role, as they are involved in initial tethering of the platelets to the vessel wall. Once activated, G-actin monomers polymerize into F-actin filaments facilitating the shape change and spreading (16.0) (Fig. 15.14). As it happens when platelets are activated in suspension, nonmuscle myosin also gets phosphorylated. Platelet activation on ECM is facilitated by or promoted by the released granule components, soluble agonists, such as ADP, and thromboxanes, glycoprotein-rich

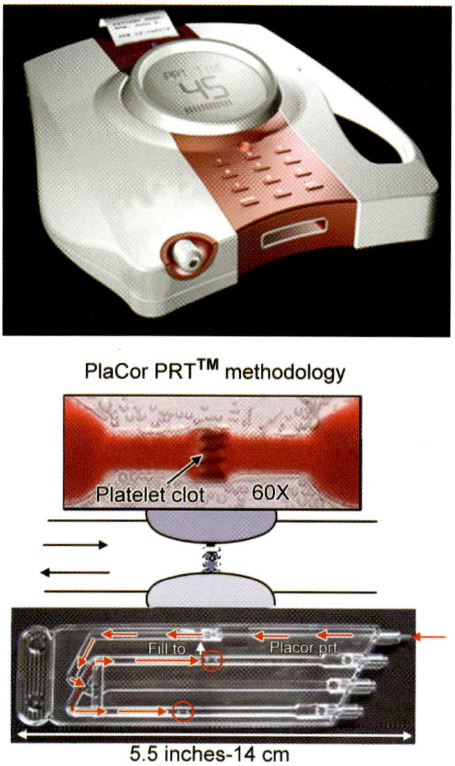

Fig. 15.15: Platelet reaction time (PRT) monitoring device developed by PlaCor, Minneapolis, MN.

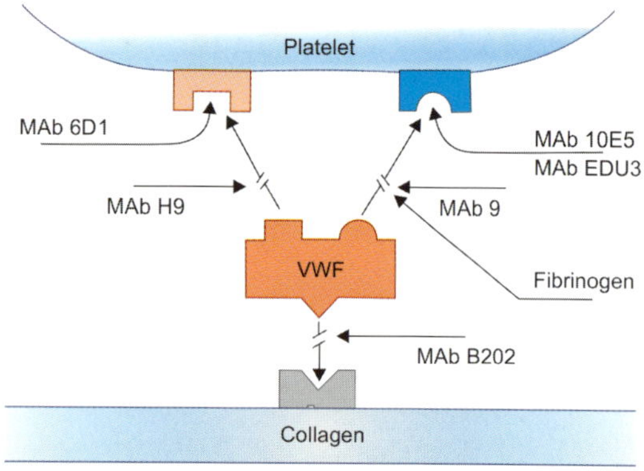

Fig. 15.16: Platelet interaction with cell- matrix components: inhibition by antibodies. (vWF, von Willebrand factor).

integrin and non-integrin receptors, and to some extent shear forces.

Platelet reaction time (PRT) monitoring device was tested at the University of Minnesota. Shear Force-mediated activation, aggregation, and clot formation was monitored.

PlaCor laboratories at Minneapolis developed a device to monitor shear force-mediated platelet activation and clot formation. The original idea for this innovation came from an observation that was made by Dr Daniel Ericson and Gundu H. R. Rao, when they were working with 3 M companies some two decades before this development. This device was validated at three independent laboratories in Minnesota. A drop of fresh blood obtained from fingerpick is introduced into capillary circulation. As the blood flows in the capillary, a stainless steel coil placed in the middle of the capillary introduces the shear force and activates platelets. Activated platelets generate thrombin and induce clot formation.[28] The time is recorded as platelet reaction time (PRT) (Fig. 15.15).

Platelet activation in suspension on surfaces, on ECM components, as well as by shear force is mediated by the same signaling events and modulated by the same biochemical pathways. By and large, aspirin and clopidogrel, commonly used antiplatelet drugs, prevent activation in suspension by soluble agonists such as AA and ADP. These drugs do not inhibit platelet interaction on vessel wall components. They will, however, inhibit thrombus growth, which is dependent on cell-cell interaction via fibrinogen binding. Our studies at the University of Minnesota have used a denuded rabbit aorta model to follow platelet-vessel wall interaction. In real-time in vivo thrombosis, platelets interact with modified endothelium surface injured subendothelium, glycocalyx, and ECM components, as such use multiple mechanisms of activation (Fig. 15.16). In view of this observation, I have provided some additional references to cover these topics.[29-98]

REFERENCES

1. Rao GHR. Physiology of blood platelet activation. Indian J Physiol Pharmacol. 1994;37: 263-75.
2. Rao GHR. Signal transduction, second messengers and platelet pharmacology. Pharmacol (Life Sci). 1994;13:39-44.
3. Rao GHR. Measurement of ionized calcium in normal human platelets. Anal Biochem. 1988;169:400-8.
4. Rao GHR. Signal transduction, second messengers and platelet function. J Lab Clin Med. 1993;121:18-22.
5. Rao GHR. Platelet hyperfunction as risk for acute coronary syndromes. In: Rao GHR, Thanikachalam S (Eds). Coronary Artery Disease: Risk Promoters, Pathophysiology and Prevention. New Delhi: JP Medical Publishers; 2004. pp. 192-201.
6. Cohn JN. Pathophysiologic and prognostic implications of measuring arterial compliance in hypertensive disease. Prog Cardiovasc Dis. 1999;41:441-50.
7. Cohn JN, Finkenstien S, McVeigh G, Morgan D, LeMay L, Robinson J, et al. Noninvasive pulse wave analysis for the early detection of vascular disease. Hypertension. 1995;26: 503-8.
8. Duprez DA, De Buyzere MM, De Bruyne L, Clement DL, Cohn JN. Small and large artery elasticity indices in peripheral arterial occlusive disease. Vasc Med. 2001;6:211-4.
9. Grey E, Bratteki C, Glasser SP, Alinder C, Finkelstein SM, Lindgren BR, et al. Reduced small artery but not large artery elasticity is an independent risk marker for cardiovascular events. Am J Hypertens. 2003;16:265-9.
10. Vallance P, Chan N. Endothelial function and nitric oxide: clinical relevance. Heart. 2001;85:342-50.
11. Ferro CJ, Webb DJ. Endothelial dysfunction and hypertension. Drugs. 1997;53:30-41.
12. Escandon JC, Cipolla M. Diabetes and endothelial dysfunction: a clinical perspective. Endocrine Rev. 2001;22:36-52.
13. Busse R, Fleming I, Hecker M. Signal transduction in endothelium-dependent vasodilation. Eur Heart J. 1993;14:2-9.
14. Sandoo A, van Zanten JJ, Metsios GS, Carroll D, Kitas GD. The endothelium and its role in regulating vascular tone. Open Cardiovasc Med J. 2010;4:302-12.
15. Rao GHR, Gandhi PG. Need for a noninvasive diagnostic platform for early detection and management of cardio-metabolic disorders. J Clin Prev Cardiol. 2014;3(3):93-8.
16. Rao GHR. Non-traditional approaches to diagnosis and management of type-2 diabetes mellitus: point of view. J Diabetes Metab. 2014;6:489.
17. Rao GHR. Platelet physiology and pharmacology: an overview. In: Rao GHR (Ed). Handbook of Platelet Physiology and Pharmacology. Boston: Kluwer Academic; 1999. pp. 1-21.
18. Kunicki TJ. Platelet membrane glycoproteins and their function: an overview. Blut. 1989;59(1):30-4.
19. Savagae B, Shatil SJ, Ruggeri ZM. Modulation of platelet function through adhesion receptors. A dual role for glycoprotein IIb-IIIa (integrin alpha and IIb beta3) mediated by fibrinogen and glycoprotein 1b-von Willebrand factor. J Biol Chem. 1992;267(16): 11300-6.
20. Rao GHR. Influence of anti-platelet drugs on platelet-vessel wall interactions. Prostaglandins Leukot Essent Fatty Acids. 1987;30:133-45.
21. Rao GHR, Escolar G, White JG. Epinephrine reverses the inhibitory influence of aspirin on platelet-vessel wall interactions. Thromb Res. 1986;44:65-74.
22. Baumgartner HR. The role of blood flow in platelet adhesion, fibrin deposition and formation of mural thrombi. Microvasc Res. 1973;5:167-79.
23. Weiss HJ, Tschopp TB, Baumgartner HR, Sussman II, Johnson MM, Egan JJ. Decreased adhesion of giant (Benard-Soulier) platelets to sub endothelium. Further implications on the role of von Willebrand factor in hemostasis. Am J Med. 1974;57:920-5.
24. Turitto VT, Baumgartner HR. Platelet interaction with sub endothelium in a perfusion system: physical role of red blood cells. Microvasc Res. 1975;9:335-44.
25. Sakariassen, KS, Muggli R, Baumgartner HR. Measurements of platelet interaction with components of the vessel wall in flowing blood. Methods Enzymol. 1989;169:37-70.

26. Escolar G, Garrido M, Aznar-Salatti J, Ordinas A, Bastida E. Comparison between human umbilical artery and rabbit abdominal aorta as substrata for platelet adhesion and platelet thrombus formation under flow conditions. Blood Vessels. 1991;28:520-31.
27. Feghi S, Sniadecki NJ. Mechanobiology of platelets: techniques to study the role of fluid flow and platelet reaction forces at the micro and nano-scale. Int J Mol Sci. 2011;12:9009-30.
28. Johnson GJ, Sharda AV, Rao GHR, Ereth MH, Laxson DD, Owen WG. Measurement of shear-activated platelet aggregate formation in no-anticoagulated blood: Utility in detection of clopidogrel and aspirin-induced platelet dysfunction. Clin Appl Thromb Hemost. 2011;17:140-9.
29. Baumgartner HR. Effects of acetylsalicylic acid, sulfinpyrazone and dipyridamole on platelet adhesion and irreversible aggregation in flowing native anticoagulated blood. Haemostasis. 1979;8:340-52.
30. Baumgartner HR, Muggli R. Adhesion and aggregation: morphological demonstration and quantitation *in vivo* and *in vitro*. In: Gordon JL (Ed). Platelets in Biology and Pathology. Amsterdam: North Holland Biomedical Press; 1976. pp. 23-60.
31. Marcum JM, McGill M, Bastida E, Ordinas A, Jamieson GA. Interaction of platelets, tumor cells and vascular endothelium. J Lab Clin Med. 1980;96:1046-53.
32. Escolar G, Bastida E, Ordinas A, Castillo R. Interaction of platelets with sub endothelium in humans treated with aspirin and dipyridamole alone or in combination. Thromb Res. 1985;40:419-24.
33. Sakariassen KS, Bolhuis PA, Blomback M. Association between bleeding time and platelet adherence to artery subendothelium. Thromb Haemost. 1984;52:144-7.
34. Weiss HJ, Turitto, VT, Vicic WJ, Baumgartner HR. Fibrin formation, fibrinopeptide A release, and platelet thrombus dimensions on sub endothelium exposed to flowing native blood. Greater in factor XII and XI than in factor VIII and IX deficiency. Blood. 1984;63:1004-14.
35. Sakariassen KS, Cattaneo M, Berg AVD, Ruggeri ZM, Mannucci PM, Sixma JJ. DDAV enhances platelet adherence and platelet aggregate growth on human artery sub endothelium. Blood. 1984;64:229-36.
36. Ruggeri ZM. Platelet adhesion under flow. Microcirculation. 2009;16(1):58-83.
37. Ruggeri ZM, Mendolicchio GL. Interaction of von Willebrand factor with platelets and the vessel wall. Hamostaseologie. 2015;35(3):211-4.
38. Hoylaerts MF. Platelet-vessel wall interactions in thrombosis and restenosis role of von Willebrand factor. Vert K Acad Geneeskd Belg. 1997;59(3):161-83.
39. Alevriadou BR, Moake JL, Turner NA, Ruggeri ZM, Folie BJ, Phillips MD, et al. Real-time analysis of shear-dependent thrombus formation and its blockade by inhibitors of von Willebrand factor binding to platelets. Blood. 1993;81(5):1263-76.
40. Chow TW, Hellums JD, Moake JL, Kroll MH. Shear stress-induced von Willebrand factor binding to platelet glycoprotein Ib initiates calcium influx associated with aggregation. Blood. 1992;80(1):113-20.
41. Rumbaut RE, Thiagarajan P. Platelet Vessel Wall Interactions in Hemostasis and Thrombosis. In: Integrated Systems Physiology: From Molecule to Function and Disease. San Rafael CA: Morgan and Claypool Life Sciences; 2010. p. 67.
42. Chen J, Lopez JA. Interactions of platelets with sub-endothelium and endothelium. Microcirculation. 2005;12(3):235-46.
43. Tailor A, Cooper D, Granger DN. Platelet-vessel wall interactions in the microcirculation. Microcirculation. 2005;12:275-85.
44. Bennett JS, Berger BW, Billings PC. The structure and function of platelet integrins. J Thromb Haemost. 2009;(7 suppl 1):200-5.
45. Bennett JS. Structure and function of platelet integrin alpha11b beta3. J Clin Invest. 2005;115:3363-9.
46. Woulfe DS. Platelet G protein-coupled receptors in hemostasis and thrombosis. J Thromb Haemost. 2005;3:2193-200.
47. Ruggeri ZM. The role of von Willebrand factor in thrombus formation. Thromb Res. 2007;120(Suppl 1):S5-9.
48. Savage B, Saldivar E, Ruggeri ZM. Initiation of platelet adhesion by arrest onto fibrinogen or translocation on von Willebrand factor. Cell. 1996;84:289-97.
49. Ruggeri ZM, Orje JN, Habermann R. Activation-independent platelet adhesion and aggregation under elevated shear stress. Blood. 2006;108:1903-10.

50. Mailhac A, Badimon JJ, Fallon JT. Effect of an eccentric severe stenosis on fibrin (ogen) deposition on severely damaged vessel wall in arterial thrombosis. Relative contribution of fibrin (ogen) and platelets. Circulation. 1994;90:988-96.
51. Sarratt KL, Chen H, Zutter MM, Santoro SA, Hammer DA, Kahn ML. GPVI and alpha-2beta1 play independent critical roles during platelet adhesion and aggregate formation to collagen under flow. Blood. 2005;106: 1268-77.
52. Jennings LK. Role of platelets in atherothrombosis. Am J Cardiol. 2009;103:4A-10A.
53. Palmer RM, Ferrige AG Moncada S. Nitric oxide release accounts for the biological activity of endothelium-derived relaxing factor. Nature. 1987;327:524-6.
54. Moncada S, Higgs EA. The discovery of nitric oxide and its role in vascular biology. Br J Pharmacol. 2006;147(Suppl 1):S193-201.
55. Dudzinxki DM, Igarashi J, Greif D, Michel T. The regulation and pharmacology of endothelial nitric oxide synthase. Annu Rev Pharmacol Toxicol. 2006;46:235-76.
56. Murad F. Shattuck lecture: nitric oxide and cyclic GMP in cell signaling and drug development. N Engl J Med. 2006;355:2003-11.
57. Radomski MW, Palmer RM, Moncada S. Endogenous nitric oxide inhibits human platelet adhesion to vascular endothelium. Lancet. 1987;2:1057-8.
58. Broeders MA, Tangelder GF, Slaaf DW, Reneman RS, Egbrink MG. Endogenous nitric oxide and prostaglandins synergistically counteract thromboembolism in venules but not in arterioles. Arterioscler Thromb Vasc Biol. 1998;18:139-45.
59. Ozuyaman B, Godecke A, Kusters S, Kirchhoff E, Scharf RE, Schrader J. Endothelial nitric oxide synthase plays a minor role in inhibition of arterial thrombus formation. Thromb Haemost. 2005;93:1161-7.
60. Naseem KM, Riba R. Unresolved roles of platelet nitric oxide synthase. J Thromb Haemost. 2008;6:1367-84.
61. Gryglewski RJ. Prostacyclin among prostanoids. Pharmacol Rep. 2008;60:3-11.
62. Mitchell JA, Ali F, Bailey L, Moreno L, Harrington LS. Role of nitric oxide and prostacyclin as vasoactive hormones released by the endothelium. Exp Physiol. 2008;93:141-7.
63. Higgs EA, Higgs GA, Moncada S, Vane JR. Prostacyclin inhibits the formation of platelet thrombi in arterioles and venules of the hamster cheek pouch. Br J Pharmacol. 1978;63:535-9.
64. Shanberge JN, Kajiwara Y, Quattrociocchi-Longe T. Effect of aspirin and iloprost on adhesion of platelets to intact endothelium *in vivo.* J Lab Clin Med. 1995;125:96-101.
65. Hantgan RR, Hindriks G, Taylor RG. Glycoprotein Ib, von Willebrand factor and glycoprotein 11b/111a are all involved in platelet adhesion to fibrin in flowing whole blood. Blood. 1990;76:345-53.
66. Reitsma S, Slaaf DW, Vink H, van Zandvoort MA, oude Egbrink MG. The endothelial glycocalyx, composition, functions, and visualization. Plfugers Arch. 2007;454:345-59.
67. Vink H, Constantinescu AA, Span JA. Oxidized lipoproteins degrade the endothelial surface layer: implications for platelet-endothelial adhesion. Circulation. 2000;101:1500-2.
68. Van den Berg BM, Vink H. Spaan JA. Endothelial glycocalyx protects against myocardial edema. Circ Res. 2003;92:592-4.
69. Smith ML, Long DS, Damiano ER, Ley K. Near-wall micro PIV reveals a hydrodynamically relevant endothelial surface layer in venules *in vivo.* Biophys J. 2003;85:637-45.
70. Baldwin AL, Winlove CP. Effects of perfusate composition on binding of ruthenium red and gold colloid to glycocalyx of rabbit aortic endothelium. J Histochem Cytochem. 1984;32:259-66.
71. Weinbaum S, Tarbell JM, Damiano ER. The structure and function of endothelial glycocalyx layer. Annu Rev Biomed Eng. 2007;9:121-67.
72. Kuijper PH, Gallaardo Tores HI, Lammers JW, Sixma JJ, Koenderman L, Zwaginga JJ. Platelet associated fibrinogen and ICAM-2 induce firm adhesion of neutrophils under flow conditions. Thromb Hemost. 1998;80:443-8.
73. Moake JL. Thrombotic microangiopathies. N Engl J Med. 2002;347:589-600.
74. Frenette PS, Denis CV, Weiss L, Jurk K, Subbarao S, Kehrel B, et al. P-Selectin glycoprotein ligand (PSGL-1) is expressed on platelets and can mediate platelet-endothelial interactions *in vivo.* J Exp Med. 2000;191:1413-22.
75. Varga-Szabo D, Braun A, Nieswandt B. Calcium signaling in platelets. J Thromb Haemost. 2009;7:1057-66.

76. Fox JE. Cytoskeletal proteins and platelet signaling. Thromb Haemost. 2001;86:198-213.
77. Goto S, Ikeda Y, Saldivar E, Ruggeri ZM. Distinct mechanisms of platelet aggregation as a consequence of different shearing flow conditions. J Clin Invest. 1998;101:479-86.
78. Povlishock JT, Rosenblum WI, Sholley MM, Wei EP. Ultrastructural analysis of endothelial change paralleling aggregation in a light/dye model of microvascular insult. Am J Pathol. 1983;110:148-60.
79. George JN, Pickett EB, Saucerman S, McEver RP, Kunicki TJ, Kieffer N, et al. Platelet surface glycoproteins. Studies on resting and activated platelets and platelet membrane microparticles in normal subjects, and observations in patients during respiratory distress syndrome and cardiac surgery. J Clin Invest. 1986;78:340-8.
80. Marten M, Pakala R, Thiagarajan P, Benedict CR. Platelet microparticles promote platelet interaction with sub endothelial matrix glycoprotein 11b/111a-dependent mechanism. Circulation. 1999;99:2577-82.
81. Afshar-Kharghan V, Thiagarajan P. Leukocyte adhesion and thrombosis. Curr Opin Hematol. 2006;13:34-49.
82. Del Conde I, Shrimpton CN, Thiagrajan P, López JA. Tissue-factor-bearing microvesicles arise from lipid rafts and fuse with activated platelets to initiate coagulation. Blood. 2005;106:1604-11.
83. Esmon CT. Basic mechanisms and pathogenesis of venous thrombosis. Blood Rev. 2009;23:225-9.
84. Franchini M, Mannucci PM. Venous and arterial thrombosis: different sides of the same coin? Eur J Intern Med. 2008;19:476-81.
85. Aird WC. Vascular bed-specific thrombosis. J Thromb Haemost. 2007;5(Suppl 1):283-91.
86. Davies MJ, Richardson PD, Woolf N, Katz DR, Mann J. Risk of thrombosis in human atherosclerotic plaque: role of extracellular lipid, macrophage and smooth muscle cell content. Br Heart J. 1993;69:377-81.
87. Badimon JJ, Lettino M, Toschi V, Fuster V, Berrozpe M, Chesebro JH, et al. Local inhibition of tissue factor reduces the thrombogenicity of disrupted human atherosclerotic plaques: effects of tissue factor pathway inhibitor on plaques thrombogenicity under flow conditions. Circulation. 1999;99:1780-7.
88. Oude Egbrink MG, van Gestel MA, Broeders MA, Tangelder GJ, Heemskerk JM, Reneman RS, et al. Regulation of microvascular thromboembolism *in vivo.* Microcirculation. 2005;12(3):287-300.
89. Oude Egbrink MG, Tangelder GJ, Slaaf DW, Reneman RS. Different roles of prostaglandins in thromboembolic processes in arterioles and venules *in vivo*. Thromb, Haemost. 1993;70:826-33.
90. Oude Egbrink MG, Tangelder GJ, Slaaf DW, Reneman RS. Fluid dynamics and the thromboembolic reaction in mesenteric arterioles and venules. Am J Physiol. 1991;260:H1826-33.
91. Lowenberg EC, Meijers JCM, Levi M. Platelet-vessel interactions in health and disease. Neth J Med. 2010;68:242-51.
92. Clemetson KJ, Clemetson JM. Platelet collagen receptors. Thromb Haemost. 2001;86:189-97.
93. Jurk K, Clemetson KJ, de Groot PG. Thrombospondin-1 mediates platelet adhesion at high shear via glycoprotein 1b (GP1b): an alternative/backup mechanism to von Willebrand factor. FASEB J. 2003;17(11):1490-2.
94. Inoue O, Suzuki-inoue K, Ozaki Y. Redundant mechanism of platelet adhesion to laminin and collagen under flow: involvement of von Willebrand factor and glycoprotein 1b-IX-V. J Biol Chem. 2008;283:16279-82.
95. Thiagarajan P, Kelly KL. Exposure of binding sites for vitronectin on platelets following stimulation. J Biol Chem. 1988;263:3035-8.
96. Ruggeri ZM. Platelets in atherothrombosis. Nat Med. 2002;8(11):1227-34.
97. Kroll MH, Hellums JD, Mcintire LV, Schafer AI, Moake JL. Platelet and shear stress. Blood. 1996;88:1525-41.
98. Falati S, Gross P, Merrill-Skoloff G, Furie BC, Furie B. Real-time in vivo imaging of platelets, tissue factor and fibrin during platelet arterial thrombus formation in the mouse. Nat Med. 2002;8(10):1175-81.

CHAPTER 16

Blood Biocompatibility Studies

BLOOD BIOCOMPATIBILITY LABORATORY (BBL), MEDICAL SCHOOL, UNIVERSITY OF MINNESOTA

Center for Interfacial Engineering (CIE), University of Minnesota, organized a brain storming session on May 17, 1995, to come up with new ideas to help to bridge the interaction between medical industries and academic health and engineering disciplines. Professor Robert Tranquillo, a faculty of the Engineering Institute, suggested organization of a workshop to discuss development of "methods and assays" for evaluating blood biocompatibility and blood material interactions. Staff that participated in this mini workshop included Ms Katherine Tweden (St Jude), Dr William Haworth (CEO, Avecor), Matthew Tirrell (HoD, Chemical Engineering), Professor Fennal Evans (Director, CIE), and Starbuck (Administrator, CIE). The group recommended the formation of a blood biocompatibility laboratory under the direction of Professor Gundu HR Rao, Director, Thrombosis, Research, Lillehei Heart Institute, University of Minnesota.

The testing facility was started at 265 Lillehei Heart Institute in 1995 under the leadership of Gundu HR Rao. Dr Thomas Chandy (an accomplished researcher in this field from Sri Chitra Tirunal Institute for Medical Sciences and Technology, Trivandrum, India), was hired as a Research Associate to help with these studies. After the new building of Basic Sciences and Biomedical Engineering (BSBE) was completed, BBL was moved to BSBE, seventh floor. Dr Rao (Director) and Dr Daniel Mooradian (Co-Director) directed the work at BBL. After Mooradian left Biomedical Engineering Institute (BMEI) for a job in the industry, BBL was moved back to Lillehei Heart Institute in 2002. Dr Rao served as the Director of BBL till his retirement in 2012.

SHORT-TERM GOALS OF BBL

To provide a platform for BMEI faculty (Robert Tranquillo; biocompatibility of small-diameter vascular bioartificial grafts) members of the Department of Medicine, Anesthesiology, and Lillehei Heart Institute, interest groups (Dr Gerald Timm; Soft Tissue Mechanics Laboratory), as well as for startup companies (Dr Thomas Chandy; CHF Solutions, Platelet interactions with membrane filters), to investigate problems associated with biocompatibility and thrombosis studies. Offer consultations to various medical device companies in the Twin Cities (Medtronic, St Jude Medical, CHF Solutions, Vascular Solutions, Biovascular, Medical CV, 3M as well as in other cities in the United States; Boston Scientific: Cardiovascular Division, MN, Stroke Division Freemont, CA).

In the early years of our existence, we trained two research fellows (Mr Michel Wolf and Dr Quin Zho) from Medtronic Inc. under a CIE-sponsored Industrial Fellow Program. We also helped Ms Katherine Tweden from St Jude Medical Inc on problems associated with biocompatibility of mechanical heart valves. In appreciation of our efforts, St Jude Medical Inc. awarded a brand new Beckman scintillation counter to Dr Rao. Dr Rao also trained Daniel Ericson of 3M Laboratories. For this effort, he received a 3M cash award. Researchers from Stroke Division of Boston Scientific, Freemont, CA, collaborated with us. Dr Rao visited their facility for consultations. A "Fee for Service Contract" was developed to facilitate collaborative studies with various industries.

BBL offered Minnesota Medical Device Companies and the staff of BMEI, the Academic Health Center University of Minnesota, a convenient central access point for testing biomaterials, medical devices, and for initiating collaborative studies in the area of blood biocompatibility and thrombosis research. With the expertise available at the University of Minnesota, we were able to customize medical device development and testing to suit the specific needs of the Medical Device Development Companies. Small startup companies made use of the testing facilities that we offered more often to improve their products. However, even larger companies were able to consult with our faculty on specific issues, Boston Scientific, Fremont, CA.

STROKE RESEARCH: PLATELET AND BLOOD CLOT STUDIES

Some of the companies which used our testing facility are St Jude Medical Inc., St Paul, (Bio-heart Valves, Mechanical Heart Valves); Bioenergy Inc., Ham Lake, MN (D-Ribose as a platelet preservative); SUBC Inc., Rochester, MN (platelet function testing system); Collagen Matrix Inc., Philadelphia, PA (perfusion studies on small diameter vascular grafts); Children's Hospital, Philadelphia, PA (indium-labeled platelet studies); CHF Solutions, Brooklyn Park, MN (platelet interactions with biopolymer filters); Medical CV, St Paul, MN (studies on omni-carbon tilting-disc heart valves); Via Cell Inc., MN (development of state-of-the-art platelet and cell preservatives for better storage); Care Point Medical, Minneapolis, Minnesota (development of point-of-Care Assays for Detection of Thrombotic State); SUBc Inc., Rochester, MN (development of medical devices; NIH-STTR Grants); Ascent Medical Technology Fund Inc, Minneapolis, MN (development of a platform for special diagnostic and clinical research in India).

Professor Gundu HR Rao served as External Examiner for PhD thesis:

P. Ravichandran: Oral Delivery of Vaccines Using Biodegradable Alginate Microspheres. Madras University, Chennai, India, 2000.

S. S Srinivasan: Preparation and Evaluation of Biodegradable Polymeric Microspheres as Carriers for Peptide and Gene Delivery. Madras University, Chennai, India, 2002.

R. L Satish, MD: Pathogenesis of Post-Surgical Adhesions in the Presence of Physical Barriers and Phospholipase A2 Inhibitors. Singapore University, Singapore, 2003.

NATIONAL INSTITUTE OF HEALTH RESEARCH GRANTS

1 R41 HL079854-01 GHR, Rao (PI)
01/19/05 to 01/18/2006

NIH-NHLBI/STTR
Rapid Detection of Bacteria in Platelet Concentrates
Goal was device development for bacteria detection.
1 R41 HL081979-01 GHR, Rao (PI)
10/01/06 to 9/30/07
NIH-NHLBI/STTR
Rapid Detection of Aspirin Resistance in Human Subjects
Goal was device development for aspirin resistance detection.

ASSAYS AVAILABLE FOR STUDIES AT BBL

Assays that were available for clients included *Parallel perfusion devices:* To test blood compatibility of flat biomaterial surfaces, membranes, and surface-modified components; *Annular perfusion devices:* These devices are used for testing various tubing used for biomedical applications, surface-modified devices, and for evaluating interaction of blood with cell matrix components.

Histology and ultrastructure: Blood cell interaction on surfaces followed by appropriate staining or specific fluorescent antibody techniques. Scanning electron microscopy for surface characterization and cell interaction studies. Ultrastructure studies for following actin assembly, cytoskeletal rearrangement, receptor mobilization, and cell activation. *Computerized morphology:* Used to assess degree of activation by monitoring surface area covered, shape change and extent of spreading, aggregation, and thrombus formation. *Immunocytochemistry:* Use of fluorescent antibodies to identify specific cell types, degree of activation, expression of activation markers, chemokines, cytokines, recruitment and rearrangement of surface membrane receptors.

Platelet Aggregation

This assay is used for the evaluation of platelet response to various agonists. It accomplishes simultaneous measurement of the kinetics of aggregation as well as release of ATP from the dense granules. Computerized system is used for studies with whole blood or cells in suspensions. *Flow cytometry:* Use of flow cytometry to follow expression of adhesion molecule, P-selectin on platelet membranes as an indicator of dense granule release. Very sensitive assay for detecting activated platelets in suspensions. Specific fluorescent antibodies were used to detect platelet-bound fibrinogen. Fibrinogen binding to platelets indicates minimal activation of these cells, without the release of granule. Platelet activation was detected by the use of antibody that detects activated IIb/IIIa receptor. Flow cytometry also was used to monitor platelet interaction on biomaterials coated on microsphere surfaces.

Surface Characterization Facility

We had access to NSF-funded surface characterization facility in the CIE, at the University of Minnesota. We have used these facilities in the past to characterize polymer, biomaterial, and medical device surfaces. We also have used their Scanning Electron Microscope for following cell–surface interactions. The Medical Device companies that used our facilities included Medtronic Inc., St Jude Medical, 3M Companies (Life Sciences Division), Medical CV, CHF Solutions, Vascular Solutions, Endocardial Solutions, Surmodics, Boston Scientific, Medical Innovations International, Rochester, MN; Bioenergy Inc., Sunnytrek Inc., Insitu Technologies, Questar, Medical Inc., ATS Medical, Terumo Heart.

Some of the materials screened at BBL for various device companies are presented in Figures 16.1 to 16.8.

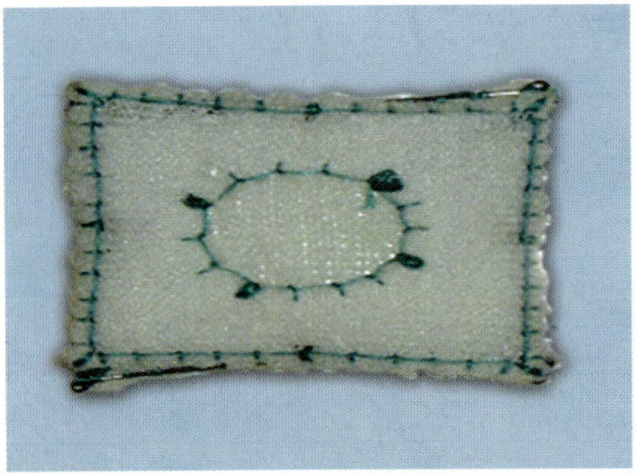

Fig. 16.1: Angel-wing closure device.

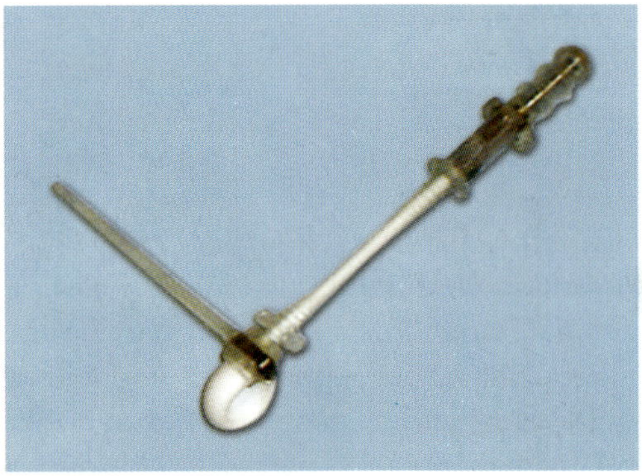

Fig. 16.2: Device for management of incontinence.

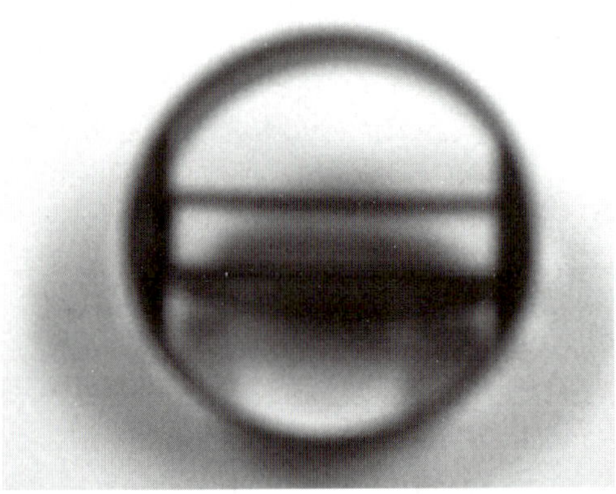

Fig. 16.3: Bileaflet heart valve.

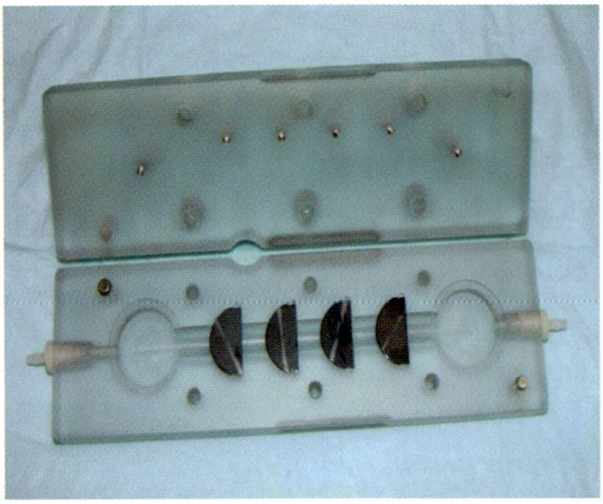

Fig. 16.4: Customized chamber for testing heart valves.

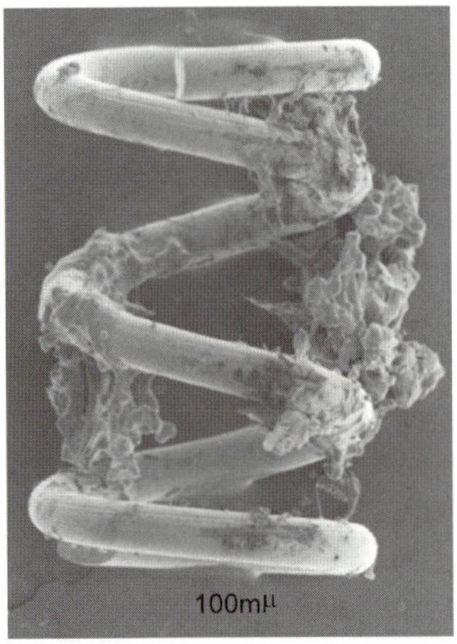

Fig. 16.5: Occluder for platelet reaction time (PRT) device.

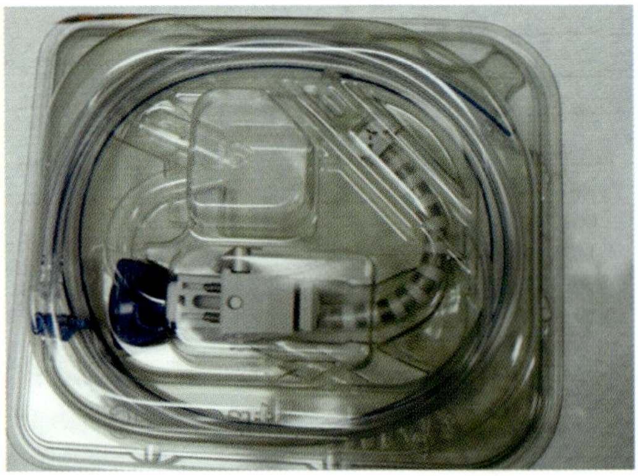

Fig. 16.6: Medtronic device used in cardiac surgery.

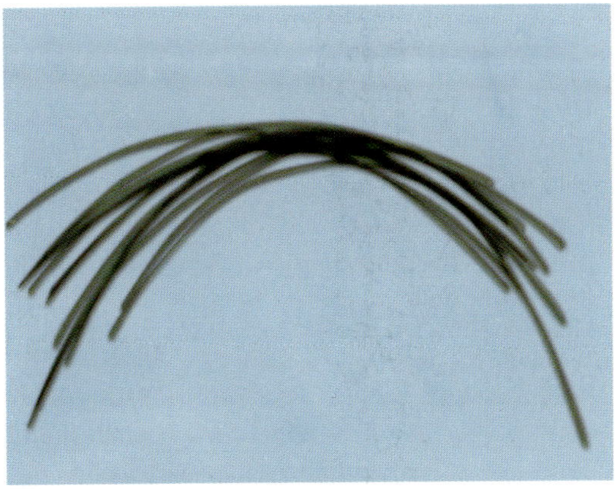

Fig. 16.7: Guidewires used in catheters.

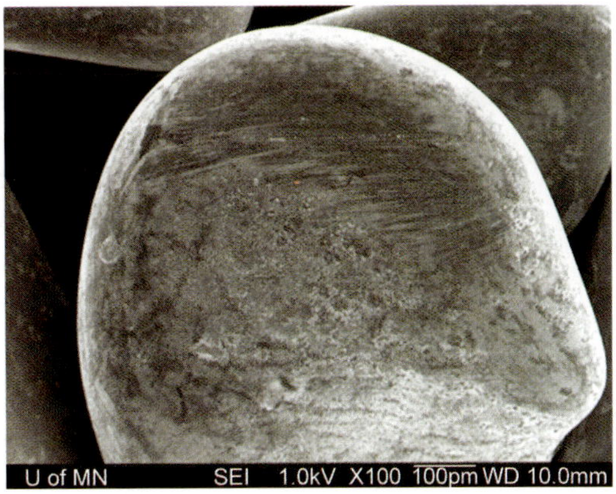

Fig. 16.8: Titanium material used for medical devices.

ROLE OF PLATELETS IN BLOOD–BIOMATERIAL INTERACTIONS

Over 2 million cardiovascular procedures are performed annually in the United States. Every one of these procedures requires some period of contact with blood with several different biomaterials used in the manufacture of assist devices or implant devices. In view of the increasing importance of the biomaterials in clinical practice, it would be timely to review briefly physiochemical characterization as well as biological evaluations. Blood compatibility encompasses a variety of events associated with blood interaction with the biomaterials used in various procedures. Two separate coagulation mechanisms are involved (arterial and venous) with different flow conditions as well as varied vessel morphology and function. At least three different interacting factors modulate normal hemostasis and the pathogenesis of thromboembolic events. They are the state of activation of coagulation pathway, circulating fibrinogen, and relative activity of platelets. When blood contacts a biomaterial surface, a variety of blood components interact with the surface. Some of the key players in platelet activation on biomaterial surface include fibrinogen and von Willebrand factor. Currently available antiplatelet drugs effectively block aggregation and secretion induced by physiological agonists such as epinephrine, adenosine diphosphate (ADP), and thromboxane in suspension. However, they do not prevent platelet interaction on biomaterial surfaces.[1]

Platelet Physiology and Function

Blood platelets play a critical role in the pathogenesis of atherosclerosis, thrombosis, and stroke. These cells interact with a variety of soluble agonists such as epinephrine, ADP, many insoluble cell matrix components, biomaterials, and medical devices.[1-20] Platelet activation on a medical device leads to adhesion, spreading, expression of adhesion molecules (P-selectin) on surface membranes, activation of prothrombin complex, tissue factor expression, fibrinogen binding, cell-cell interaction, cell-surface interaction, thrombus growth, thrombin generation, and clot formation. Medical device industry, by and large to a great extent, has relied heavily on the use of animal models such as bovine and ovine for the research and development of their devices. Early work on the development of artificial heart was exclusively done using calf and cow models. Similarly, much of the research and development work on heart valves was done using sheep and goat models. In the 80s, studies from our laboratory demonstrated that platelets from bovine and ovine models are not very reactive.[21,22] Based on our studies, we concluded that these animal models were not suitable for testing medical devices for their thrombogenic properties. We expressed our views on this subject both at meetings of the National Institutes of Heart (NIH) and Food and Drug Administration (FDA). Furthermore, we also demonstrated a fundamental difference in cell-cell interaction versus cell-surface interaction. Cell-cell interaction is mediated by the activation of GPIIb/IIIa receptor and fibrinogen binding. Activated cells recognize the amino acid sequence RGD on the surface of soluble fibrinogen in circulating blood and bind these molecules. However, surface-bound fibrinogen does not need activation of GPIIb/IIIa receptor for this process. Studies from our laboratory using a novel blood perfusion system demonstrated that cell-cell interaction can be inhibited by antiplatelet drugs, whereas cell-surface interaction cannot be inhibited by commonly used antiplatelet drugs.[23-25] In view of these observations, surface modification studies on medical devices have relied heavily on the use of polymers and heparin for achieving blood compatibility of the devices.[26-98]

Michael F. Wolf Joined as the first industrial research fellow under the new CIE program to work on biomaterials for characterizing how blood- and vascular tissue contacting devices/materials interact with the body. The loop material he tested in our BBL facility consisted of tubular test materials with and without surface modifications formed into valved Chandler loops (Fig. 16.9).[27] The components of the test circuit were connected with 9.5 × 2.4 mm or 6.4 × 1.6 mm noncoated medical-grade PVC tubing and 9.5 or 6.4 mm polycarbonate connectors to form a closed loop system. Using a BP-50 pediatric BioPump (Medtronic, Eden Prairie, MN) test system was primed with 1 L of priming solution.

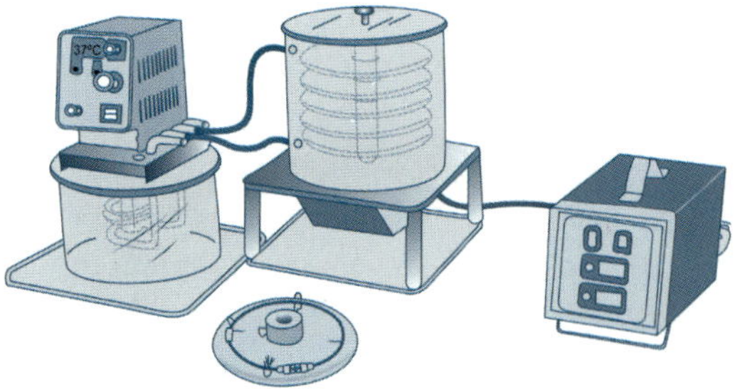

Fig. 16.9: Chandler loop system.
Courtesy: Dr Michael F Wolf, Medtronic Inc., Minneapolis, MN.

Priming solution consisted of 950 mL Ringer lactate, 20 mL 5% dextrose solution, and 30 mL of 8.4% sodium bicarbonate buffer. Five hundred milliliter of heparinized freshly drawn human blood was obtained from healthy volunteers, who had not taken any aspirin in the last 1 week before blood drawing. In order to avoid any blood-air interface, the blood bag was directly connected to the experimental reservoir blood bag, and blood was allowed to enter the test loop by gravity to replace the priming buffer. Recirculation was maintained for 90 minutes at a flow rate of 1.5 L/min^{-1} and a temperature of 30°C. Samples were taken at 0, 1, 5, 10, 20, 30, 60, and 90 minutes after starting recirculation. Blood samples were gently mixed with a mixture of citrate, theophylline, adenosine and dipyridamole (CTAD) anticoagulant (1:9 parts whole blood), centrifuged for 30 minutes at 2,000 g. After centrifugation, aliquots of the plasma were transferred to 1.5 mL Eppendorf tubes and stored at –70°C until further analysis. Standard blood analysis was conducted in accordance to recommendations of ISO standards.[28] The specific enzyme-linked immunosorbent assay (ELISA) used included thrombin–antithrombin III TAT complex, polymorphonuclear elastase, and complement C3a formation. Differential blood cell count was done using a Coulter counter. Michael Wolf and associates at Medtronic Inc., Minneapolis, Minnesota, have utilized this and other complex loop tests for evaluating blood material interactions using Carbameda bioactive heparin as well as Duraflo II heparin. They also have tested heparin-coated as well as noncoated oxygenators.[26]

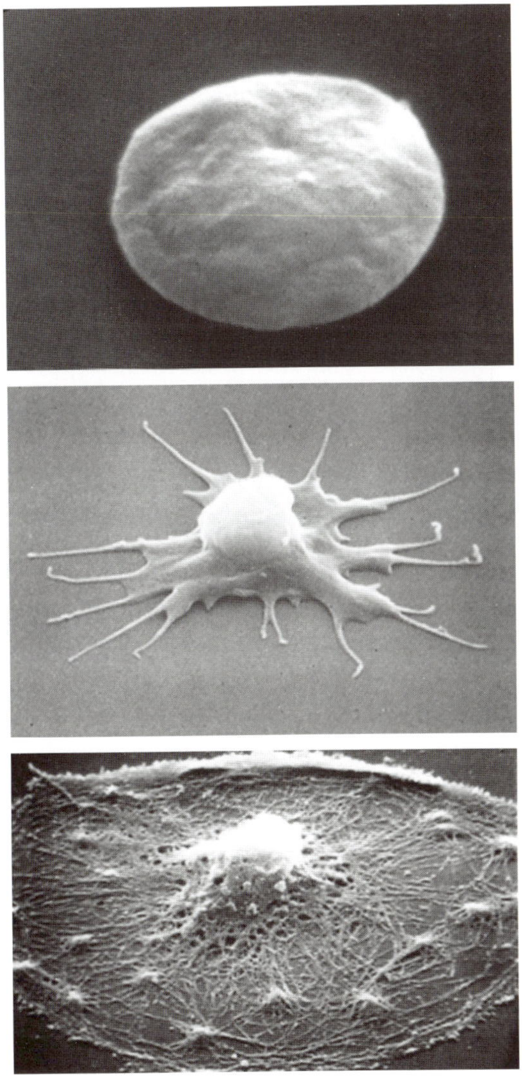

Fig. 16.10: Platelets in various stages of activation.

The compatibility of polymers used for medical devices, which facilitate the storage of blood and blood products is important, especially in device contacting blood will be reintroduced into a patient. In such cases, standard biocompatibility testing conducted in accordance with the ISO 10993, as mentioned in the previous paragraph, not only includes hemocompatibility, but also interaction of platelets on surfaces (Fig. 16.10). That is direct examination by the electron microscope (SEM/TEM). Platelet activation after adhesion to blood-contacting materials occurs with various activation steps starting with the initial attachment of cells, the spreading of the cells, and the final release of granule contents. The nonactivated state describes platelet in which platelets retain their disk-like state. The second phase occurring subsequently is the partially activated state where the pseudopods have become visible. The final phase is fully activated state, where the pseudopods have disappeared and F-actin is assembled.

VALIDATION OF BLOOD–BIOMATERIAL INTERACTIONS WITH PYROLYTIC CARBON BILEAFLET HEART VALVES

Human heart is a very efficient muscular pump with four chambers, each closed off by a one-way valve, which controls the flow of blood into these chambers. A heart valve acts like the doors of a floodgate, opening and closing to control the flow of blood in the heart. This mechanism operates over 100,000 times a day allowing flow of over 2,000 gallons equivalent circulating blood. By opening and closing in fine-tuned synchronized manner, these valves keep the blood flowing in one direction. More than 250,000 bioprosthetic heart valves are implanted annually. In the United States, more than 80,000 adults undergo procedures to replace damaged heart valves. If the prosthetic valve is made of titanium or pyrolytic carbon, the patients require lifelong anticoagulation. Complications associated with mechanical heart valves center around this kind of anticoagulation therapy. If the blood gets too much of this drug, patients may experience bleeding complications. If they get too little of this drug, then clots may form on the valve leading to acute vascular events. This situation mandates close monitoring of the blood levels of anticoagulation periodically, so that appropriate level of anticoagulation could be administered. Existing heart valve technology has not been able to find ways to avoid the problems associated with blood clotting and protein build up on the device's surface over a long period.

However, there is considerable interest in developing improved mechanical heart valves, which may not need anticoagulation therapy following implant in patients. One idea that is under active pursuit by the St Jude researchers is to develop a suitable coating that will prevent platelet activation on the carbon surface of the valves. Anja Mueller, Professor, Central Michigan University, Mt. Pleasant, MI, is trying to develop surface modification of the valve with a nonadhesive drug-coated formulation to prevent platelet and bacteria from sticking to the heart valves postimplantation. Researchers in this field also are trying to develop heart valves with plastic material that is flexible and may not require any anticoagulants. Similarly, ATS medical Inc., Minnesota is trying to improve the technology used for the design and development of the bileaflet heart valves as well as find appropriate surface modifications to prevent platelet and protein interactions on the valve surface. In this "White Paper," (Cutting edge technologies and research to improve the function of mechanical valves. Gundu HR Rao, University of Minnesota and Brian Pederson, ATS Medical Inc., Minneapolis, MN). We will describe briefly the improvements made in the development of mechanical heart valves, testing procedures, and newer techniques of surface modification of the carbon surface of the valve.

After almost three decades, pyrolytic carbon remains the most widely used material for the construction of mechanical heart valves. Mechanical heart valves have been implanted in more than 4 million patients globally in more than 25 different designs. Based on the mechanism, there are three major types of mechanical heart valves: a reciprocating ball, a tilting disk, or bileaflet valve. About 200,000 of the reciprocating ball types have been implanted. Whereas, 360,000 of the tilting disks and 600,000 of the bileaflet valves have been implanted. According to the published reports, in all, there have been only 50 failures out of the more than 1 million heart valves in use.

Most mechanical valves are made of titanium, graphite, pyrolytic carbon, pure carbon, and polyester. The titanium is used for making the housing for the valve assembly, graphite coated with pyrolytic carbon or pure carbon is used for leaflets. Pyrolytic carbon is sometimes impregnated with tungsten for visualizing postimplantation. The sewing cuff used for attaching the valve to the heart is made of double velour polyester. Till the late 90s, majority of mechanical heart valves consisted of silicon carbide-alloyed pyrolytic carbon. Pyrolytic carbon coatings were made by co-deposition of carbon and silicon carbide (3–8 wt% silicon) onto a suitable substrate using chemical vapor deposition processes. Deposition was carried out in a fluidized bed furnace supplied with silicon carrier gas and a hydrocarbon.

Pyrolytic carbon is a form of carbon coating, originally developed for nuclear fuel industry by heating a hydrocarbon gas to release carbon atoms onto a solid hardness without compromising material. In 1996, Dr Bokors and his team formed General Atomic Company, introduced pure carbon-based technology for coating heart valves. In recent years, Vincent Gott and others have compared the clotting tendencies of silicon carbide, pyrolytic carbon alloyed with silicon carbide, and pure pyrolytic carbon and found that pure carbon was least thrombogenic. Based on their results, they developed On-X-carbon heart valve with pure carbon coating. Several researchers have worked on the development of pyrolytic carbon heart valves.[29-35] Future researchers may use graphene for developing nonreactive surfaces for medical applications.

Materials and Methods

The Internal Review Board (IRB) of the Medical School, University of Minnesota, approved device material blood compatibility studies done at the BBL. Blood for these studies was obtained from volunteer donors after informed consent at the Donor Center at the University Fairview Hospital. Blood was drawn into approved sterile bags containing appropriate anticoagulant [citrate, acid-citrate-dextrose (ACD), or heparin]. Freshly collected blood was used for these studies within 2 hours after collection from volunteer donors. Blood from animals was collected from the Experimental Surgery Services at University of Minnesota.

EXPOSURE OF MECHANICAL PYROLYTIC CARBON LEAFLETS TO HUMAN BLOOD UNDER FLOW CONDITIONS

Blood perfusion system (BPS) was custom designed to meet the requirements for these specific studies (Figs. 16.11 and 16.12). For testing individual carbon leaflets, less than 100 mL of blood was used and the leaflets exposed to circulating blood in custom-developed perfusion chambers. For these studies, Watson-Marlow-Bredel Pumps (Boston, MA) were used for perfusing blood at an appropriate flow rate. After circulating blood

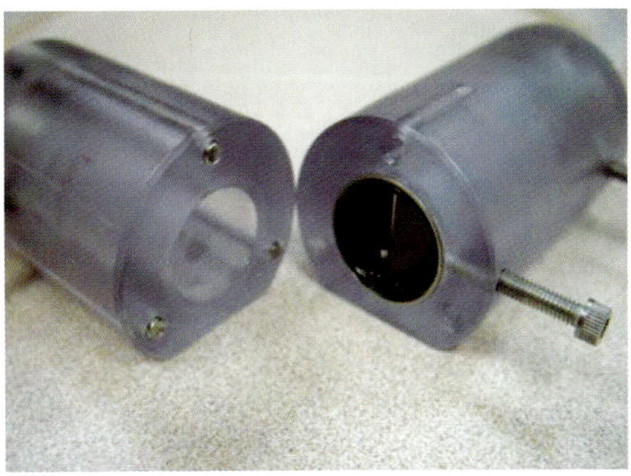

Fig. 16.11: Customized chambers for screening valves.

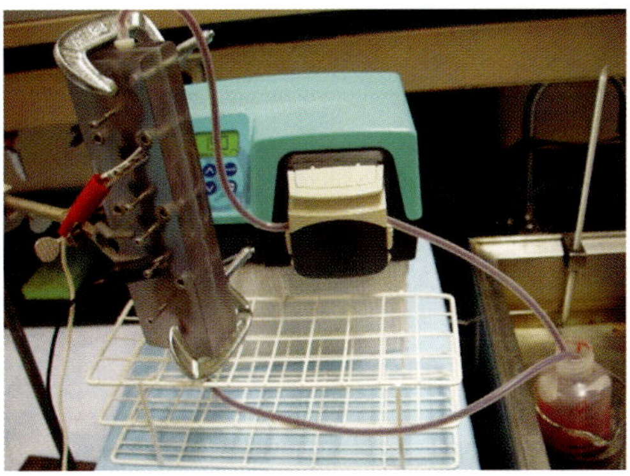

Fig. 16.12: Testing heart valves under flow conditions.

for various periods of time over the test surface the perfusion was stopped, surfaces washed with buffer and fixed for scanning electron microscopy.

EXPOSURE OF FULLY ASSEMBLED HEART VALVES TO HUMAN BLOOD UNDER FLOW CONDITIONS

For testing fully assembled valves, "MOX-100" Oxygenator (Waters Instruments, Rochester, MN) was used. Fully assembled heart valves manufactured from different companies were tested in custom-designed chambers using freshly obtained human blood as well as animal blood. Desired flow rate of blood was obtained using a diaphragm pump. After perfusing blood over the test valves for various periods of time, the valve assembly was washed with buffer, fixed with glutaraldehyde for further processing the heart valves for characterization of the surfaces by scanning electron microscopy.

Blood biocompatibility laboratory has evaluated both pyrolytic carbon (PC) leaflets as well as fully assembled heart valves manufactured by different companies using customized blood perfusion system. Although pyrolytic carbon is supposed to be very inert, all PC surfaces tested were very reactive and attracted fibrinogen and platelets onto their highly polished surfaces. Blood obtained from donors who had ingested aspirin (350 mg), clopidogrel (75 mg), or Coumadin were less reactive (10–30% less reactive) compared to control (100%). As expected, blood obtained from animals (sheep, pig) were relatively nonreactive with the valve surfaces. Significant finding from these studies was that application of "force field" current on PC surface virtually eliminated platelet interaction on charged surfaces (<5% interaction) compared to the control untreated heart valves (>90% reaction) (Figs. 16.13 and 16.14).

Slaughter and associates from the Division of Thoracic Surgery, University of Louisville, KY and Brian Pederson of ATS Medical Inc., Minneapolis, MN, evaluated the efficacy of this novel technique of electrically modifying surface of conductive biomaterials for the prevention of thrombogenesis. (This novel technique was developed at BBL with fundings from ATS Medical Inc., Minneapolis, MN). A modulated low-voltage current is

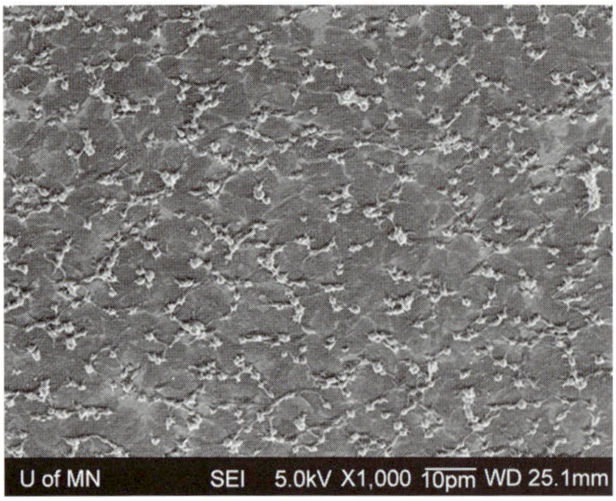

Fig. 16.13: SEM of control untreated surface.

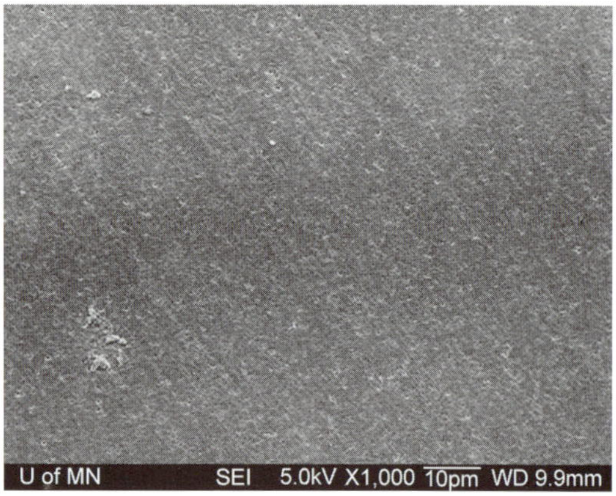

Fig. 16.14: SEM of force field treated surface.

directly applied to pyrolytic carbon surfaces to stimulate adherence of a layer of proteins form circulating blood components that are resistive to platelet deposition.[36]

For the first time in decades of research on platelet interactions, we find a breakthrough in finding a procedure that significantly prevents platelet interaction on PC surface. However, this raises lots of pertinent questions. Can we translate these findings made from a short-term exposure of devices to human blood, to human clinical conditions where one needs continued protection for the entire life? How reliable and reproducible these results are in clinical conditions? How long will force field keep the blood proteins and platelets from interacting on the charged surface? Can we develop the needed technology, using this information for human use in a variety of conditions where platelet activation will lead to acute vascular events? If our preliminary observations can be reproduced in human clinical studies without any ill effects, this procedure may have potential cardiovascular application.

The above mentioned studies on PC surfaces using pulsed force field of electric current were done at BBL, University of Minnesota, by Brain Pederson of ATS Medical, Minneapolis, MN, with help from Mrs. Debra Cocking-Johnson, Laboratory Manager, BBL, University of Minnesota.

Left ventricular-assist devices (LVADs) have been used with great clinical success as a bridge to transplant therapy. The improving reliability of next-generation LVAD technology in response to the growing shortage of donor organs has led to the application of LVADs as destination therapy (i.e. permanent implantation) as a viable alternative for treating end-stage congestive heart failure in patients with a contraindication to transplantation. This new technology, with the rotary blood pumps, is significantly smaller in size, weight, and power consumption making them easier to implant than the first-generation pulsatile devices (i.e. Heart Mate XVE), with the promise of greater longevity and reliability, leading to improved quality of life and patient outcomes. A significant challenge toward widespread clinical acceptance of these new rotary blood pumps (i.e. HeartMate II, Jarvik 2000, Heartware, etc.) is the risk of bleeding, pump thrombosis, and thromboembolic events that could lead to permanent neurocognitive dysfunction. To avoid platelet activation and minimize this risk, physicians typically prescribe varying doses of aspirin, Coumadin, Plavix, and/or Persantine. There has been no general consensus due to a lack of empirical scientific data for physicians to determine the optimal antiplatelet therapy to effectively treat LVAD patients.

LVADs are increasingly being used to treat patients with advanced cardiac failure as a bridge to transplant (BTT) or destination therapy (DT). The benefits of an LVAD in supporting patients are clear, but there are still substantial risks of complications not only during the implant period, but throughout their duration of support. Some of the most devastating complications are related to bleeding and thromboembolic events, which can lead to increased morbidity and mortality. The mechanisms behind these adverse events include platelets and the complex activation cascades that cause their activation and production. Currently, next-generation LVADs with axial or centrifugal flow rotary pump designs are in clinical trials. Many investigators believe these smaller LVADs may be more appropriate for their patients than current pulsatile devices due to their size and durability. These rotary pumps also offer the advantage of having a smaller total blood contacting surface area and lack valves.

These pumps shown below generally use titanium alloys for interior pump surfaces and expose blood to transient shear stresses from rotors that spin in the 5,000–12,000 rpm range. However, these high-speed rotary pumps can generate shear stresses that may lead to platelet activation. Thus, an LVAD patient-specific anticoagulation therapy is required to reduce platelet activation and avoid bleeding complications while minimizing the risk of thromboembolic and hemorrhagic events that may lead to permanent neurocognitive dysfunction (Fig. 16.15).

An exploratory investigation was conducted as a contract research between Dr Mark Slaughter's group at the Christ Medical Center, Chicago, IL, and BBL, University of Minnesota, to determine the level of platelet activation and the efficacy of antiplatelet therapy in LVAD patients. The IRB at Advocate Christ Medical Center (ACMC, Oak Lawn, IL) approved this exploratory study. A single blood sample (7.2 mL, EDTA tube) from 34 ambulatory heart failure patients being supported by a HeartMate II continuous axial flow pump (Thoratec, Pleasanton, CA) was collected to obtain the preliminary data on degree of platelet activation for each patient at one point in time. These single sample points for each patient were collected at different (1) lengths of LVAD support, (2) age of patient, and (3) anticoagulation therapy. Parameters for collection of data included information about age and gender of the patients, anticoagulation therapy (aspirin and Coumadin), platelet activation (sP-selectin and sCD40L),

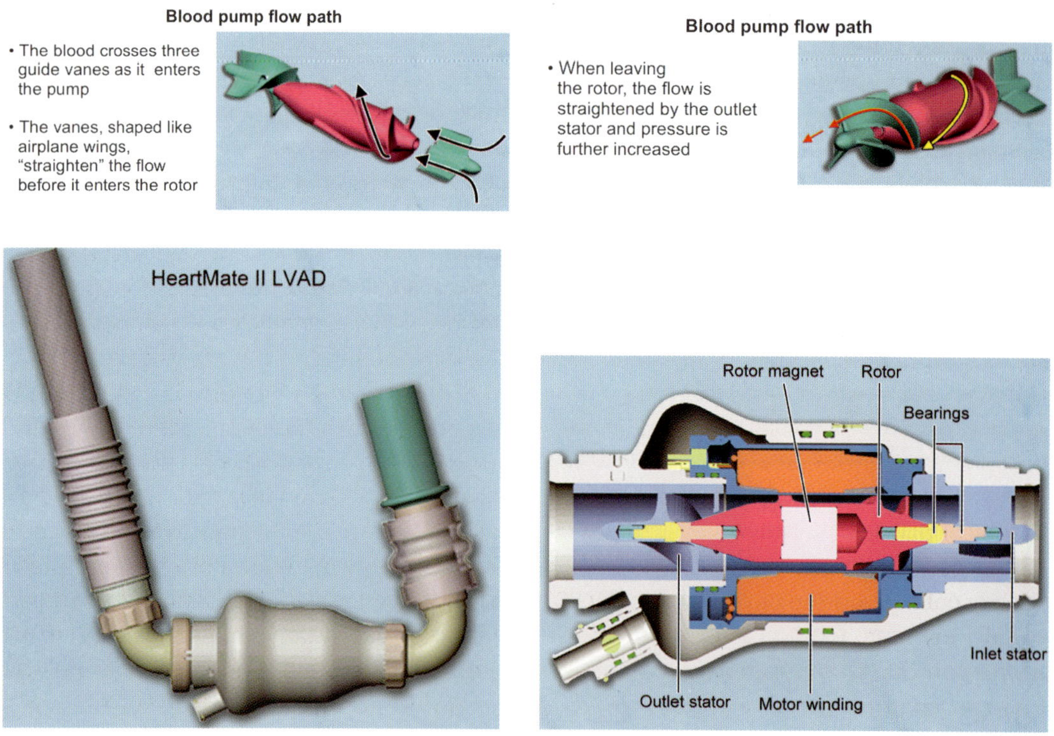

Fig. 16.15: HeartMate pumps are used as temporary vascular-assist devices to prevent end-stage congestive heart failure. These pumps are made of titanium alloys and expose blood to transient shear force stress from rotors that spin at 5,000 to 12,000 rpm range.
Courtesy: THORATEC Corp, St Jude Medical, USA.

hematological [hematocrit (Hct), hemoglobin (Hgb), international normalized ratio (INR), and platelet count], and renal [creatinine (Cr), blood urea nitrogen (BUN)] markers. A single blood sample was used to calculate these parameters, which was collected during different lengths of LVAD support (time of current device). Blood samples were analyzed at the BBL facilities at the University of Minnesota. Plasma supernatant was extracted from the blood samples following centrifugation (15 minutes, 1,000 × g) to quantify levels of platelet activation using sP-selectin and Quantikine CD40 Ligand immunoassay test at R&D Systems, Inc (Minneapolis, MN). The Hct, Hgb, INR, platelet count, Cr, and BUN were determined using standard laboratory practices. In formulating meaningful hypotheses toward determining whether current anticoagulation therapies for pulsatile LVAD (i.e. HeartMate XVE) are suitable for these new rotary blood pumps (i.e. HeartMate II), the platelet activation marker data (sP-selectin and sCD40) were pooled by (1) length of LVAD support (<6 months, 6–12 months, 12–18 months, and >18 months), (2) patient's age (<50 years, 50–65 years, and >65 years), and (3) anticoagulation therapy (aspirin or Coumadin dose). The preliminary data suggested an age effect for sCD40L; time on LVAD effect for sP-selectin and sCD40L; aspirin effect for sCD40l, and Coumadin dose effect for sP-selectin. Statistical interpretation of these findings is limited due to small number of patients, use of single data point, absence of control data, and the fact that data were not collected at the same length of LVAD support or time intervals. For additional information on this topic, readers are urged to refer recent reviews by the experts.[37,38]

Innovative and novel medical technologies will have the potential to greatly improve the public health in many different areas. FDA believes that by addressing and clarifying regulatory uncertainty, development of new technologies will be expedited and the predictability in product development will be increased. This should allow more of these products to reach the marketplace in a timely manner. As part of a broad effort to increase the development of novel medical technologies, FDA recently conducted a public workshop entitled, "Innovative Systems for Delivery of Drugs and Biologics: Scientific, Clinical and Regulatory Challenges." The workshop was held in July 2003 in Bethesda, Marriott. Speakers included outstanding researchers and product developers from academia and industry as well as regulatory authorities and experts from the FDA and outside government. The workshop provided a forum for the academic, clinical, and industry communities and the FDA to discuss the latest scientific and clinical developments for drug and biological delivery systems as well as the perceived regulatory concerns and challenges.[39]

Combination products are therapeutic and diagnostic products that combine drugs, devices, and/or biological products. FDA expects to receive large numbers of combination products for review as technological advances continue to merge product types and blur the historical lines of separation between FDA's medical product centers, which are made up of the Center for Biologics Evaluation and Research (CBER), the Center for Drug Evaluation and Research (CDER), and the Center for Devices and Radiological Health (CDRH). Because combination products involve components that would normally be regulated under different types of regulatory authorities and frequently by different FDA Centers, they raise concerns relating to regulatory policy and review management challenges. Differences in regulatory pathways for each component can impact the regulatory processes for all aspects of product development and management, including preclinical testing, clinical investigation, marketing applications, manufacturing and quality control, adverse event reporting, promotion and advertising, and postapproval modifications.

As a part of our effort in the newly established Blood Biomaterial Compatibility Laboratory, we started a series of investigations leading to the development of polymer-based targeted drug delivery systems for cardiovascular and other therapeutic applications.[40-51] As we mentioned in earlier chapters, any material or device that comes in contact with blood needs to be evaluated for the blood compatibility. In view of these regulatory requirements, many of the polymer-based drugs for targeted delivery also needed thorough evaluation in our blood biocompatibility facility. Much of the work on polymer-based drug development used nano or microspheres of polymers or lipid lysosomes for dispensing drugs. Nanoparticles and microparticles are colloidal drug carriers in the micro- and submicron range. Targeting the delivery of drugs to the diseased areas using suitable drug carriers is one of the important aspects of drug delivery system. Nano- and microparticle carriers have important potential applications for the administration of therapeutic molecules to the diseased lesions.

Controlled drug delivery technology represents one of the frontier areas of science, which involves multidisciplinary scientific approach contributing to human health care. These delivery systems offer numerous advantages compared to conventional dosage forms, which include improved efficacy, reduced toxicity, and improved patient compliance and convenience. Controlled drug delivery occurs when a polymer, whether natural or synthetic, is judiciously combined with a drug or other active agent in such a way that the active agent is released from the material in a predesigned manner. The release of the active agent may be constant over a long period, it may be cyclic over a long period, or it may be triggered by the environment milieu or other external events. Other advantages of using controlled-delivery systems include the maintenance of drug levels within a desired range, the need for fewer administrations, optimal use of the drug in question.

A wide range of polymers have been employed to control the release of drugs and other active agents. To be successfully used in controlled drug delivery formulations, a material must be chemically inert and free of leachable impurities. It must also have an appropriate physical structure with minimal undesired aging and be readily processable. However, in recent years, additional polymers designed primarily for medical applications have entered the arena of controlled release. Many of these materials are designed to degrade within the body. The greatest advantage of these degradable polymers is that they are broken down into biologically acceptable molecules that are metabolized and removed from the body via normal metabolic pathways. However, biodegradable materials do produce degradation byproducts that must be tolerated with little or no adverse reactions within the biological environment.

Platelet Adhesion on Biomaterials

Activation of platelets by contact with synthetic surfaces is a key event in the thromboembolic complications of prosthetic devices in contact with blood. It is known that a film of plasma protein adsorbs on the surface of biomaterials exposed to blood and this event precedes interaction of the surface with platelets. As mentioned before in our writing, platelet adhesion to the surfaces occurs via various stages of activation, adhesion, shape change, pseudopod formation, spreading, signal transduction, calcium mobilization, generation of second messengers, contraction, and secretion of granule contents. These changes are collectively termed surface-mediated platelet activation. Platelets under flow conditions are seen to adhere rapidly to various surfaces upon contact either as a monolayer or as aggregates and this process is influenced by a combination of factors including surface texture, surface charge, wettability, surface tension, and the flow conditions (vessel wall shear stress).

Immediately following implantation, the prosthetic surface is exposed to flowing blood, and plasma proteins are adsorbed on the surface of the synthetic surface. The proteins such as albumin, fibrinogen, and globulins are rapidly deposited on exposed surfaces and are partially replaced over time by high-molecular-weight kininogen, Hageman factor, fibronectin, hemoglobin, and von Willebrand factor. The platelet–surface interaction can be described as consisting of three consecutive events. An initial platelet-to-surface adhesion occurs between platelet membrane receptors and adsorbed matrix proteins on the biomaterial surface. The information provided by the interactive domains of cell matrix components dictates the degree of activation. For instance, laminin induces only focal adhesion of platelets onto the surface. Whereas, fibronectin promotes spreading on the surface and triple helical collagen supports aggregation and secretion of granule contents. Thrombus formation and thrombus growth result from the deposition of additional blood elements and recruitment of additional platelets.

Fibrinogen appears to be an important component of the adsorbed protein film and may be an essential player in the early events of platelet activation adsorbing preferentially on many surfaces in a concentration relatively higher than in the bulk plasma. One should remember that the platelet adhesion to fibrinogen on surface does not require activation of GPIIb/IIIa receptor on platelets. On the other hand, in suspension agonist-mediated signal transduction and activation of GPIIb/IIIa receptor are essential for activation of GPIIb/IIIa and fibrinogen binding.

We have studied platelet activation and spreading on glass surfaces under high shear (1,000 s^{-1}) using washed platelets, platelets in plasma, and whole blood using fluorescence optima's imaging system and software. The studies demonstrated that the platelet adhesion and spreading was higher with fibrinogen, fibronectin, and von Willebrand factor-coated glass surfaces and least on albumin-coated surfaces. The variations in platelet adhesion and spreading on albuminated glass and other adhesive proteins-coated glass may be due to the status and availability of platelet and other protein molecules in solution at the interface. Adhesive proteins, in general, possess tripeptide sequence of amino acids arginine-glycine-aspartic acid (RGD), binding sites, which interact with GPIIb/IIIa and induce signal transduction events such as calcium mobilization, actin assembly, contraction, and secretion. The plasma proteins such as fibrinogen and von Willebrand factor are unable to bind their respective receptors on platelets in suspension, yet once adsorbed on a surface, the proteins become active and are capable of receptor–ligand coupling.

The in vitro study of the hemocompatibility of biomaterials requires the consideration of many parameters such as static or dynamic contact, flow rate, wall shear rate, form of biomaterial to be tested, various stages of platelet activation to be monitored, and duration of contact. For surface modification of biomaterials, synthetic polyelectrolytes (SPEs) are used. Polyelectrolytes are synthetic analogs having sulfamate and carboxyl groups arranged in a steric manner as that of heparin. The SPEs have been shown to enhance surface binding of albumin and to reduce binding of fibrinogen and γ globulins. The observations that SPE reduces platelet-surface attachments may partly be due to the reduced availability of platelet receptors for fibrinogen on the modified biomaterial surfaces.

In clinical conditions, foreign surfaces represent only one of the factors influencing the blood-biomaterial interactions. These interactions also are influenced by the presence of antithrombotic agents, the blood condition (status of coagulability), and the nature of the device. The increasing use of biomaterials in cardiovascular and other applications underlies the need for a better understanding of the blood-biomaterial interactions. Since various theranostic applications include the use of polymers as substrates (nano/microspheres) for drug delivery to the targeted sites, one needs to evaluate the compatibility of these drugs/devices for hemocompatibility. Indeed, even the synthetic bioresorbable vascular grafts are considered as devices for regulatory purposes. A recent comparative review of bioresorbable stents with drug-eluting stents (DESs) has been published in the *New England Journal of Medicine* (March 2017, DOI 10.1056/NEJMoa1614954).

In order to overcome the shortcomings of DESs, bioresorbable (BIOR) vascular grafts were developed for use in percutaneous coronary interventions (PCI). In this study reported in *New England Journal of Medicine* (1845), patients were given a choice between BIOR and DES stents. The median follow-up was 707 days. The authors concluded, "In this preliminary report of a trial undergoing PCI, there was no significant difference in the rate of target-vessel failure between the patients who received BIOR and DES." The bioresorbable scaffold was associated with a higher incidence of device thrombosis than in the metallic stent through 2 years of follow-up. The study was funded by Abbott Vascular AIDA Clinical Trials (gov. number NCT01858077). Based on the results of this study, the US FDA has asked the manufacturers of the BIOR to use a warning label on their product. This demonstrates the need for robust hemocompatibility studies for all implantable devices. In view of the fact that this is a very important topic, I have included additional references at the end of this article.[52-98]

NOVEL NANOPARTICLE-BASED THERANOSTICS: EXPECTATIONS AND LIMITATIONS

I was invited by the Indian Institute of Technology (IIT), Guwahati, Assam, in February of this year (2017) to participate in a workshop on nanotechnology. I was asked to discuss novel uses of nanotechnology for theranostics. Theranostic nanomedicine using nanosystems capable of diagnosis targeted drug delivery and monitoring therapeutic responses are becoming important for developing personalized medicine. Emerging technologies have enabled construction of such function-integrated systems for therapeutic applications. For instance, in the development of theranostic therapies for cancer, one should have an immunotoxin and an antibody that is specific for the tumor to be treated, if not, the delivery of the toxin would be nonspecific. One such system of clinical relevance is targeted delivery of bioactive molecules to tumor cells.

Nanoparticles were first developed in the 70s and were initially used for delivering vaccine and anticancer drugs. Nanoparticles are roughly defined as submicron-sized colloidal systems (varying in size from 10 to 1,000 nm), biodegradable or nondegradable, and have a matrix-like structure. The active compounds are firmly adsorbed at the nanoparticle surface, entrapped/encapsulated, or dissolved in their matrix. Microspheres are spherical microscopic particles that range in size from 1 to 1,000 µm and are developed from degradable or nondegradable polymers. Microspheres can be synthesized via two different strategies. The spheres can be produced from linear preexisting polymer chains or can be formed during the polymerization process starting from a monomer solution.[52]

In micro- or nanocapsules, the drug can be present in a liquid form, it can be dissolved or suspended in a liquid or solid core, or it may be present in the core itself. Figure 16.16 indicates the various forms of drug loadings to nanospheres. Microspheres are monolithic particles possessing a porous or solid polymer matrix, whereas microparticles consist of a polymeric membrane surrounding a solid or liquid drug reservoir.[51]

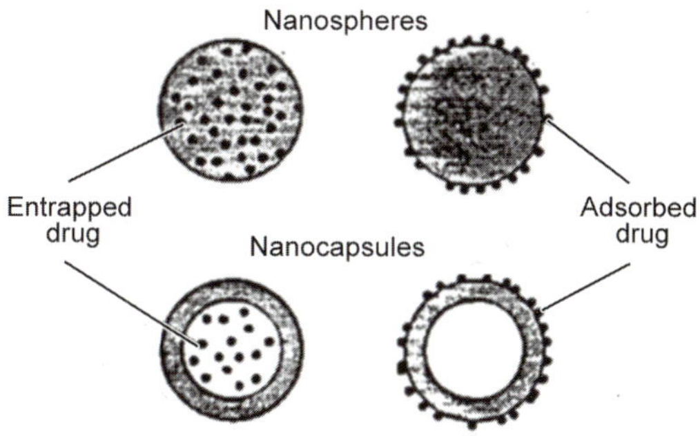

Fig. 16.16: Various types of drug-loaded nanoparticles.
Courtesy: Chandy and Rao[52]

NANO- AND MICROPARTICLES IN CARDIOVASCULAR DRUG DELIVERY

Smooth muscle cell proliferation plays a major role in the genesis of restenosis after angioplasty or vascular injury. Controlled release of appropriate drugs alone and in combinations is one approach for treating coronary obstructions, balloon angioplasty, restenosis associated with thrombosis, and calcification.[52-60] Restenosis or pathological narrowing of newly opened coronary arteries remains the major limitation of percutaneous transluminal coronary angioplasty in treating coronary artery disease. Despite intense experimental and clinical efforts, the incidence of restenosis remains at greater than 30–40% of treated patients after balloon angioplasty and 20–30% after coronary stent implantation. To inhibit vascular smooth muscle cell proliferation, drugs must be used at a high concentration for a prolonged time. Applying local drug delivery techniques in treating restenosis with antiproliferative agents is a novel strategy in enhancing drug efficacy while minimizing systemic toxicity.[59,60] Thus, an urgent need exists to prevent restenosis using newer methods of targeting and using combinations of pharmacologic agents.

In a collaborative study Chandy et al. demonstrated the possibility of entrapping an antiproliferative agent, Taxol, in polyethylene glycol (PEG)-coated, biodegradable PLA microspheres with a mean diameter of 1–6 µm. The release of the drug was sustained over 4 weeks in vitro. The amount of drug release was much higher initially (25–30%); this was followed by a constant slow release for a 30-day period of study.[58] This PEG-coated PLA microsphere formulation has shown potential for the targeted delivery of antiproliferative agents to treat restenosis.[58] This study also indicated the possibility of encapsulating Taxol-loaded PLA microspheres within heparin–chitosan spheres to

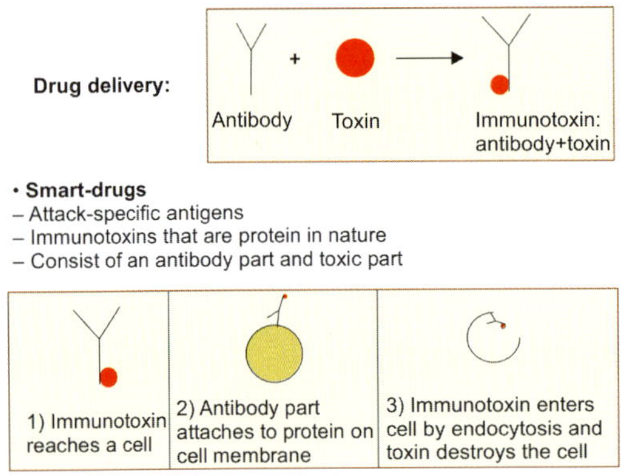

Fig. 16.17: Targeted delivery of anticancer molecules.

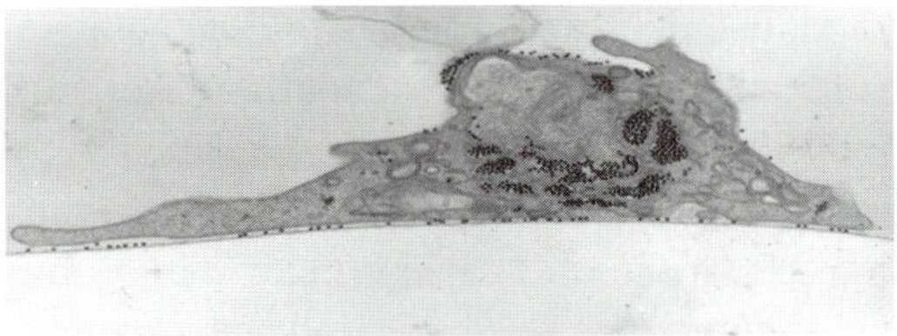

Fig. 16.18: Receptor-mediated internalization of nanogold by platelets.

develop prolonged release co-matrix form. The initial burst release of Taxol (15.8%) and heparin (32.7%) from the co-matrix was further modified with PEG coatings (13.5 and 25.4%), respectively, for 24 hours. This study showed the release of drug combinations having synergistic effects for prolonged periods for treating restenosis. Dr Ronald Shebuski, a close associate of mine (PI of our collaborative project at Questar Inc., Minneapolis, MN) has also done similar studies and reached the same conclusion about the prevention of restenosis using targeted delivery of antiproliferative drugs to the site of injury.[60]

Dr Shebuski and associates investigated biodegradable nanoparticles (100 ± 39 nm in diameter, mean ± SD) for the local intra-arterial drug delivery. The specific purpose of this study was to investigate nanoparticle surface modifications to enhance their arterial uptake. They used polylactic polyglycolic acid copolymer (PLGA) nanoparticles formulated by an oil-in-water emulsion solvent evaporation technique, using a 2-aminochromone (U-86983, Upjohn and Pharmacia) (U-86) as a model antiproliferative agent. They used various formulations of nanoparticles to validate the arterial wall uptake by using an ex vivo dog femoral artery model. The selected formulations were also tested in vivo in acute dog femoral artery and pig coronary artery models. In these studies, nanoparticles' surface modified with a cationic compound, didodecyldimethylammonium bromide (DMAB), demonstrated 7- to 10-fold greater arterial U-86 levels, compared to the unmodified nanoparticles in different ex vivo and in vivo studies.

Use of a novel theranostic has been described in which thiolated siRNA has been incorporated onto aminated dextran particles using N-succinimidyl-3-(2-pyridylthio) propionate (SPDP) with a near-infrared dye Cy5.5 and myristoylated polyarginine peptide (MPAP), a membrane translocation peptide. These probes were equipped with siRNA that target green fluorescence protein (GFP) and the conjugates were tested against mouse bilateral 9LGFP and 9LRFP tumors (Fig. 16.17). These conjugates have been successfully tested against human colorectal carcinoma xenograft model. Since my area of interest is cardiometabolic diseases, I will share some of our research efforts related to the management of these chronic disorders using novel cellular, molecular, and theronastic therapies.

Studies from our laboratory also demonstrated the use of nanoparticles of gold to follow the receptor-mediated internalization of fibrinogen in platelets (Fig. 16.18). We further explored the use of micro- and nanospheres for targeted drug delivery as well as for encapsulation of cells for use as bioartificial organs.

We demonstrated the possibility of entrapping an antiproliferative agent, Taxol, in PEG-coated biodegradable polylactic acid microspheres with a mean diameter of 2–6 µm. This was one of the very early studies in which we demonstrated that PEG-coated formulation might have potential for the targeted delivery of antiproliferative agents to treat restenosis. Currently, we are working on the development of targeted delivery of "clot busters" using biodegradable nanoparticles coupled with thrombolytic drugs.

The efficiency of cytotoxic siRNA delivery using carbon nanotubes has been shown to be greater than using cationic DOTAP: cholesterol liposomes. Prostate-specific membrane antigen (PSMA) offers a great promise for targeting prostate cancer imaging and therapy. PSMA is a transmembrane carboxypeptidase with cell surface expression of several orders magnitude higher in malignant cells and is internalized. Studies have demonstrated the ability of aptamer siRNA chimeras to kill PSMA-expressing cells with cytotoxicity upon injection. When clustered nanoparticles (PH-sensitive) of cisplatinum reach the acidic pH near the tumor, microenvironment releases nanoparticles of cisplatinum. We, in India, are developing silver nanoparticles, which when tweaked with infrared waves become activated and raise temperature inside the cells to toxic levels. Currently, we are working with in vitro conditions to develop specificity and safety for such therapies.

We would like to develop methods to produce particles that are all between 20 and 40 nm in size (a nanometer is one billionth of a meter), a range best able to elude macrophages (how about platelets?). Also coat them with a polyethylene glycol shell, which helps them survive longer in blood circulation and enter target cells. Finally, incorporate powerful light-absorbing chlorine-based molecules that turn these nanoparticles into tumor killers. As an example, it has been shown that Zn-pyrophosphate (ZnP) nanoparticles loaded with the photosensitizer pyrolipid (ZnP@pyro) can kill tumor cells upon irradiation with light directly by inducing apoptosis and/or necrosis and indirectly by disrupting tumor vasculature and increasing tumor immunogenicity. In our laboratory in Bengaluru (www.stellixir.org), we are investigating the mechanism by which these nanoparticles exert their toxicity.

REFERENCES

1. Rao GHR, Chandy T. Role of platelets in blood-biomaterial interactions. Bull Mater Sci. 1999;22(3):633-39.
2. Rao GHR. Physiology of blood platelet activation. Indian J Physiol Pharmacol. 1993; 37(4):263-75.
3. Marcus AJ, Zucker MB. The Physiology of Blood Platelets. New York: Crune and Stratton; 1965. p. 162.
4. Caen J. Platelet Aggregation. Paris: Masson and Cie; 1971. p. 228.
5. Brinkhous KM, Sherman RW, Mostof FK. The Platelet. Baltimore: Williams and Wilkinson Co.; 1971. p. 420.
6. Johnson SA. The Circulating Platelet. New York: Academic Press; 1971. p. 601.
7. Weiss HJ. Platelets and their role in hemostasis. Annu Re. N Y Acad Sci. 1972;201:1-450.
8. Ciba Foundation. Biochemistry and Pharmacology of Platelets. New York: Elsevier; 1975. p. 352.
9. Caen JP, Cronberg S, Kubisz P. Platelet Physiology and Pathology. New York: Stratton International Medical Book Co; 1977. p. 136.
10. de Gaetano G, Garattini S. Platelets: A Multidisciplinary Approach. New York: Raven Press; 1977. p. 485.
11. Kwan HC, Bowie EJW. Thrombosis. Philadelphia: W. B. Saunders; 1982. p. 331.
12. Phillips DR, Shuman MA. Biochemistry of Platelets. New York: Academic Press; 1986. p. 462.

13. Coleman RW, Hirsch J Marder VJ, Salzman EW. Hemostasis and Thrombosis: Basic Principles and Clinical Practice. Philadelphia: JB Lippincott Co.; 1987. p. 1507.
14. Bloom AL, Thomas DP. Hemostasis and Thrombosis. London: Churchill Livingstone; 1987. p. 1022.
15. Marguerie, G, Zawaal RFA. Biochemistry and physiology of platelet membrane. London: John Libbey; 1988. p. 189.
16. Corriveau DM, Fritsma GA. Haemostasis and thrombosis in the clinical laboratory. Philadelphia: JB Lippincott Co; 1988. p. 443.
17. Crawford N, Scrutton MC. Biochemistry of the blood platelet. In: Bloom AL,Thomas DP (Eds). Hemostasis and thrombosis. Eddinburgh: Churchill and Livingstone, 1987: 47-77.
18. Nachman RL. Thrombosis and atherogenesis: molecular connections. Blood. 1992;79: 1897-906.
19. Seiss W. Molecular mechanisms in platelet activation. Physiol Rev. 1989;69:59-178.
20. Michelson AD. Platelets, 3rd edition. New York: Elsevier; 2013.
21. Weiss DJ, McClay CB, Smith CM, Rao GHR, White JG. Platelet function in the racing thoroughbred, implications of exercise-induced pulmonary hemorrhage in the equine athlete. Vet Clin Pathol. 1990;19(2):35-9.
22. Grouse LH, Rao GHR, Weiss DJ. Surface activated bovine platelets do not spread, they unfold. Am J Pathol. 1990;136:369-408.
23. Rao GHR, White JG. Disaggregation and reaggregation of "irreversibly" aggregated platelets: a method for more complete evaluation of antiplatelet drugs. Agents Actions. 1985;16(5):425-34.
24. Rao GHR, Escolar G, White JG. Epinephrine reverses the inhibitory influence of aspirin on platelet-vessel wall interactions. Thromb Res. 1986;44:65-74.
25. Rao GHR. Influence of anti-platelet drugs on platelet-vessel wall interactions. Prostaglandins Leukot Med. 1987;30:133-45.
26. Munch K, Wolf MF, Gruffaz P, Ottenwaelter C, Bergan M, Schroeder P, et al. Use of simple and complex *in vitro* models for multiparameter characterization of human blood-material/device interactions. J Biomater Sci Polym Ed. 2000;11(11):1147-63.
27. Chandler AB. In vitro thrombotic coagulation of the blood: a method for producing a thrombus. Lab Invest. 1958;7(2):110-4.
28. International Standard ISO 10993-4-2017. Biological evaluation of medical devices—part 4: selection of tests for interactions with the blood. 1992. https://www.iso.org/standard/32086.html.
29. Gott VL, Alejo DE, Cameron DE. Mechanical heart valves: 50 years of evolution. Ann Thorac Surg. 2003;76:S2230-9.
30. Goodman SL, Tweden KS, Albrecht TA. Platelet interaction with pyrolytic carbon heart valves. J Biomed Mater Res. 1996;32:249-58.
31. Goodman AL, Scranton VL, Brendzel AM. Platelet responses to silicon-alloyed with pyrolytic carbons. J Biomed Mater Res. 2007;83:64-9.
32. Mantero D, Piuri D, Montevecchi S, Vesentini S, Ganazzoli F, Raffaini G. Albumin adsorption onto pyrolytic carbon: a molecular mechanics approach. J Biomed Mater Res. 2002;59:329-39.
33. Tsai CC, Huo HH, Kulkarni P, Eberhart RC. Biocompatible coatings with high albumin affinity. ASAIO Trans. 1990;36:M307-10.
34. Zhang J, Blackmore PF, Hargrave BY, Xiao S, Beebe SJ, Schoenbach KH. Nanosecond pulse electric field (nanopulse): a novel non-ligand agonist for platelet activation. Arch Biochem Biophys. 2008;471:240-8.
35. Chin JA, Phillips RE, Lew KR, Horbett TA. Tenacious binding of fibrinogen and albumin to pyrolytic carbon and biomer. J Colloid Interface Sci. 1996;184:11-9.
36. Slaughter MS, Pederson B, Graham JD, Sobieski MA, Koenig SC. Evaluation of new forcefield technology: reducing platelet adhesion and cell coverage of pyrolytic carbon surfaces. J Thorac Cardiovasc Surg. 2011;142:921-5.
37. Black MC, Schumer EM, Trivedi JR, Slaughter MS. Recent advances in assist devices. In: Rao GHR (Ed). Coronary Artery Disease. New Delhi: Macmillan Medical Communications; 2017. pp. 293-7.
38. Kamdar F, John R. Mechanical circulatory support devices. In: Rao GHR (Ed). Coronary Artery Disease. New Delhi: Macmillan Medical Communications; 2017. pp. 297-309.
39. Guidance for industry and FDA Staff: Current Good Manufacturing Practice Requirements

for Combination Products 2015. https://www.fda.gov/CombinationProducts/MeetingsConferencesWorkshops/ucm118247.htm.
40. Chandy T, Vasudev SC, Rao GHR. Changes in pericardial calcification due to antiplatelet agents: in vitro studies. Artif Organs. 1998;22:666-71.
41. Chandy T, Mooradian DL, Rao GHR. Chitosan/polyethylene glycol-alginate microcapsules for oral delivery of hirudin. J Appl Polym Sci. 1998;70:2143-53.
42. Chandy T, Mooradian DL, Rao GHR. Platelet adhesion and spreading on protein-coated surfaces. Variations in behaviour in washed cells, PRP and whole blood. J Biomater Appl. 1998;13:46-65.
43. Chandy T, Vasudev SC, Rao GHR, Sharma CP. Pericardial calcification: changes due to antiplatelet agents. Cardiovasc Eng. 1998;3:79-85.
44. Chandy T, Das GS, Wilson RF, Rao GHR. Surface immobilized biomolecules on albumin modified porcine pericardium for preventing thrombosis and calcification. Intern J Artif Organs. 1999;22:547-58.
45. Chandy T, Mooradian DL, Rao GHR. Evaluation of modified alginate-PEG microcapsules for cell encapsulation. Artif. Organs. 1999;23:894-903.
46. Chandy T, Rao GHR. Platelet biomaterial interactions. In: Rao GHR (Ed). Platelet Physiology and Pharmacology. USA: Kluwer Academic Publishers; 1999.
47. Chandy T, Das GS, Rao GHR. 5 Fluorouracil-loaded chitosan-coated polylactic acid microspheres as biodegradable drug carriers for cerebral tumors. J Microencapsulation. 2000;17:625-38.
48. Chandy T, Wilson RF, Rao GHR, Das GS. Changes in cisplatin delivery due to surface-coated poly (lactic acid) /poly (e-carpolactone) microspheres. J Biomater. Appl. 2002;16:275-92.
49. Chandy T, Rao GHR. Preparation of surface-engineered elastin/laminin nerve guide tubes of poly (lactic acid)/poly (ethylene vinyl acetate). J. Bioacitve Comp Polym. 2002;17:183-95.
50. Chandy T, Rao GHR, Wilson RF, Das GS. The development of porous alginate/PEG/composite for cardiovascular engineering. J Biomate Appl. 2003;17:287-363.
51. Chandy T, Rao GHR. Comparison of nano- and microparticles for targeted drug delivery. In: Rao GHR, Reddy M (Eds). Handbook of Biotechnology, Bioengineering, and Biomedical Applications. Bangalore: National Design Research Foundation, Institution of Engineers; 2017.
52. Takahashi H, Letourneur D, Grainger DW. Delivery of large biopharmaceuticals for cardiovascular stents: a review. Biomacromolecules. 2007;8:3281-93.
53. Faxon DP, Currier JW. Prevention of post-PTCA restenosis. Ann NY Acad Sci. 1995;748: 410-28.
54. Sheth S, Litvack F, Dev V. Substrate thrombosis and vascular injury resulting from slotted-tube nitinol and stainless stents in a rabbit carotid artery model. Circulation. 1996;94:1733-40.
55. Schaltz RA. A view of vascular stents. Circulation. 1989;79:445-57.
56. Suh H, Jeong R, Rathi R, Kim SW. Regulation of smooth muscle cell proliferation using paclitaxel-loaded poly (ethylene oxide)-poly (lactide/glycolide) nanospheres. J Biomed Mater Res. 1995;42:231-338.
57. Das GS, Rao GHR, Wilson RF, Chandy T. Controlled delivery of taxol from poly (ethylene glycol)-coated (lactic acid) microspheres. J Biomed Mater Res. 2001;55:96-103.
58. Chandy T, Rao GHR, Wilson RTF, Das GS. Development of poly (lactic acid)/chitosan comatrix microspheres: controlled release of taxol-heparin for preventing restenosis. Drug Deliv. 2001;8:77-88.
59. Lubhasetwar V, Song C, Humphrey W, Shebuski E, Levy RL. Arterial uptake of biodegradable nanoparticles: effect of surface modifications. J Pharm Sci. 1998;87(10):1229-34.
60. Humphrey WR, Erickson LA, Simmons CA, Northup JL Wishika DG et al. The effect of intramural delivery of polymeric nanoparticles loaded with the antiproliferative 2-aminochromone U-86983 on neointimal hyperplasia development in balloon-injured porcine coronary arteries. Adv Drug Del Rev. 1997;24:87-108.
61. Wykrzykowska JJ, Kraak RP, Hofma SH, van der Schaaf RJ, Arkenbout EK, IJsselmuiden AJ, et al. Bioresorbable scaffolds versus metallic stents in routine PCI. N Engl J Med. 2017;376(24):2319-28.

62. Serruys PW, Garcia-Garcia HM, Onuma Y. From metallic cages to transient bioresorbable scaffolds: change in paradigm of coronary revascularization in the upcoming decade. Eur Heart J. 2012;33:16-25.
63. Puricel S, Cuculi F, Weissner M, Schmermund A, Jamshidi P, Nyffenegger T, et al. Bioresorbable coronary scaffold thrombosis: multicenter comprehensive analysis of clinical presentations, mechanisms, and predictors. J Am Coll Cardiol. 2016;67:921-31.
64. Kolandaivelu K, Swaminathan R, Gibson EJ, Kolachalama VB, Nguyen-Ehrenreich KL, Giddings VL. Stent thrombogenicity early in high-risk interventional settings is driven by stent design and deployment and protected by polymer drug coatings. Circulation. 2014;123:1400-9.
65. Bourantas CV, Papafaklis MI, Kotsia A, Farooq V, Muramatsu T, Gomez-Lara J, et al. Effect of the endothelial shear stress patterns on neointimal proliferation following drug-eluting bioresorbable vascular scaffold implantation: an optical coherence tomography study. JACC Cardovasc Interv. 2014;7:315-24.
66. Sotomi Y, Suwannasom P, Serruys PW, Onuma Y. Possible mechanical causes of scaffold thrombosis: insights from case reports with intracoronary imaging. Eurointervention. 2017;12:1746-56.
67. Mauri L, Kereiakes DJ, Yeh RW, Driscoll-Shempp P, Cutlip DE, Steg PG, et al. Twelve or 30 months of dual antiplatelet therapy after drug eluting-stents. N Engl J Med. 2014;371:2155-66.
68. Chesterman, CN, Bendt MC. Platelet and vessel wall interaction and the genesis of atherosclerosis. Clin Haematol. 1986;15:323-53.
69. Salzman EW, Lindon J, Brier D, Merrill EW. Surface-induced platelet adhesion, aggregation and release. Ann NY Acad Sci. 1977;283:114-24.
70. Park K, Park H. Application of video-enhanced interference reflection microscopy to the study of platelet-surface interactions. Scanning Microsc Suppl. 1989;3:137-46.
71. Goodman SL, Cooper SL, Albrecht RM. The effect of substrate-adsorbed albumin on platelet spreading. J Biomater Sci Polym Ed. 1990;2:147-59.
72. Feurstein LA, Sheppard JI. Stats in adherent platelet morphology and the adsorbed protein on biomaterials. Biomaterials. 1993;14:137-46.
73. Friedman LL, Liem H, Grabowski EF, Leonard EF, McCord CW. Inconsequentiality of surface properties for initial platelet adhesion. Trans Am Soc Artif Intern Organs. 1970;16:63-73.
74. Lewis JC, White MS, Prater T, Porter KR, Steele RJ. Cytoskeletal changes during adhesion and release: a comparison of human and nonhuman primate platelets. Scann Electron Microsc. 1986;1:199-209.
75. Mohammad SF, Hardison MD, Glenn CH, Morton BD, Bolan JC, Mason RG. Adhesion of blood platelets to glass and polymer surfaces. Haemostasis. 1974;3:257-70.
76. Baier RE, Depalma VA, Goupil D, Cohen E. Human platelet spreading on substrate of known surface chemistry. J Biomed Mater Res. 1985;19:1157-67.
77. Difazio LT, Stratouias C, Greco RS, Haimovich B. Multiple platelet surface receptors mediate platelet adhesion to surfaces coated with plasma proteins. J Surg Res. 1994;57:133-7.
78. Brash J, Suniyal S. Dependence of albumin-fibrinogen simple and competitive adsorption on surface properties of biomaterials. J Polym Sci. 1979;66:377-89.
79. Bailly AL, Laurent A, Lu H, Elalami I, Jacob P, Mundler O, et al. Fibrinogen binding and platelet retention: relationship with thrombogenicity of catheters. J Biomed Mater Res. 1996;39:101-8.
80. Peerschke EI, Zucker MB, Grant RA, Egan JJ, Johnson MM. Correlation between fibrinogen binding to human platelets and platelet aggregability. Blood. 1980;55:841-7.
81. Margurie GA, Plow EF, Edgungton TS. Human platelets possess an inducible and saturable receptor specific for fibrinogen. J Biol Chem. 1979;254:5357-63.
82. Tomikawa M, Iwamoto M, Olson P, Söderman S, Blombäck B. On the platelet fibrinogen interactions. Thromb Res. 1988;19:869-76.
83. Andrews RK, Fox JEB. Platelet receptors in hemostasis. Curr Opin Cell Biol. 1991;2:894-903.
84. Goodman SL, Cooper SL, Albrecht RM. Integrin receptors and platelet adhesion to synthetic surfaces. J Biomater Res. 1993;27:683-95.

85. Phillips RD, Jennings LK, Edwards HH. Identification of membrane proteins mediating the interaction of human platelets. J Cell Biol. 1980;86:77-86.
86. Roth GL. Developing arterial platelet adhesion, glycoprotein Ib and leucine-rich glycoproteins. Blood. 1991;77:5-18.
87. Lindon JN, McManama G, Kushner L. Does the conformation of adsorbed fibrinogen dictate platelet interactions. Blood. 1986;68:355-62.
88. Park K, Mosher DE, Cooper SL. Acute surface-induced thrombosis in the canine *ex vivo* model: importance protein composition of the initial monolayer and platelet activation. J Biomed Mater Res. 1986;20:589-612.
89. Ryu G, Han D, Kim Y, Min B. Albumin immobilized polyurethane and its blood compatibility. ASAIO J. 1992;38:M644-50.
90. Rhodes NP, Kumary TV, Williams DF. Influence of wall shear rate on parameters of blood compatibility of intravascular catheters. Biomaterials. 1996;17:1995-2002.
91. Harker LA, Slichter SJ. Arterial and venous thromboembolism: kinetic characterization and evaluation of therapy. Thromb Diath Haemorrh. 1996;31:188-203.
92. Salzman EW. Role of platelet in blood-surface interactions. Fed Proc. 1971;30:1503-9.
93. Stewart GJ, Lynch PR, Reichle FA. The adhesion of leukocytes, erythrocytes and non-cellular material to the luminal surface of natural and artificial blood vessels *in vivo*. Ann NY Acad Sci. 1977;283:179-207.
94. Courtney JM, Forbes CD. Thrombosis on foreign surfaces. Br Med Bull. 1994;4:966-81.
95. Bolz A, Schaldach M. Artificial heart valves: improved blood compatibility by PECVD a-Si:H coating. Artif Organ. 1990;14(4):260-9.
96. Bjork VO. The pyrolytic carbon occluder for the Bjork-Shiley tilting disc valve prosthesis. Scand J Thorac Cardiovasc Surg. 2009;6(2):109-13.
97. Smith KL, Black KM. Characterization of the threated surfaces of silicon-alloyed pyrolytic carbo and SiC. J. Vaccum Sci Technol. 1984;2:744.
98. Behzadi S, Imani M, Yousefi M, Galinetto P, Simchi A, Amiri H, et al. Pyrolytic carbon coating for cytocompatibility of titanium oxide nanoparticles: a promising candidate for medical applications. Nantotechnology. 2012;23(4):045102.

Afterword

When I started putting together this monograph on Platelets, I did a literature search on articles published by my mentor, Dr. James G. White. In his obituary, published in Minneapolis Star and Tribune, his associates, Dr. Gerhard Johnson and Dr. Gregory Vercellotti mentioned over 700 articles to his credit. However, when I Googled for his published articles, in Google Scholar, I could only find a few hundred references. This indicates, two different problems associated with such a search. Firstly, not all of our published articles are indexed. Secondly, the way Google algorithm works, it pulls out those references that are frequently used or cited. I will give here another example, as to what I mean by this. One of my major collaborator and mentor is Professor (Sir) Vijay V. Kakkar (VJ), ex-director of Thrombosis Research Institute (TRI), London. I was trying to do a write-up on his work and did a literature search. Google Scholar pulled up more work of Dr. (Lord) Baron, Ajay Kakkar, his son and current director of TRI, than of his father. What this experiment tells us is, that pretty soon the name of Ajay will pull out more references to his work, than Vijay V. Kakkar. I also did a search on Mendeley (https://www.mendeley.com) and Researchgate (https://www.researchgate.net), but failed to get significant number of articles of Dr. White on these sites.

Since I was not able to access all his articles on the web, I contacted the Laboratory Medicine and Pathology, University of Minnesota for a copy of his CV. They too did not have a copy and told me, that his son cleared all his stuff from his office, soon after the death of Jim White. Finally, I was able to get hold of my associates, who wrote the obituary and obtain a copy of his CV. In view of the fact that I had such a hard time getting his CV, I decided to include complete Bibliography of our work at the end of this chapter, so that those who are interested in accessing any of our work, should not have to go through the same hardship.

What are the salient discoveries of Platelet Research Laboratory and Thrombosis Research Laboratory at the University of Minnesota? White described muscular system of the blood platelets and noticed that such a system did not exist in any other blood cells, except the muscle cells. He also discovered the role of ionized calcium in platelet signaling pathways, as well as its regulation of platelet contractile proteins and cytoskeletal rearrangements. Using calcium sensitive ionophore, we demonstrated the role of transmembrane calcium flux in platelet activation. We also demonstrated using phorbol ester (PMA), that one can bypass the classical diglyceride-mediated PKC activation, as PMA can directly activate the PKC and initiate cytoskeletal rearrangements. Using Trifluoperazine, a calmodulin antagonist, we were able to demonstrate the role of calmodulin, in platelet aggregation. We were able to demonstrate the localization of prostaglandin synthesizing enzymes, in the dense tubular system of platelets. We also demonstrated the role of cyclic nucleotides, cAMP and cGMP in the modulation of platelet cytosolic calcium levels. Our laboratory demonstrated the agonist binding to specific receptors, receptor internalization and their distribution in activated platelets, both by ultrastructure studies as well as by flow cytometry. We also demonstrated the existence of a phenomenon called, "membrane modulation" capable of restoring the response of drug induced refractory platelets to the action of dual agonists. Our studies for the first time, demonstrated that the release of ADP or synthesis of prostaglandin second messengers, were not essential for achieving irreversible aggregation.

Using denuded aorta and flow conditions, we were able to demonstrate the platelet-vessel wall interactions. Our studies demonstrated, that the agents that inhibit cell-cell interaction (aggregation) were not able to inhibit cell surface-interactions (platelet vessel-wall). Our laboratory was one of the few laboratories in the world, which developed capabilities to study blood-biocompatibility under a variety of flow conditions, using freshly harvested human blood. We also developed polymer based targeted drug delivery systems. In collaboration with my ex-student and associate, Dr. Daniel Ericsson of SUBc, Inc. Rochester, Minnesota, we developed STTR grants, to National Institute of Health (NIH) for the development of prototypes of medical devices, for monitoring pathogens in blood bags. Using the same technology, we developed a device for monitoring platelet activity. IBM Rochester developed the prototypes of these devices under a research contract. Dr. Rao was the principal instigators for these two research grants.

Bibliography

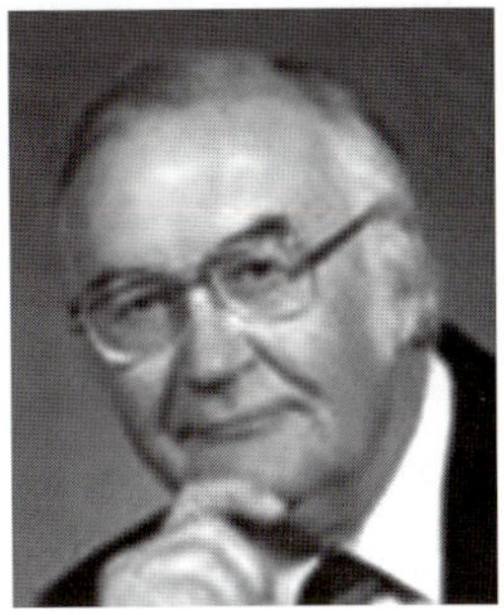

Collected Works of Platelet Research Laboratory, University of Minnesota

James G White MD

Professor of Pediatrics, Laboratory Medicine and Pathology
Director, Platelet Research Laboratory
University of Minnesota (1959–2014)
Regents Professor Emeritus, University of Minnesota, Minneapolis, Minnesota

Dr James White was nominated for the Hemostasis and Thrombosis Research Society: Lifetime Achievement Award for his contributions to the understanding of platelets. He is recognized worldwide as an icon in electron microscopy (EM) and its application to understanding disease. His use of electron microscopy has shed light on the ultrastructure of platelets. His work has uncovered the details of many platelet processes such as activation, aggregation, and secretion and contributed greatly to the understanding of several platelet disorders. As a prominent figure in hemostasis, he has published more than 700 manuscripts, been active in numerous organizations, and served on the editorial board of several journal. He received his medical degree from the University of Minnesota. After completing an internship at Detroit Receiving Hospital and service in the US Army at Ft. Mead, he completed training in Pediatrics at the University of Minnesota. He began his long journey with electron microscopy during his fellowship the University of Minnesota, where he has remained for the duration of his career. He is currently a Regents Emeritus Professor, Departments of Pediatrics and Laboratory Medicine and Pathology, University of Minnesota.

1. Abdel Galil M Abdel Gader, Abeer K Al Ghumlas, Mansour F Hussain, et al. The Ultrastructure of Camel Blood Platelets: A Comparative study with Human, Bovine, and Equine Cells. Platelets. 2008;19:51-8.
2. Abel J, White JG, Kelly W, et al. Management of spontaneous splenic rupture in AHG deficient hemophilia. Lancet. 1965;85:71-5.
3. Allen DW, Burgoyne CF, Groat JD, et al. Comparison of hemoglobin Koln erythrocyte membranes with normal erythrocyte membranes. Blood. 1984;64:1263-9.
4. Anderson PD, Huizing M, Claassen DA, et al. Hermansky-Pudlak syndrome type 4 (HPS-4): Clinical and molecular characteristics. Hum Genet. 2003;113:10-17.
5. Anikster Y, Huizing M, White JG, et al. Mutation of a new gene causes a unique form of Hermansky-Pudlak syndrome in a genetic isolate of central Puerto Rico. Nature Genetics. 2001;28:376-80.
6. Arderiu G, Pérez-Pujol S, Escolar G, et al. External calcium facilitates signaling, contractile and secretory mechanisms induced after activation of platelets by collagen. Platelets. 2008;19(3):172-81.
7. Ayoub EM, White JG. Intraphagocytic degradation of group A streptococci: electron

microscopic studies. J Bacteriol. 1969;98(2): 728-36.
8. Aznar-Salatti J, Escolar G, Arnau C, et al. An intermediate-purity factor VIII concentrate supports platelet adhesion under flow conditions. Hemophilia. 1997;3(1):14-20.
9. Bravo ML, Escolar G, White JG. Dextran does not inhibit the hemorheological mechanisms of blood platelet function. Clin Hemorhol. 1991;11:339-49.
10. Bravo ML, Escolar G, White JG. Dextrans "in vitro" do not inhibit the hemorheological mechanisms of platelet function. Clinical Hemorheology. 1991;11:339-49.
11. Brodie HA, Chole RA, Griffin GC, et al. Macrothrombocytopenia and progressive deafness: a new genetic syndrome. Am J Otol. 1992;13(6):507-11.
12. Brown JE, White JG, Hockett RD Jr, et al. Functional studies of Platelet aggregation inhibition by fab monomers of BA-2. Leukocyte Typing II. Human B Lymphocytes. EL Reinherz, BF Haynes, LM Nadler and ID James Bernstein, (Eds), Springer-Verlag, New York, Inc. 1986;2:541-50.
13. Brunso L, Segura D, Monreal L, et al. The secretory mechanisms in equine platelets are independent of cytoskeletal polymerization and occur through membrane fusion. Platelets. 2010;21(8):658-66.
14. Burns WA, Zimmerman HJ, Hammond J, et al. The clinician's view of diagnostic electron microscopy. Hum Path. 1975;6:467-78.
15. Burris S, White JG, Eaton JW. Calcium-induced erythrocyte shape change. Proceedings of the Second International Symposium on Red Blood Cells and Lens Metabolism: Developments in Biochemistry (SK Srivastava, Ed.), Elsevier/North Holland Inc. 1980;9:49-54.
16. Burris SM, Eaton JW, White JG. Evaluation of the role of diacylglycerol in calcium-induced erythrocyte shape change and rigidity. J Lab Clin Med. 1980;96(4):749-56.
17. Burris SM, Smith CM, Rao GHR, et al. Aspirin treatment reduces platelet resistance to deformation. Arteriosclerosis. 1987;7(4):385-8.
18. Burris SM, Smith CM, Tukey D, et al. Micropipette aspiration of human platelets: influence of rewarming on deformability of chilled cells. J Lab Clin Med. 1986; 107(3):238-43.
19. Burris SM, Smith CM, Tukey DT, et al. Micropipette aspiration of human platelets after exposure to aggregating agents. Arteriosclerosis. 1986;6(3):321-5.
20. Butler AM, Gerrard JM, Peller J, Stoddard SF, Rao GHR, White JG. Vitamin E inhibits the release of calcium from a platelet membrane fraction in vitro. Prostaglandins Med. 1979; 2(3):203-16.
21. Carmona-Rivera C, Hess RA, O'Brien K, et al. Novel Mutations in the HPS1 gene among Puerto Rican patients. Clin Genet 2010.
22. Castaneda JP, White JG, Williams RC Jr. Antinuclear antibodies in normal human subjects. Arthritis Rheum. 1967;10(5):431-43.
23. Catalfamo JL, Raymond SL, White JG, et al. Defective platelet-fibrinogen interaction in hereditary canine thrombopathia. Blood. 1986;67(6):1568-77.
24. Challey CH, Caperton EM Jr, White JG, et al. Antinuclear antibodies—attempts at ultrastructural localization. Proc Soc Exp Biol Med. 1968;128(2):520-4.
25. Chen B, Polunovsky V, White J, et al. Mesenchymal cells isolated after acute lung injury manifest an enhanced proliferative phenotype. J. Clin. Invest. 1992;90(5):1778-85.
26. Christopher MM, Perman V, White JG, et al. Propylene glycol-induced Heinz body formation and D-lactic acidosis in cats. Prog Clin Biol Res. 1989;319:69-87; discussion 88-92.
27. Christopher MM, White JG, Eaton JW. Erythrocyte pathology and mechanisms of Heinz body-mediated hemolysis in cats. Vet Pathol. 1990;27(5):299-310.
28. Clawson CC, Nesbit ME, White JG, et al. Quantification of chemotaxis and maximal bacterial capacity of mature neutrophils in chronic myelogenous leukemia. J Reticuloendothel Soc. 1979;26(5):515-23.
29. Clawson CC, Parins DJ, White JG, et al. Interactions of blood with solid and porous platinum endocardial electrodes for cardiac pacemakers. Scan Electron Microsc. 1980;(3): 211-8, 226.
30. Clawson CC, Rao GHR, White JG. Platelet interaction with bacteria. IV. Stimulation of

the release reaction. Am J Pathol. 1975;81(2): 411-20.
31. Clawson CC, Repine JE, White JG. The Chediak-Higashi syndrome: quantitation of a deficiency in maximal bactericidal capacity. Am J Pathol. 1979;94(3):539-47.
32. Clawson CC, White JG, Herzberg MC. Platelet interaction with bacteria. VI. contrasting the role of fibrinogen and fibronectin. Am J Pathol. 1980;9(1):43-53.
33. Clawson CC, White JG, Repine JE. The Chediak-Higashi syndrome. Evidence that defective leukotaxis is primarily due to an impediment by giant granules. Am J Pathol. 1978;92(3):745-53.
34. Clawson CC, White JG. Development of giant granules in platelets during prolonged storage. Am J Pathol. 1980;101(3):635-46.
35. Clawson CC, White JG. Platelet interaction with bacteria. I. Reaction phase and effects of inhibitors. Am J Pathol. 1971;65(2):367-80.
36. Clawson CC, White JG. Platelet interaction with bacteria. II. Fate of the bacteria. Am J Pathol. 1971;65(2):381-97.
37. Clawson CC, White JG. Platelet interaction with bacteria. V. Ultrastructure of congenital afibrinogenemic platelets. Am J Pathol. 1980; 98(1):197-205.
38. Cohen I, Burk DL, White JG. The effect of peptides and monoclonal antibodies that bind to platelet glycoprotein IIb-IIIa complex on the development of clot tension. Blood. 1989; 73(7):1880-7.
39. Cohen I, Gerrard JM, Bergman RN, et al. The role of contractile filaments in platelet activation. Protides of the Biological Fluids. Pergammon Press, Oxford and New York. 1979; 555-66.
40. Cohen I, Gerrard JM, White JG. Ultrastructure of clots during isometric contraction. J Cell Biol. 1982;93(3):775-87.
41. Cohen I, Lim CT, Kahn DR, et al. Disulfide-linked and transglutaminase-catalyzed protein assemblies in platelets. Blood. 1985; 66(1):143-51.
42. Condie RM, White JG, Najarian JS. Platelet activity of antilymphocyte serum (ALS) preparations. Transplant Proc. 1973;5(1):555-9.
43. Cox AC, Carroll RC, White JG, et al. Recycling of platelet phosphorylation and cytoskeletal assembly. J Cell Biol. 1984;98(1):8-15.
44. Cox AC, Rao GH, Gerrard JM, et al. The influence of vitamin E quinone on platelet structure, function and biochemistry. Blood. 1980; 55(6):907-11.
45. Craddock PR, Hammerschmidt D, White JG, et al. Complement (C5-a)-induced granulocyte aggregation in vitro. A possible mechanism of complement-mediated leukostasis and leukopenia. J Clin Invest. 1977;60(1): 260-4.
46. Craddock PR, White JG, Jacob HS. Potentiation of complement (C5a)-induced granulocyte aggregation by cytochalasin B. J Lab Clin Med. 1978;91(3):490-9.
47. Craddock PR, White JG, Weisdorf DJ, et al. Digital integration of granulocyte aggregation responses. A simple and reproducible method for the quantitation of granulocyte adhesiveness. Inflammation. 1980;4(4):381-95.
48. Cragg A, Einzig S, Castenedo-Zuniga W, et al. Vessel wall arachidonate metabolism after angioplasty: possible mediators of prostaangioplasty vasospasm. Am J Cardiol. 1983; 51(8):1441-5.
49. Cullinane AR, Curry JA, Carmona-Rivvera C, et al. A Bloc-1 mutation screen reveals that PLDN is mutated in Hermansky-Pudlak Syndrome Type 9. American Journal of Human Genetics. 2011;88:778-87.
50. Cullinane AR, Curry JA, Golas G, et al. A BLOC-1 mutation screen reveals a novel BLOC1S3 mutation in Hermansky-Pudlak Syndrome type 8. Pigment Cell & Melanoma Research. 2012;25:584-91.
51. Daniels TM, Foss DN, White JG, et al. Platelet storage pool deficiency in pigs. Blood. 1986; 67(4):1043-7.
52. Dascombe WH, Hong C, Garrett KO, et al. Artificial microvascular graft thrombosis: the consequences of platelet membrane glycoprotein Ib inhibition and thrombin inhibition. Blood. 1993;82(1-2):126-34.
53. Davis RB, White JG. Localization of 5-hydroxytryptamine in blood platelets: an autoradiographic and ultrastructural study. Br J Haematol. 1968;15(1):93-9.
54. Dent PB, Fish LA, White JG, et al. Chediak-Higashi syndrome. Observations on the nature of the associated malignancy. Lab Invest. 1966;15(10):1634-42.

55. Díaz-Ricart M, Arderiu G, Estebanell E, et al. Inhibition of cytoskeletal assembly by cytochalasin B prevents signaling through tyrosine phosphorylation and secretion triggered by collagen but not by thrombin. Am J Pathol. 2002;160(1):329-37.
56. Diaz-Ricart M, Brunso L, Pino M, et al. Preanalytical treatment of EDTA-anticoagulated blood to ensure stabilization of the mean platelet volume and component measured with the ADVIA counters. Thromb Res. 2010;126(1):e30-5.
57. Diaz-Ricart M, Estebanell E, Lozano M, et al. Thrombin facilitates primary platelet adhesion onto vascular surfaces in the absence of plasma adhesive proteins: studies under flow conditions. Haematologica. 2000;85(3):280-8.
58. Diaz-Ricart M, Palomo M, Fuste B, et al. Inhibition of tyrosine kinase activity prevents adhesive and cohesive properties of platelets and the expression of procoagulant activity in response to collagen. Thromb Res. 2008;121 (6):873-83.
59. Dodds WJ, White JG. Coagulation and platelet function. 1. The normal hemostatic mechanism. Proceedings of First International Symposium on Equine Hematology H Kitcher, JD Krehbiel (Eds.) Am Assoc Equine Practitioners, Golden, Colorado. 1975;197-9.
60. Donna S Woulfe, Joanne Klimas Lilliendahl, Shelley August, et al. Serglycin proteoglycan deletion induces defects in platelet aggregation and thrombus formation in mice. Blood. 2008;111:3458-67.
61. Dreher KL, Eaton JW, Breslawec KP, et al. Calcium-induced erythrocyte rigidity: the roles of cellular metabolism, hydration, and ionic balance. Am J Pathol. 1980;101(3):543-55.
62. Dreher KL, Eaton JW, Kuettner JF, et al. Retention of water and potassium by erythrocytes prevents calcium-induced membrane rigidity. Am J Pathol. 1978;92(1):215-25.
63. du Credt RF, Adkins MC, Hunter DW, et al. Therapeutic embolization: enhanced radiolabeled monitoring. Radiol. 1990;177:571-5.
64. Durante W, Schini VB, Kroll MH, et al. Platelets inhibit the induction of nitric oxide synthesis by interleukin-1 beta in vascular smooth muscle cells. Blood. 1994; 83(7):1831-8.
65. Eaton JW, Berger E, Nelson D, et al. Intracellular calcium: lack of effect on ovine red cells. Proc Soc Exp Biol Med. 1978;157(3):506-10.
66. Eaton JW, Berger E, White JG, et al. Calcium-induced damage of haemoglobin SS and normal erythrocytes. Br J Haematol. 1978; 38(1): 57-62.
67. Eaton JW, Berger E, White JG, et al. Effects of calcium on hemoglobin SS erythrocytes: Evidence that calcium accumulation underlies formation of irreversibly sickled cells. Proceedings, Symposium on Molecular and Cellular Aspects of Sickle Cell Disease (Hercules JI, Cottam GL, ME Watterman and AN Schechter, Eds.), Dept. of HEW, Publication No. 76-1007 (NIH). 1976;327-42.
68. Eaton JW, Berger E, White JG, et al. Interspecies variation in erythrocyte calcium response. Prog Clin Biol Res. 1978;20:37-49.
69. Eaton JW, Berger E, White JG, et al. Metabolic and morphologic effects of intraerythrocytic calcium: implications for pathogencsis of sickle cell disease. Prog Clin Biol Res. 1977;14:275-98.
70. Eaton JW, Jacob HS, White JG. Membrane abnormalities of irreversibly sickled cells. Semin Hematol. 1979;16(1):52-64.
71. Eaton JW, Konzen DK, White JG. Cellular and molecular aspects of aging: the red cell as a model: proceedings of a conference held in Minneapolis, Minnesota, September 8-11, 1984. Progress in clinical and biological research. 1985;195.
72. Edson JR, Blaese RM, White JG, et al. Defibrination syndrome in an infant born after abruption placentae. J Pediatr. 1968;72(3): 342-6.
73. Edson JR, Krivit W, White JG, et al. Intravascular coagulation in acute stem cell leukemia successfully treated with heparin. J Pediatr. 1967;71(3):342-50.
74. Edson JR, Krivit W, White JG. Kaolin partial thromboplastin time: high levels of procoagulants producing short-clotting times or masking deficiencies of other procoagulants of low concentrations of anticoagulants. J Lab Clin Med. 1967;70(3):463-70.
75. Edson JR, White JG, Krivit W. The enigma of severe factor XI deficiency

without hemorrhagic symptoms: distinction from Hageman factor and "Fletcher factor" deficiency; family study; problems of diagnosis. Thromb Diath Haemorrh. 1967;18(3-4):342-8.

76. Einzig S, Noren GR, Staley NA, et al. Arachidonic acid metabolism in thrombocytes and vascular tissues of turkeys. Prostaglandins. 1985;30(6):999-1017.

77. Einzig S, Rao GHR, Pierpont ME, et al. Acute effects of amrinone on regional myocardial and systemic blood flow distribution in the dog. Canad J Physiol Pharmacol. 1982;60(6): 811-8.

78. Einzig S, Rao GHR, White JG. Differential sensitivity of regional vascular beds in the dog to low-dose prostacyclin infusion. Canad J Physiol Pharmacol. 1980;58(8): 940-6.

79. Einzig S, Sotomara R, Rao GHR, et al. Effect of low dose prostacyclin infusion on blood flow in acutely ischemic canine myocardium. Prostaglandins Med. 1980; 5(3):209-21.

80. Ekaterini T, Tsilou ET, Rubin BI, et al. Milder Ocular Findings in Hermansky-Pudlak Syndrome Type-3 Compared with Hermansky-Pudlak Syndrome Type-1. Ophthalmology. 2004;111:1599-1603.

81. Erlandsen SL, Bitterman AG, White JG, et al. High-resolution cryo-FESEM of individual cell adhesion molecules (CAM) in the glycocalyx of human platelets: Detection of P-selectin (CD62P), GPIb/IX complex (CD42a/CD42α, bβ), and integrin GPIIb/IIIa (CD41/CD61) by immunogold labeling and stereo imaging. J Histochem Cytochem. 2001;49:809-19.

82. Erlandsen SL, Bittermann A, Krumweide M, et al. High-resolution backscatter electron detection of cell surface molecules on human platelets using double layer coating method and cryo field emission scanning electron microscopy. Scanning. 1997;19(5):356-60.

83. Escolar G, Clemetson K, White JG. Persistence of mobile receptors on surface- and suspension-activated platelets. J Lab and Clin Med. 1994;123(4):536-46.

84. Escolar G, Diaz-Ricart M, Cases A, et al. Abnormal cytoskeletal assembly in platelets from uremic patients. Am J Pathol. 1993; 143(3):823-31.

85. Escolar G, Diaz-Ricart M, White JG. Talin does not associate exclusively with alpha 2b beta 3 integrin in activated human platelets. J Lab Clin Med. 1995;125(5):597-607.

86. Escolar G, Hagert-Whiting K, Bravo ML, et al. Interaction of long-term stored platelets with vascular subendothelium. J Lab Clin Med. 1987;109(2):147-54.

87. Escolar G, Krumwiede M, White JG. Organization of the actin cytoskeleton of resting and activated platelets in suspension. Am J Pathol. 1986;123(1):86-94.

88. Escolar G, Leistikow E, White JG. The fate of the open canalicular system in surface and suspension-activated platelets. Blood. 1989; 74(6):1983-8.

89. Escolar G, Lopez-Vilchez I, Diaz-Ricart M, et al. Internalization of tissue factor by platelets. Thrombosis Research. 2008;122:537-41.

90. Escolar G, Lozano M, Diaz-Ricart M, et al. Modifications in accessibility of membrane glycoproteins, binding of specific ligands and coagulation factor V during the activation of platelets in blood emerging from bleeding time wounds. Am J Hematol. 1999; 60(4): 260-7.

91. Escolar G, Mazzara R, White JG, et al. Contribution of perfusion techniques to the evaluation of the hemostatic effectiveness of platelet concentrates. Blood Cells. 1992;18:403-15; discussion 416-20. Review.

92. Escolar G, Rao GHR, Nieuwenhuis HK, et al. Ultrastructural expression of P-selection on surface-activated platelets. Platelets. 1996;7: 297-301.

93. Escolar G, Sauk JJ, Bravo ML, et al. Development of a simple embedding procedure allowing immunocytochemical localization at the ultrastructural level. J Histochem Cytochem. 1988;36(12):1579-82.

94. Escolar G, Sauk JJ, Bravo ML, et al. Immunogold staining of microtubules in resting and activated platelets. Am J Hematol. 1987;24(2): 177-88.

95. Escolar G, White JG. Changes in glycoprotein expression after platelet activation:

differences between in vitro and in vivo studies. Thromb Haemost. 2000;83(3):371-86. Review.

96. Escolar G, White JG. Combined use of immunocytochemical techniques and ligand-gold complexes for investigation of platelet membrane responses to surface activation. Microsc Res Tech. 1994;28(4):308-26.
97. Escolar G, White JG. Distribution of GPIb on and in resting platelets. Blood. 1998;92(12):4874-7.
98. Escolar G, White JG. Organization of von Willebrand factor on surface-activated platelets. Arterioscler Thromb. 1993;13(12):1852-8.
99. Escolar G, White JG. The platelet open canalicular system: a final common pathway. Blood Cells. 1991;17(3):467-85.
100. Estensen RD, White JG, Holmes B. Specific degranulation of human polymorphonuclear leukocytes. Nature. 1974;248(446):347-8.
101. Estensen RD, White JG. Ultrastructural features of the platelet response to phorbol myristate acetate. Am J Pathol. 1974;74(3):441-52.
102. Evangelista V, Piccardoni P, White JG, et al. Cathepsin G-dependent platelet stimulation by activated polymorphonuclear leukocytes and its inhibition by antiproteinases: role of P-selectin-mediated cell-cell adhesion. Blood. 1993;81(11):2947-57.
103. Evangelista V, Rajtar G, de Gaetano G, et al. Platelet activation by fMLP-stimulated polymorphonuclear leukocytes: the activity of cathepsin G is not prevented by antiproteinases. Blood. 1991;77(11): 2379-88.
104. Fabbro S, Kahr WH, Hinckley J, et al. Homozygosity mapping with SNP arrays confirms 3p21 as a recessive locus for gray platelet syndrome and narrows the interval significantly. Blood. 2011;117:3430-34.
105. Falik-Zaccai TC, Anikster Y, Rivera CE, et al. A new genetic isolate of gray platelet syndrome (GPS): clinical, cellular, and hematologic characteristics. Mol. Genet Metab. 2001; 74(3):303-13.
106. Fiddler MB, Hudson LD, White JG, et al. Enzyme therapy XIV. Comparison of methods for enzyme entrapment in human erythrocytes. J Lab Clin Med. 1980;96(2):307-17.
107. Flynn TP, Allen DW, Johnson GJ, et al. Oxidant damage of the lipids and proteins of the erythrocyte membranes in unstable hemoglobin disease. Evidence for the role of lipid peroxidation. J Clin Invest. 1983; 71(5):1215-23.
108. Fong JS, White JG, Good RA. Inhibition of endotoxic lipopolysaccharide-mediated platelet aggregation by cobra venom anticomplementary factor. Blood. 1974;44(3):399-409.
109. Fradera J, Velez-Garcia E, White JG. Acute lymphoblastic leukemia with unusual cytoplasmic granulation: a morphologic, cytochemical and ultrastructural study. Blood. 1986;68(2):406-11.
110. Frojmovic MM, Wong T, White JG. Platelet plasma membrane is equally distributed between surface and osmotically-evaginable surface-connecting membrane, independent of size, subpopulation or species. Nouv Rev Fr Hematol. 1992;34:99-110.
111. Fuste B, Diaz-Ricart M, Jensen MK, et al. TRAP induces more intense tyrosine phosphorylation than thrombin with differential ultrastructural features. Am J Pathol. 2002; 160(6):2245-52.
112. Fuste B, Krogh-Jensen M, Ordinas A, et al. Differential effect of TRAP (14 mer peptide) and thrombin on platelet activation. Am J Path. 2002;160:2245-52.
113. Gader AGMA, Ghomlas AKA, Hussain MF, et al. Effects of Heat on Camel Platelet Structure and Function: A Comparative Study with Humans. Platelets. 2009;20(7):528.
114. Garry VF, Nesbit M, White JG, et al. Histological and cytological technique for the quantitation of cultured human bone marrow cells: Formations of aggregates. In Vitro. 1978;14: 495-501.
115. Gartner TK, Gerrard JM, White JG, et al. Fibrinogen is the receptor for the endogenous lectin of human platelets. Nature. 1981;289(5799):688-90.
116. Gartner TK, Gerrard JM, White JG, et al. The endogenous lectin of human platelets as an alpha-granule component. Blood. 1981; 58(1):153-7.
117. Ge S, White JG, Haynes CL. Cytoskeletal F-actin, not the circumferential of

microtubules, regulates platelet dense body secretion. Platelets. 2012;23:259-63.

118. Ge S, White JG, Haynes CL. Critical role of membrane cholesterol in exocytosis revealed by single platelet study. ACS Chem Biol. 2010; 5(9):819-28.

119. Ge S, Woo E, White JG, et al. Electrochemical measurement of endogenous serotonin release from human blood platelets. Analytical Chemistry. 2011;83:2598-604.

120. Gerrard JM, Butler AM, Graff G, et al. Prostaglandin endoperoxides promote calcium release from a platelet membrane fraction in vitro. Prostaglandins Med. 1978;1(5):373-85.

121. Gerrard JM, Butler AM, Peterson DA, et al. Phosphatidic acid releases calcium from a platelet membrane fraction in vitro. Prostaglandins Med. 1978;1(5):387-96.

122. Gerrard JM, Clawson CC, White JG. Lysophosphatidic acids: III. Enhancement of neutrophil chemotaxis. Am J Pathol. 1980;100(3): 609-18.

123. Gerrard JM, Graff G, Dedon PC, et al. 1-Arachidonyl-monoglyceride causes platelet aggregation—implications for an acyl glycerol achy hydrolase involvement in control of prostaglandin synthesis. Prog Lipid Res. 1981;20:575-8.

124. Gerrard JM, Kindom SE, Peterson DA, et al. Lysophosphatidic acids. Influence on platelet aggregation and intracellular calcium flux. Am J Pathol. 1979;96(2):423-38.

125. Gerrard JM, Kindom SE, Peterson DA, et al. Lysophosphatidic acids. II. Interaction of the effects of adenosine diphosphate and lysophosphatidic acid in dog, rabbit and human platelets. Am J Pathol. 1979;97(3):531-47.

126. Gerrard JM, Peller JD, Krick TP, et al. Cyclic AMP and platelet prostaglandin synthesis. Prostaglandins. 1977;14(1):39-50.

127. Gerrard JM, Peller JD, White JG. The role of cyclic AMP in platelet physiology. Proceedings of the workshop on "The Significance of Platelet Function Tests in the Evaluation of Hemostatic and Thrombotic Tendencies." Philadelphia, PA. Platelet Function (HJ Day, J Holmsen and MB Zucker, Eds.) DHEW Pub. No. 78-1087 (NIH), 1978;522-31.

128. Gerrard JM, Perry GS, Shapiro RS, et al. Further studies of a metabolic stress test in Wiskott-Aldrich syndrome carriers. Am J Ped Hematol Oncol. 1980;2:25-30.

129. Gerrard JM, Peterson DA, Glover SM, et al. Epinephrine reduction of heme: Implication for understanding the transmission of an agonist stimulus. Science. 1982;215:71-3.

130. Gerrard JM, Peterson DA, Rao GHR, et al. Some recent advances in understanding the tangle of biochemical events involved in thromboxane dependent and independent aggregation. Proceedings of the International Workshop on Regulation of Coagulation. KG Mann and FB Taylor, (Eds). The Regulation of Coagulation. New York, Elsevier/North Holland. 1980;399-408.

131. Gerrard JM, Peterson DA, White JG. Calcium mobilization. Platelets II (JL Gordon, Ed.), London, Elsevier, North-Holland, Biomedical Press. 1981; 407-36.

132. Gerrard JM, Phillips DR, Rao GHR, et al. Biochemical studies of two patients with the gray platelet syndrome. Selective deficiency of platelet alpha granules. J Clin Invest. 1980; 66(1):102-9.

133. Gerrard JM, Rao GHR, Stuart MJ, et al. Alterations in the balance of thromboxane and prostacyclin synthesis in platelets and the vessel wall in a diabetic model. The Effect of Platelet Active Drugs on the Cardiovascular System. J Hirsch, PP Steele, RL Vernier, (Eds), University of Colorado Press. 1981;207-23.

134. Gerrard JM, Rao GHR, White JG. The influence of reserpine and ethylenediaminetetracetic acid (EDTA) on serotonin storage organelles of blood platelets. Am J Pathol. 1977;87(3): 633-46.

135. Gerrard JM, Schollmeyer JV, Phillips DR, et al. Alpha-Actinin deficiency in thrombasthenia: possible identity of alpha-actin and glycoprotein III. Am J Pathol. 1979; 94(3):509-28.

136. Gerrard JM, Schollmeyer JV, White JG. The role of contractile proteins in the function of the platelet surface membrane. Cytoskeletal elements and plasma membrane organization. Elsevier/North-Holland. 1981;218-51.

137. Gerrard JM, Stoddard SF, Shapiro RS, et al. Platelet storage pool deficiency and prostaglandin synthesis in chronic granulocytic leukemia. Br J Haematol. 1978; 40(4):597-607.

138. Gerrard JM, Stuart MJ, Rao GHR, et al. Alteration in the balance of prostaglandin and thromboxane synthesis in diabetic rats. J Lab Clin Med. 1980;95(6):950-8.
139. Gerrard JM, Townsend D, Stoddard S, et al. The influence of prostaglandin G2 on platelet ultrastructure and platelet secretion. Am J Pathol. 1977;86(1):99-115.
140. Gerrard JM, White JG, Krivit W. Labile aggregation stimulating substance, free fatty acids, and platelet aggregation. J Lab Clin Med. 1976;87(1):73-82.
141. Gerrard JM, White JG, Krivit W. Platelet function in health and disease. Practice of Pediatrics. 1975;3(69):1-17.
142. Gerrard JM, White JG, Krivit W. Platelet function in health and disease. Pract Peds. 1980; 69:1-20.
143. Gerrard JM, White JG, Krivit W: Effects of pH on arachidonic acid induced platelet aggregation. Thromb Diath Haemorrh. 1975;34(2): 560.
144. Gerrard JM, White JG, Peterson DA. The platelet dense tubular system: its relationship to prostaglandin synthesis and calcium flux. Thromb Haemost. 1978;40(2):224-31. Review.
145. Gerrard JM, White JG, Rao GHR, et al. Labile aggregation stimulating substance (LASS): the factor from storage pool deficient platelets correcting defective aggregation and release of aspirin treated normal platelets. Br J Haematol. 1975;29(4):657-65.
146. Gerrard JM, White JG, Rao GHR, et al. Localization of platelet prostaglandin production in the platelet dense tubular system. Am J Pathol. 1976;83(2):283-98.
147. Gerrard JM, White JG, Rao GHR. Effects of the ionophore A23187 on blood platelets II. Influence on ultrastructure. Am J Pathol. 1974; 77(2):151-66.
148. Gerrard JM, White JG. Prostaglandins and thromboxanes: "middlemen" modulating platelet function in hemostasis and thrombosis. Prog Haemost Thromb. 1978;4:87-125. Review.
149. Gerrard JM, White JG. The influence of aspirin and indomethacin on the platelet contractile wave. Am J Pathol. 1976;82(3):513-26.
150. Gerrard JM, White JG. The influence of prostaglandin endoperoxides on platelet ultrastructure. Am J Pathol. 1975;80(2): 189-202.
151. Gerrard JM, White JG. The structure and function of platelets, with emphasis on their contractile nature. Pathobiol Annu. 1976;6:31-59.
152. Gerritsen SM, Akkerman JWN, Nijmeier B, et al. The Hermansky-Pudlak syndrome: Evidence for a lowered 5-hydroxytryptamine content in platelets of heterozygotes. Scand J Haematol. 1977;18:249-56.
153. Gibson BE, Buchanan MR, Barr RD, et al. Primary thrombocythaemia in childhood: symptomatic episodes and their relationship to thromboxane A2, 6-keto-PGE1 and 12-hydroxy-eicosatetraenoic acid production: a case report. Prostaglandins Leukot Med. 1987;26(3):221-31.
154. Gilman AL, Sloand E, White JG, et al. A novel hereditary macrothrombocytopenia. J Pediatr Hematol Oncol. 1995;17(4):296-305.
155. Ginsberg MH, Wencel JD, White JG, et al. Binding of fibronectin to alpha-granule-deficient platelets. J Cell Biol. 1983;97(2):571-3.
156. Glass DB, Gerrard JM, Townsend D, et al. The involvement of prostaglandin endoperoxide formation in the elevation of cyclic levels during platelet aggregation. J Cyc Nucleotide Res. 1977;3(1):37-44.
157. Goldberg ND, Haddox MK, Estensen RD, et al. Evidence for a dualism between cyclic GMP and cyclic AMP in the regulation of cell proliferation and other cellular processes. Cyclic AMP in Immune Response and Tumor Growth. (Ed. By Lichtenstein L, and Parker C). Springer-Verlag, in the press.
158. Good RA, Quie PG, Windhorst DB, et al. Fatal (chronic) granulomatous disease of childhood: a hereditary defect of leukocyte function. Sem Hematol. 1968;5(3):215-54.
159. Greenberg-Sepersky SM, Simons ER, White JG. Studies of platelets from patients with the gray platelet syndrome. Br J Haematol. 1985; 59(4):603-9.
160. Greinacher A, Bux J, Kiefel V, et al. May-Hegglin anomaly: a rare cause of thrombocytopenia. Eur J Pediatr. 1992;151(9):668-71.
161. Greinacher A, Nieuwenhuis HK, White JG. The Sebastian platelet syndrome. A new form of hereditary thrombocytopenia with

giant thrombocytes and inclusion bodies in granulocytes. Blut. 1990;26:383-5.
162. Greinacher A, Potzsch B, Kiefel V, et al. Evidence that DDAVP transiently improves haemostasis in Bernard-Soulier syndrome independent of von Willebrand-factor. Ann Hematol. 1993;67(3):149-50.
163. Grouse LH, Rao GHR, Weiss DJ, et al. Surface-activated bovine platelets do not spread, they unfold. Am J Pathol. 1990;136(2):399-408.
164. Grouse LH, White JG. Gold-labeled bovine fibrinogen for study of human platelets. Thromb Haemost. 1989;62(4):1112-5.
165. Gunay-Aygun Meral, Falik-Zaccai Tzipora C, Vilboux Thierry, et al. Nature Genetics. 2011;43(8):732-4.
166. Gunning W, Dole M, Brecher M, et al. The Medich giant platelet syndrome: two new cases. Platelets. 2013;24:107-12.
167. Guo Y, Krumwiede M, White JG, et al. HOCl effects on the tight junctions of rabbit tracheal epithelium. Am J Physiol. 1996;270(2 Pt 1): L224-31.
168. Haddox MK, Stephenson JH, Moser ME, et al. Ascorbic acid modulation of splenic cell cyclic GMP metabolism. Life Sci. 1979;24:1555-6.
169. Haga JH, Beaudoin AJ, White JG, et al. Quantification of the passive mechanical properties of the resting platelet. Ann Biomed Eng. 1998; 26(2):268-77.
170. Haire RN, Tisel WA, White JG, et al. On the precipitation of proteins by polymers: the hemoglobin—polyethylene glycol system. Biopolymers. 1984;23(12):2761-79.
171. Ham TH, Grauel JA, Dunn RF, et al. Physical properties of red cells as related to effects in vivo. IV. Oxidant drugs producing abnormal intracellular concentration of hemoglobin (eccentrocytes) with a rigid-red-cell hemolytic syndrome. J Lab Clin Med. 1973;82(6): 898-910.
172. Hamilton RW, Shaikh BS, Ottie JN, et al. Platelet function, ultrastructure, and survival in the May-Hegglin anomaly. Am J Clin Pathol. 1980;74:663-8.
173. HammerschmidtDE, WhiteJG, CraddockPR, et al. Corticosteroids inhibit complement-induced granulocyte aggregation. A possible mechanism for their efficacy in shock states. J Clin Invest. 1979;63(4):798-803.
174. Harmon KR, Witkop CJ, White JG, et al. Marinelli WA, Bitterman PB. Pathogenesis of pulmonary fibrosis: Platelet-derived growth factor precedes structural alterations in the Hermansky-Pudlak syndrome. J Lab Clin Med. 1994;123(4):617-27.
175. Hayward CPM, Moffat KA, Spitzer E, et al. Results of an external proficiency testing exercise on platelet dense-granule deficiency testing by whole mount electron microscopy. American J Clin Path. 2009;131: 671-5.
176. Hazelwood S, Shotelersuk V, Wildenberg SC, et al. Evidence for locus heterogeneity in Puerto Ricans with Hermansky-Pudlak syndrome. Am J Hum Genet. 1997;61(5): 1088-94.
177. Heath KE, Campos-Barros A, Toren A, et al. Non-muscle myosin heavy chain IIA mutations define a spectrum of autosomal dominant macrothrombocytopenias: May-Hegglin anomaly and Fecthner, Sebastian, Epstein, and Alport-like syndromes. Am J Hum Genet. 2001;69(5):1033-45.
178. Hebbel RP, Eaton JW, Steinberg MH, et al. Erythrocyte/endothelial interactions and the vasocclusive severity of sickle cell disease. Prog Clin Biol Res. 1981;55:145-62.
179. Hebbel RP, Eaton JW, Steinberg MH, et al. Erythrocyte/endothelial interactions in the pathogenesis of sickle cell disease: a "real logical" assessment. Blood Cells. 1982;8(1): 163-73.
180. Hebbel RP, Yamada O, Moldow CF, et al. Abnormal adherence of sickle erythrocytes to cultured vascular endothelium: a possible mechanism for microvascular occlusion in sickle cell disease. J Clin Invest. 1980;65(1): 154-60.
181. Hester JP, White JG. [Effect of plasmacytapheresis on thrombocyte ultrastructure] Gematol Transfuziol. 1985;30(1):39-41. Russian.
182. Hill TD, White JG, Rao GHR. Platelet hypersensitivity induced by 1-chloro-2, 4-dinitrobenzene, hydroperoxides and inhibition of lipoxygenase. Thromb Res Suppl. 1989; 53(5): 447-55.

183. Hill TD, White JG, Rao GHR. Role of glutathione and glutathione peroxidase in human platelet arachidonic acid metabolism. Prostaglandins. 1989;38(1):21-32.
184. Hill TD, White JG, Rao GHR. The influence of glutathione depleting agents on human platelet function. Thromb Res Suppl. 1989; 53(5):457-65.
185. Hoak JC, White JG, Day HJ, Kaplan KL, Smith JB. Platelet measurements: Methods, interpretation of results and their value. A. Platelet size and morphology. Hematology 1981 (San Antonio). Am Soc Hematol, 1981; pp. 32-6.
186. Hoidal J, White JG, Repine JE. Influence of cationic local anesthetics on the metabolism and ultrastructure of human alveolar macrophages. J Lab Clin Med. 1979;93:857-66.
187. Hoidal JR, Repine JE, Beall GD, et al. Comparison of the metabolism of alveolar macrophages from humans, rats, and rabbits: phorbol myristate acetate. J Lab Clin Med. 1978;92(5):787-94.
188. Hoidal JR, Repine JE, Beall GD, et al. The effect of phorbol myristate acetate on the metabolism and ultrastructure of human alveolar macrophages. Am J Pathol. 1978; 91(3): 469-82.
189. Hoidal JR, White JG, Repine JE. Impairment of human alveolar macrophage oxygen consumption, and superoxide anion production by local anesthetics used in bronchoscopy. Chest. 1979;75(2 Suppl):243-6.
190. Holmes B, Page AR, Windhorst DB, et al. The metabolic pattern of phagocytic function of leukocytes from children with chronic granulomatous disease. Ann N Y Acad Sci. 1968; 155:888-901.
191. Holmes BH, Page AR, Windhorst DB, et al. Fatal granulomatous disease: a genetic defect of phagocytic function. Birth Defects. Original Article Series. 1968;4:433-42.
192. Horns DJ, Gerrard JM, Rao GHR, et al. Smoking and platelet labile aggregation stimulating substance (LASS) synthesizing activity. Thromb Res Suppl. 1976;9(6):661-8.
193. Horowitz H, White JG. In vivo and in vitro studies on the effect of guanidino-succinic acid on platelet structure and function. Thromb Diath Haemorrh, 2006.
194. Horowitz HI, Stein IM, Cohen BD, et al. Further studies on the platelet-inhibitory effect of guanadinosuccinic acid and its role in uremic bleeding. Am J Med. 1970;49(3):336-45.
195. Huizing M, Anikster Y, Fitzpatrick DL, et al. Hermansky-Pudlak syndrome type 3 in Ashkenazi Jews and other non-Puerto Rican patients with hypopigmentation and platelet storage pool deficiency. Am J Hum Genet. 2001;69:1022-32.
196. Huizing M, Anikster Y, White JG, et al. Characterization of the murine gene corresponding to human Hermansky-Pudlak syndrome type 3: exclusion of the Subtle gray (sut) locus. Mol Genet Metab. 2001; 74(1-2):217-25.
197. Huizing M, Hess R, Dorward H, et al. Cellular, Molecular, and Clinical Characterization of Patients with Hermansky-Pudlak Syndrome Type 5. Traffic 2004;5:711-22.
198. Huizing M, Parkes JM, White JG, et al. Platelet alpha granules in BLOC-2 and BLOC-3 subtypes of Hermansky-Pudlak Syndrome. Platelets. 2007;18(2):150-7.
199. Hussain N, Quezado M, Geho D, et al. Intestinal Disease in Hermansky-Pudlak Syndrome: Prevalence of Colitis and Association with Genotype. J. Clin Gastroenterology and Hepatology. 2006;4(1):73-80.
200. I Ninkovic, JG White, A Rangel-Filho, et al. The role of Rab38 in platelet dense granule defects. Thromb Haemost. 2008;6:2143-51.
201. Ikeda M, White JG, Mizuno H, et al. A morphological study of platelets from stroke-prone spontaneously hypertensive rat and Wistar Kyoto rat. Pathophysiology. 1998; 5:119-24.
202. Irene Lopez-Vilchez, Gines Escolar, Maribel Diaz-Ricart, et al. Tissue factor-enriched vesicles are taken up by platelets and induce platelet aggregation in the presence of factor Vlla. Thromb Haemost. 2007;97:202-11.
203. Jacob H, Amsden T, White JG. Membrane microfilaments of erythrocytes: alteration in intact cells reproduces the hereditary spherocytosis syndrome. Proc Nat Acad Sci. 1972;69:471-4.
204. Jacob HS, Yawata Y, Matsumota N, et al. Cyclic nucleotide-membrane interaction in the regulation of erythrocyte shape and survival: defect in hereditary spherocytosis.

Ann Arbor Symp (George G. Brewer, Ed.) Alan R. Liss, Inc., New York, Erythrocyte Structure and Function. 1975;235-47.
205. Jamieson GA, Agrawal AK, Greco NJ, et al. Phencyclidine binds to blood platelets with high affinity and specifically inhibits their activation by adrenaline. Biochem J. 1992;285: 35-9.
206. Johnson GJ, Allen DW, Cadman S, et al. Red-cell-membrane polypeptide aggregates in glucose-6-phosphate dehydrogenase mutants with chronic hemolytic disease. A clue to the mechanism of hemolysis. N Engl J Med. 1979; 301(10):522-7.
207. Johnson GJ, Allen DW, Flynn TP, et al. Decreased survival in vivo of diamide-incubated dog erthrocytes. A model of oxidant-induced hemolysis. J Clin Invest. 1980;66(5): 955-61.
208. Johnson GJ, Leis LA, Rao GHR, et al. Arachidonate-induced platelet aggregation in the dog. Thromb Res Suppl. 1979;14(1):147-54.
209. Johnson GJ, Rao GHR, Leis LA, et al. Effect of agents that alter cyclic AMP on arachidonate-induced platelet aggregation in the dog. Blood. 1980;55(5):722-9.
210. Johnson GJ, Rao GHR, White JG. Platelet dysfunction induced by parenteral carbenicillin and ticarcillin. Studies of the dose-response relationship and mechanism of action in dogs. Am J Pathol. 1978;91(1):85-106.
211. Johnson GJ, White JG. Proceedings: platelet dysfunction induced by parental administration of carbenicillin and ticarcillin. Thromb Diath Haemorrh. 1975;34(1):341-2.
212. Johnson, GJ, Leis LA, Krumwiede MD, et al. The Critical Role of Myosin IIA in Calcium-Independent Platelet Internal Contraction. J Thromb Haemost. 2007; 5: 1516-29.
213. Kahmann RD, Donohue JM, Bradford DS, et al. Platelet function in adolescent idiopathic scoliosis. Spine. 1992;17(2):145-8.
214. Kahmann RD, Donohue JM, Bradford DS, et al. Platelet function in adolescent scoliosis. 1992;17:145-8.
215. Keuttner JF, Dreher KL, Rao GHR, et al. Influence of the ionophore A23187 on the plastic behavior of normal erythrocytes. Am J Pathol. 1977;88(1):81-94.
216. King RA, Townsend D, Oetting W, et al. Temperature-sensitive tyrosinase associated with peripheral pigmentation in oculocutaneous albinism. J Clin Invest. 1991;87(3): 1046-53.
217. King RA, Wiesner GL, Townsend D, et al. Hypopigmentation in Angelman syndrome. Am J Med Genet. 1993;46(1):40-4.
218. Kotasek D, Vercellotti GM, Ochoa AC, et al. Mechanism of cultured endothelial injury induced by lymphokine-activated killer cells. Cancer Res. 1988;48(19):5528-32.
219. Kourelis TV, Chen D, White JG, et al. Myeloid malignancy presenting with a platelet storage pool disorder. Leukemia & Lymphoma 2013; 54:1800-1.
220. Krishnamurti L, Neglia JP, Nagarajan R, et al. Paris-Trouseau syndrome platelets in a child with Jacobsen's syndrome. Am J Hematol. 2001;66(4):295-9.
221. Krivit K, Tate D, White JG, Robison LL. Idiopathic thrombocytogenic purpura and intracranial hemorrhage. Pediatrics. 1981; 67(4): 570-1.
222. Krivit W, White JG. A simplified approach for the detection of coagulation disorders. Lancet. 1965;85:381-4.
223. Krivit W, Yunis E, White JG. Platelet survival studies in Aldrich syndrome. Pediatrics. 1966;37(2):339-41.
224. Langer F, Obser T, Oyen F, et al. Characterization of the pA1461D mutation causing von Willebrand disease type 2B with severe thrombocytopenia, circulating giant platelets, and defective alpha-granule secretion. Thromb Haemost. 2014;111:777-9.
225. Lasslo A, White JG. The effect of alpha'-bis [3-(N,N-diethylcarbamoyl) piperidino]-p-xylene on human blood platelet structural physiology. Biochim Biophys Acta. 1984; 777(1):37-40.
226. Lederer DJ, Kawut SM, Sonett JR, et al. Successful bilateral lung transplantation for pulmonary fibrosis associated with the hermansky-pudlak syndrome. Journal of Heart and Lung Transplantation. 2005;24:1697-9.
227. Lefebvre P, White JG, Krumwiede MD, et al. Role of actin on platelet function. Eur J Cell Biol. 1993;62:194-204.

228. Leistikow EA, Barnhart MI, Albrecht RM, et al. Redistribution of fibrinogen receptors on surface-activated platelets. Fibrinogen 3. Biochemistry, Biological Functions, Gene Regulation and Expression. MW Mosesson et al, (Eds), Elsevier Science Publishers. 1988; 215-20.
229. Leistikow EA, Barnhart MI, Escolar G, et al. Receptor-ligand complexes are cleared to the open canalicular system of surface-activated platelets. Br J Haematol. 1990; 74(1):93-100.
230. Levine AS, Lemieux B, Brunning R, et al. Ceroid accumulation in a patient with progressive neurological disease. Pediatrics. 1968;42(3): 583-91.
231. Levine AS, Nesbit ME, White JG, et al. Effects of fractionated histones on nucleic acid synthesis in 6C3HEB mouse ascites tumor cells and in normal spleen cells. Cancer Res. 1968;28(5):831-44.
232. Lockman LA, Kennedy WA, White JG. The Chediak-Higashi syndrome: electrophysiologic and electron microscopic observations on the peripheral neuropathy. J Pediatr. 1967;70(6):942-51.
233. Lopez-Vilchez I, Escolar G, Diaz-Ricart M, et al. Isolated platelets internalize human tissue factor and become fully activated in the presence of factor VIIA. Thromb Res. 2008;122: S37-S41.
234. Lopez-Vilchez I, Galan AM, Diaz-Ricart M, et al. Serotonin enhances the procoagulant properties and platelet activation induced during uptake of tissue factor. Cardiovascular Research. 2009;84:309-16.
235. Lopez-Vilchez I, Galan AM, Hernandez MR, et al. Platelet-associated tissue factor enhances platelet reactivity and thrombin generation in experimental studies in vitro. Thrombosis Research. 2012;130:294-300.
236. Lozano M, Escolar G, Mazzara R, et al. Effects of the addition of second-messenger effectors to platelet concentrates separated from whole-blood donations and stored at 4 degrees C or -80 degrees C. Transfusion. 2000; 40(5):527-34.
237. Lozano M, Escolar G, White JG, et al. Redistribution of membrane glycoproteins in platelets activated under flow conditions. Blood Coagul Fibrinolysis. 1996;7(2):214-7.
238. Luckasen JR, White JG, Kersey JH. Mitogenic properties of a calcium ionophore, A23187. Proc Natl Acad Sci USA. 1974; 71(12):5088-90.
239. Lyman BT, Johnson GJ, White JG. Dose-dependent inhibition of experimental arterial thrombosis by carbenicillin and ticarcillin. Am J Pathol. 1978;92(2):473-90.
240. Manoli I, Golas G, Westbroek W, et al. Chediak-Higashi syndrome with early developmental delay resulting from paternal heterodisomy of chromosome 1. Am J Med Genet Part A 152A:1474-83.
241. Huizing M, Pederson B, Hess RA, et al. Clinical and Cellular Characterization of Hermansky-Pudlak Syndrome Type-6. J Med Genet. 2009;46: 803-10.
242. Matzdorff AC, White JG, Malzahn K, et al. Perioperative management of a patient with the Fechtner syndrome. Ann Hematol. 2001; 80(7):436-9.
243. Maynard DM, Heijnen H, Horne MK, et al. Proteomic analysis of platelet alpha granules using mass spectrometry. Journal of Thrombosis and Haemostasis. 2008; 5:1945-55.
244. Mazharian A, Wang YJ, Mori J, et al. Mice Lacking the ITIM-Containing Receptor G6b-B Exhibit macrothrombocytopenia and aberrant platelet function. Science Signaling 5:2012.
245. McBane RD, Elliot MA, White JG, et al. Fechtner syndrome: physiologic analysis of macrothrombocytopenia. Blood Coagul. Fibrinolysis. 2000;11(3):243-7.
246. McDonald RJ, Berger EM, White CW, et al. Effect of superoxide dismutase encapsulated in liposomes or conjugated with polyethylene glycol on neutrophil bactericidal activity in vitro and bacterial clearance in vivo. Am Rev Respir Dis. 1985;131(4):633-7.
247. McGuire SM, Cooley LD, Wicklaud BM, et al. Platelet disorders in Jacobsen syndrome. Genetics in Medicine. 2003;5:231.
248. Miles LA, Ginsberg MH, White JG, et al. Plasminogen interacts with human platelets through two distinct mechanisms. J Clin Invest. 1986;77(6):2001-9.
249. Miller JL, Sheridan JD, White JG. Electrical responses by guinea pig megakaryocytes. Nature. 1978;272(5654):643-5.

250. Mills EL, Gerrard JM, Filipovich D, et al. The chemiluminescence response of human platelets. J Clin Invest. 1978;61:807-14.
251. Milstein JM, White JG, Swaiman KF. Oxidative phosphorylation in mitochondria of developing rat brain. J Neurochem. 1968;15(5):411-5.
252. Milton JG, Frojmovic MM, Tang SS, et al. Spontaneous platelet aggregation in a hereditary giant platelet syndrome (MPS). Am J Pathol. 1984;114(2):336-45.
253. Moxey-Mims MM, Young G, Silverman A, et al. End-stage renal disease in two pediatric patients with Fletchner syndrome. Pediatr. Nephrol. 1999;13(9):782-6.
254. Mundschenk DD, Connelly DP, White JG, Brunning RD. An improved technique for the electronic measurement of platelet size and shape. J Lab Clin Med. 1976; 88(2):301-15.
255. Mundschenk DD, Connelly DP, White JG, et al. An improved technique for the electronic measurement of platelet size and shape. J Clin Lab Med. 1975;88:301-15.
256. Murray KJ, White JG Douglas SD. Comparative biochemical and ultrastructural studies of capillaries from normal humans, normal mice, and human astrocytomas. Surgical Neurology. 1980;14:53-8
257. Murray KJ, White JG, Douglas SD. Albuminal surface topographical studies on human brain capillary isolates in normal and neoplastic states. Scan Elec Micros. 1978;2:907-10.
258. Nichols KE, Crispino JD, Poncz M, et al. Familial dyserythropoietic anemia and thrombocytopenia due to an inherited mutation in GATA1. Nat Genet. 2000;24(3): 266-70.
259. Nickerson DS, White JG, Kronvali G, et al. Indirect visualization of Staphylococcus aureus protein A. J Exp Med. 1970; 131(5):1039-47.
260. NinkovicI, White JG, Rangel-Filho A, et al. The role of Rab38 in platelet dense granule defects. J Thromb and Haemosta. 2008; 6:2143-51.
261. Nyberg SL, Shatford RA, Peshwa MV, et al. Evaluation of a hepatocyte-entrapment hollow fiber bioreactor: A potential bioartificial liver. Biotech Bioeng. 1993;41:194-203.
262. Oetting WS, Handoko HY, Mentink MM, et al. Molecular analysis of an extended family with type IA (tyrosinase-negative) oculocutaneous albinism. J Invest Dermatol. 1991;97(1):15-9.
263. Oetting WS, Mentink MM, Summers CG, et al. Three different frameshift mutations of the tyrosinase gene in type IA oculocutaneous albinism. Am J Hum Genet. 1991;49(1): 199-206.
264. Ordinas A, Escolar G, White JG. Ultrastructure of platelets and platelet-surface interactions (Fissirlis YF and Name J-L (eds.), The Role of Platelets in Blood-Biomaterial Interactions. The Netherlands, Kluwer Academic Publishers. 1993;3-13.
265. Panella TJ, Peters W, White JG, et al. Platelets acquire a secretion defect after high-dose chemotherapy. Cancer. 1990;65(8):1711-6.
266. Parker MS, Rosado Shipley W, de Christenson ML, et al. The Hermansky-Pudlak syndrome. Ann Diagn Pathol. 1997;1(2):99-103.
267. Parker RI, Bray GL, McKeown LP, et al. Failure to mobilize intracellular calcium in response to thrombin in a patient with familial thrombocytopathy characterized by macrothrombocytopenia and abnormal platelet membrane complexes. J Lab Clin Med. 1993;122(4):441-9.
268. Perez-Pujol S, Aras O, Cocking-Johnson D, et al. Stored platelets contain residual amounts of tissue factor. Studies on platelet concentrates stored for prolonged periods. Transfusion. 2005;45(4):572-9.
269. Peterson DA, Gerrard JM, Glover SM, et al. Epinephrine reduction of heme: implication for understanding the transmission of an agonist stimulus. Science. 1982;215(4528):71-3.
270. Peterson DA, Gerrard JM, Peller J, et al. Interactions of zinc with arachidonic acid. Prostaglandins Med. 1981;6(1):91-9.
271. Peterson DA, Gerrard JM, Rao GHR, et al. Epinephrine and other activators of prostaglandin endoperoxide synthetase can reduce Fe3+-heme to Fe2+-heme. Prostaglandins Med. 1980;5(5):357-64.
272. Peterson DA, Gerrard JM, Rao GHR, et al. Ferrous iron mediated oxidation of arachidonic acid: studies employing nitroblue

tetrazolium (NBT). Prostaglandins Med. 1978; 1(4): 304-17.
273. Peterson DA, Gerrard JM, Rao GHR, et al. Inhibition of ferrous iron induced oxidation of arachidonic acid by indomethacin. Prostaglandins Med. 1979;2:97-108.
274. Peterson DA, Gerrard JM, Rao GHR, et al. Interaction of arachidonic acid and heme iron in the synthesis of prostaglandins. Adv Prostaglandin Thromboxane Res. 1980;6: 157-61.
275. Peterson DA, Gerrard JM, Rao GHR, et al. Reduction of ferric heme to ferrous by lipid peroxides: possible relevance to the role of peroxide tone in the regulation of prostaglandin synthesis. Prostaglandins Med. 1980;4(2):73-8.
276. Peterson DA, Gerrard JM, Rao GHR, et al. Reduction of heme by lipid peroxides and its potential relevance to understanding control of cyclo-oxygenase activity. Prog Lipid Res. 1981;20:299-301.
277. Peterson DA, Gerrard JM, Rao GHR, et al. Salicylic acid inhibition of the irreversible effect of acetylsalicylic acid on prostaglandin synthetase may be due to competition for the enzyme cationic binding site. Prostaglandins Med. 1981;6(2):161-4.
278. Peterson LA, Rao KV, Crosson JT, et al. Renal transplantation in Epstein syndrome. Am J Hematol. 1987;24(1):113.
279. Peterson LC, Dampier C, Coetzer T, et al. Clinical and laboratory study of two Caucasian families with hereditary pyropoikilocytosis and hereditary elliptocytosis. Am J Clin Path. 1987;88:58-65.
280. Peterson LC, Rao KV, Crosson JT, et al. Fechtner syndrome: a variant of Alport's syndrome with leukocyte inclusions and macrothrombocytopenia. Blood. 1985; 65(2):397-406.
281. Pfueller SL, Howard MA, White JG, et al. Shortening of bleeding time by 1-deamino-8-argenine vasopressin (DDAVP) in the absence of platelet von Willebrand factor in Gray platelet syndrome. Thromb Heamost. 1987;58(4):1060-3.
282. Polunovsky VA, Rosenwald IB, Tan AT, et al. Translational control of programmed cell death: eukaryotic translation initiation factor 4E blocks apoptosis in growth-factor-restricted fibroblasts with physiologically expressed or unregulated Myc. Molec Cell Biol. 1996;16(11):6573-81.
283. Portoghese PS, Larson DL, Dunham EW, et al. A novel prostaglandin endoperoxide mimic, prostaglandin F2 acetal. J Med Chem. 1977; 20:320-1.
284. Potter WT, Rong S, Griffith J, et al. Phosphine-mediated Heinz body formation and hemoglobin oxidation in human erythrocytes. Toxicol Lett. 1991;57:37-45.
285. Quie PG, White JG, Holmes B. In vitro bactericidal capacity of human polymorphonuclear leukocytes: diminished activity in chronic granulomatous disease of childhood. J Clin Invest. 1967;46(4):668-79.
286. Radha E, Hill TD, Rao GHR, et al. Glutathione levels in human platelets display a circadian rhythm in vitro. Thromb Res Suppl. 1985; 40(6):823-31.
287. Rao GH, Cox CA, Gerrard JM, et al. Alpha tocopherol quinone (alpha TQ): a potent inhibitor of platelet function. Prog Lipid Res. 1981;20:549-52.
288. Rao GH, Radha E, Johnson GJ, et al. Enteric-coated aspirin, platelet cyclooxygenase activity and function. Prostaglandins Leukot Med. 1984;13(3):341-7.
289. Rao GHR, Burris SM, Gerrard JM, et al. Inhibition of prostaglandin (PG) synthesis in sheep vesicular gland mircrosomes (SVGM) by nitroblue tetrazolium (NBT) and vitamin E (VE). Prostaglandins Med. 1979;2(2):111-21.
290. Rao GHR, Cox AC, Gerrard JM, et al. Effects of 2, 2'-dipyridyl and related compounds on platelet prostaglandin synthesis and platelet function. Biochim Biophys Acta. 1980;628(4):468-79.
291. Rao GHR, Cox CA, Witkop CJ Jr, et al. Influence of UV light (250 nm) on platelet activation. International Conference on Prostaglandin and Lipid Metabolism in Radiation Injury. 1986 Oct.
292. Rao GHR, Einzig S, Johnson GJ, et al. Effect of amrinone, a cardiotonic drug, on hemodynamics and platelet function. Prostaglandins Med. 1981;6(1):51-64.

293. Rao GHR, Einzig S, Reddy KR, et al. Tranylcypromine-induced hypertension is not mediated by the inhibition of prostacyclin synthesis. Prostaglandins Med. 1979;3(4): 201-10.
294. Rao GHR, Ericson DG, Weiss DJ, et al. Influence of aspirin and carbacyclin on bovine platelet function. ASAIO J. 1992;38(4):830-4.
295. Rao GHR, Escolar G, White JG. Biochemistry, physiology and function of platelets stored as concentrated. Transfusion. 1993;33(9): 767-78.
296. Rao GHR, Escolar G, White JG. Epinephrine reverses the inhibitory influence of aspirin on platelet-vessel wall interactions. Thromb Res Suppl. 1986;44(1):65-74.
297. Rao GHR, Escolar G, White JG. Monitoring signal transduction and cytoskeletal alterations by fluorescent imaging and confocal microscopy. Ann N Y Acad Sci. 1994;714:297-9.
298. Rao GHR, Escolar G, White JR, et al. Differential response of human and bovine platelets to bovine von Willebrand factor and vascular subendothelium. Platelets. 2001;12:150-55.
299. Rao GHR, Escolar G, Zavoral J, et al. Influence of adrenergic receptor blockade on aspirin-induced inhibition of platelet function. Platelets. 1990;1:145-50.
300. Rao GHR, Fareed J, White JG. Influence of heparins on inositol 1,4,5-trisphosphate-induced calcium mobilization in permeabilized human platelets. Biochem Med Metab Biol. 1991;45(2):171-80.
301. Rao GHR, Fields CG, White JG, et al. Promotion of human platelet adhesion and aggregation by a synthetic, triple-helical "mini-collagen". J Biol Chem. 1994;269(19): 13899-903.
302. Rao GHR, Friedland M, Gerrard JM, et al. The influence of metabolites on the assay of platelet serotonin. Thromb Res Suppl. 1977;10(6):791-802.
303. Rao GHR, Gerrard JM, Cohen I, et al. Origin and role of calcium in platelet activation-contraction-secretion coupling. Cell Calcium Metabolism (Fiskum G, Ed), Plenum Pub Corp. 1989;411-25.
304. Rao GHR, Gerrard JM, Cohen I, et al. Origin and role of calcium in platelet activation-contraction secretion coupling. Cell Calcium Metabolism (Ed): Fiskum, Plenum publishing Corporation. 1989; pp. 411-20.
305. Rao GHR, Gerrard JM, Eaton JW, et al. Arachidonic acid peroxidation, prostaglandin synthesis and platelet function. Photochem Photobiol. 1978;28(4-5):845-50.
306. Rao GHR, Gerrard JM, Eaton JW, et al. The role of iron in prostaglandin synthesis: ferrous iron mediated oxidation of arachidonic acid. Prostaglandins Med. 1978;(1):55-70.
307. Rao GHR, Gerrard JM, Murthy M, et al. Possible mechanisms of epinephrine actions in quin-2-loaded platelets refractory to arachidonic acid. Biochem Med Metab Biol. 1993;50(3):322-37.
308. Rao GHR, Gerrard JM, Witkop CJ, et al. Platelet aggregation independent of ADP release or prostaglandin synthesis in patients with Hermansky-Pudlak syndrome. Prostaglandins Med. 1981;6(4):459-72.
309. Rao GHR, Hordinsky M, Witkop CJ Jr, et al. Influence of psoralen and ultraviolet therapy on platelet function and arachidonic acid metabolism in patients with vitiligo. Prostaglandin and Lipid Metabolism in Radiation Injury. TL Wolden Jr, HN Hughes, (Eds), Plenum Press, New York. 1987;179-84.
310. Rao GHR, Jachimowicz AA, White JG. Rapid separation of tumor-promoting agents, phorbol and phorbol myristate acetate (12-o-tetradecanoylphorbol-13-acetate) by high pressure liquid chromatography. J Chromatogr. 1974;96(1):151-4.
311. Rao GHR, John V, Hill TD, et al. Inhibition of platelet aggregation by novel triphenylethylene analogs. Thromb Res Suppl. 1986;44(4): 527-38.
312. Rao GHR, Johnson GG, Reddy KR, et al. Ibuprofen protects platelet cyclooxygenase from irreversible inhibition by aspirin. Arteriosclerosis. 1983;3(4):383-8.
313. Rao GHR, Johnson GJ, Reddy RK, et al. Rapid return of cyclo-oxygenase active platelets in dogs after a single oral dose of aspirin. Prostaglandins. 1981;22(5):761-72.
314. Rao GHR, Johnson GJ, White JG. Influence of epinephrine on the aggregation response of aspirin-treated platelets. Prostaglandins Med. 1980;5(1):45-58.

315. Rao GHR, Kishore NP, Peller JD, et al. Influence of polyenoic acids on arachidonic acids metabolism and platelet function. Cardiovascular Disease. Plenum Pub. Corp., New York. 1987;495-505.
316. Rao GHR, Kishore NP, White JG. Differential effects of putative inhibitors on cytosolic and membrane associated platelet lipoxygenase. Prostaglandins Leukot Med. 1987;26(3): 281-90.
317. Rao GHR, Krishnamurthi S, Raij L, et al. Influence of nitric oxide on agonist-mediated calcium mobilization in platelets. Biochem Med Metab Biol. 1990;43(3):271-5.
318. Rao GHR, Mahadevappa VG, Hill TD, et al. Arachidonic acid oxidation and platelet function. In: Biological Oxidation Systems, C Reddy, Ed., Academic Press, New York. 1990;779-91.
319. Rao GHR, Peller JD, Knopman DS, et al. Physiology and function of platelets from patients with Alzheimer's disease. Indian J Physiol Pharmacol. 1996;40(1):5-14.
320. Rao GHR, Peller JD, Richards KL, et al. Rapid separation of nucleotides from granulocytes by isocratic, reversed-phase high-performance liquid chromatography. J Chromatogr. 1982;229(1):205-10.
321. Rao GHR, Peller JD, Semba CP, et al. Influence of the calcium-sensitive fluorophore, Quin 2, on platelet function. Blood. 1986; 67(2): 354-61.
322. Rao GHR, Peller JD, White JG. Influence of ionized calcium on thrombin-induced down regulation of GPIb/IX receptors on human platelets. Thromb Res. 1997;85(1):23-31.
323. Rao GHR, Peller JD, White JG. Measurement of ionized calcium in blood platelets with a new generation calcium indicator. Biochem Biophys Res Commun. 1985;132(2):652-7.
324. Rao GHR, Peller JD, White JG. Rapid separation of platelet nucleotides by reverse-phase, isocratic high-pressure liquid chromatography with a radially compressed column. J Chromatogr. 1981;226(2):466-70.
325. Rao GHR, Radha E, White JG. Effect of docosahexaenoic acid (DHA) on arachidonic acid metabolism and platelet function. Biochem Biophys Res Commun. 1983; 117(2):549-55.
326. Rao GHR, Radha E, White JG. Irreversible platelet aggregation does not depend on lipoxygenase metabolites. Biochem Biophys Res Commun. 1985;131(1):50-7.
327. Rao GHR, Raij L, Lester B, et al. Inhibition of agonist-induced human platelet activation by nitric oxide. Roy Soc Proc. Moncada S and Higgs EA, (Eds), Elsevier Pub. Co., Inc., New York. 1990;355-67.
328. Rao GHR, Rao AS, White JG. Aspirin in ischemic heart disease—an overview. Indian Heart J. 1993;45(2):73-9.
329. Rao GHR, Rao AS, White JG. Influence of low dose enteric-coated aspirin on platelet function. Indian Heart J. 1992;44(6):365-70.
330. Rao GHR, Ratnammal K Reddy KR, White JG. Low dose aspirin, platelet function and prostaglandin synthesis: influence of epinephrine and alpha adrenergic blockade. Prostaglandins Med. 1981;6(5):485-94.
331. Rao GHR, Reddy KR, Hagert K, et al. Influence of pH on the prostacyclin (PGI2) mediated inhibition of platelet function. Prostaglandins Med. 1980;4(4):263-73.
332. Rao GHR, Reddy KR, White JG. Effect of acetaminophen and salicylate on aspirin-induced inhibition of human platelet cyclooxygenase. Prostaglandins Leukot Med. 1982;9(1): 109-15.
333. Rao GHR, Reddy KR, White JG. Influence of trifluorperazine on platelet aggregation and disaggregation. Prostaglandins Med. 1980; 5(3):221-34.
334. Rao GHR, Reddy KR, White JG. Modification of human platelet response to sodium arachidonate by membrane modulation. Prostaglandins Med. 1981;6(1):75-90.
335. Rao GHR, Reddy KR, White JG. Penicillin induced human platelet dysfunction and its reversal by epinephrine. Prostaglandins Leukot Med. 1983;11(2):199-11.
336. Rao GHR, Reddy KR, White JG. Simple method for the separation of monohydroxy fatty acid metabolites of arachidonate metabolism. J Chromatogr. 1982;232(1): 176-9.
337. Rao GHR, Reddy KR, White JG. The influence of epinephrine on prostacyclin (PGI2) induced dissociation of ADP aggregated platelets. Prostaglandins Med. 1980;4(6): 385-97.

338. Rao GHR, Schmidt HH, Reddy KR, et al. Human platelet activation by an alkylacetyl analogue of phosphatidylcholine. Biochim Biophys Acta. 1982;715(2):205-14.
339. Rao GHR, Smith CM, Doni MG, et al. Intracellular calcium in adherent human platelets. Arterioscl Thromb. 1994;5:95-103.
340. Rao GHR, Smith CM, Escolar G, et al. Influence of heat on platelet biochemistry, structure and function. J Lab Clin Med. 1993;122(4):455-64.
341. Rao GHR, Smith CM, White JG. Influence of calcium antagonists on thrombin-induced calcium mobilization and platelet-vessel wall interactions. Biochem Med Metab Biol. 1992; 47(3):226-31.
342. Rao GHR, Tate MR, Murthy M, et al. Influence of antioxidants on arachidonic acid metabolism and platelet function. Biochem Med Metab Biol. 1994;51(1):74-9.
343. Rao GHR, White JG, Cox CA. Influence of a calcium dependent protease inhibitor on platelet activation and secretion. Thromb Res Suppl. 1987;47(6):625-37.
344. Rao GHR, White JG, Jackimowicz AA, et al. An improved method for the extraction of endogenous platelet serotonin. J Lab Clin Med. 1976;87(1):129-37.
345. Rao GHR, White JG, Jackimowicz AA, et al. Nucleotide profiles of normal and abnormal platelets by high pressure liquid chromatography. J Lab Clin Med. 1974;84:839-50.
346. Rao GHR, White JG. An improved method for measuring endogenous serotonin in platelets of patients with Hermansky-Pudlak syndrome. Thromb Res Suppl. 1988; 51(2):225-7.
347. Rao GHR, White JG. Aspirin, prostaglandin E1 and Quin-2 AM-induced platelet dysfunction: restoration of function by noradrenalin. Prostaglandins Leukot Essent Fatty Acids. 1990;39(2):141-6.
348. Rao GHR, White JG. Comparative pharmacology of cyclooxygenase inhibitors in platelet function. Prostaglandins Leukot Med. 1985;18(1):119-31.
349. Rao GHR, White JG. Coronary artery disease: an overview of risk factors. Indian Heart J. 1993;45(3):143-53. Review.
350. Rao GHR, White JG. Disaggregation and reaggregation of "irreversibly" aggregated platelets: a method for more complete evaluation of anti-platelet drugs. Agents Actions. 1985;16(5):425-34.
351. Rao GHR, White JG. Epinephrine and platelet function. J Lab Clin Med. 1997; 130(3):238-9.
352. Rao GHR, White JG. Epinephrine potentiation of arachidonate-induced aggregation of cyclooxygenase-deficient platelets. Am J Hematol. 1981;11(4):355-66.
353. Rao GHR, White JG. Epinephrine-induced platelet membrane modulation. Platelet Amine Storage Granules (Myers K, Ed.), Academic Press. 1989;117-47.
354. Rao GHR, White JG. Heme-polyenoic acid interaction and prostaglandin synthesis. In: Prostaglandins, Leukotrienes and Lipoxins: Biochemistry Mechanisms of Action and Clinical Applications. MJ Bailey, (Ed), Plenum Publishing Co. 1985;357-69.
355. Rao GHR, White JG. Influence of esterase inhibitors on platelet aggregation induced by phorbol myristate acetate. Biochem Pharmacol. 1975;24(2):293-5.
356. Rao GHR, White JG. Influence of GDP(B)S on agonist-induced calcium mobilization and platelet function. Biology of Cellular Transducing Signals. J Franklin, (Ed), Plenum Pub. 1989;343-52.
357. Rao GHR, White JG. Influence of phospholipase A2 on human blood platelet alpha adrenergic receptor function. Thromb Res Suppl. 1989;53(5):427-34.
358. Rao GHR, White JG. Influence of various doses of aspirin (in vivo) on platelet arachidonic acid metabolism (ex vivo) and function. Prostaglandins Leukot Essent Fatty Acids. 1994;51(1):63-7.
359. Rao GHR, White JG. Platelet activating factor (PAF) causes human platelet aggregation through the mechanism of membrane modulation. Prostaglandins Leukot Med. 1982;9(4): 459-72.
360. Rao GHR, White JG. Role of arachidonic acid metabolism in human platelet activation and irreversible aggregation. Am J Hematol. 1985; 19(4):339-47.
361. Rao GHR, Wilson RF, White CW, et al. Influence of thrombolytic agents on platelet function. Thromb Res Suppl. 1991;62(4):319-34.

362. Rao, GHR, Krick PT, White JG. Preparation, separation and characterization of vitamin E quinone. J Chromatog. 1980;196:506-11.
363. Ratliff NB, Gerrard JM, White JG. Platelet-leukocyte interactions following arterial endothelial injury. Am J Pathol. 1979;96(2):567-80.
364. Repine JE, Clawson CC, Burchell HB, et al. Reversible neutrophil defect in patients with bacterial endocarditis. J Lab Clin Med. 1976; 88(5):780-7.
365. Repine JE, Clawson CC, White JG, et al. Spectrum of function in neutrophils from carriers of sex-linked chronic granulomatous disease. J Pediatr. 1975;87(6 Pt 1):901-7.
366. Repine JE, Hoidal JR, Beall GD, et al. The effect of temperature on the chemiluminescence response of polymorphonuclear leukocytes in vitro. Biochemical and Clinical Aspects of Oxygen. WS Caughey, (Ed). Academic Press, New York. 1979;725-36.
367. Repine JE, Rao GH, Beall GD, et al. Inhibition of human neutrophil oxidative metabolism and degranulation in vitro by nitroblue tetrazolium and vitamin E. Am J Pathol. 1978;90(3):659-74.
368. Repine JE, Rasmussen B, White JG. An improved nitroblue tetrazolium test using phorbol myristate acetate-coated coverslips. Am J Clin Pathol. 1979;71(5):582-5.
369. Repine JE, White JG, Clawson C, et al. The influence of phorbol myristate acetate on the metabolism of neutrophils from carriers of sex-linked chronic granulomatous disease. J Lab Clin Med. 1975;85(1):82-6.
370. Repine JE, White JG, Clawson CC, et al. Effects of phorbol myristate acetate on the metabolism and ultrastructure of neutrophils in chronic granulomatous disease. J Clin Invest. 1974;54(1):83-90.
371. Repine JE, White JG, Clawson CC, et al. The influence of phorbol myristate acetate on oxygen consumption by polymorphonuclear leukocytes. J Lab Clin Med. 1974; 83(6):911-20.
372. Ringeisen AL, Schimmenti LA, White JG, et al. Hermansky-Pudlak syndrome (HPS5) in a nonagenarian. J. AAPOS. 2013;17:334-6.
373. Roder JC, Haliotis T, Laing L, et al. Further studies of natural killer cell function in Chediak-Higashi patients. Immunology. 1982; 46(3):555-60.
374. Rodriguez V, Nichols WL, Charlesworth JE, et al. Sebastian platelet syndrome, a hereditary macrothrombocytopenia: case report and review. Mayo Clinic Journal of Medicine. Mayo Clin Proc. 2003;78:1416-21.
375. Rubin CM, Burke BA, McKenna RW, et al. The accelerated phase of Chediak-Higashi syndrome. An expression of the virus-associated hemophagocytic syndrome? Cancer. 1985; 56(3):524-30.
376. Ruska E. The development of electron microscopy Bioscience Reports. 1986;7: 607-29.
377. Sauk JJ Jr, White JG, Witkop CJ Jr. Alteration in the surface morphology of synchronized B-16 melanoma cell during the cell cycle. Acta Derm Venereol. 1975;55(5):331-6.
378. Sauk JJ Jr, White JG, Witkop CJ Jr. Influence of prostaglandin E1, E2 and arachidonate on melanosomes in melanocytes and keratinocytes of analgen hair bulbs in vitro. J Invest Dermatol. 1975;64(5):332-7.
379. Sauk JJ, Krumwiede M, Cocking-Johnson D, et al. Alterations in lipid fluidity by cholesterol and cholesterol hemisuccinate modulate the organization of microtubule skeletons in epithelial cells. J Oral Pathol. 1987;16(2):69-74.
380. Sauk JJ, Krumwiede M, Cocking-Johnson D, et al. Reconstitution of cytokeratin filaments in vitro: further evidence for the role of nonhelical peptides in filament assembly. J Cell Biol. 1984;99(5):1590-7.
381. Schattner M, Lefebvre P, Mingolelli SS, et al. Thrombopoietin-stimulated ex vivo expansion of human bone marrow megakaryocytes. Stem Cells. 1996;14(2):207-14.
382. Schmaier AH, Smith PM, Purdon AD, et al. High molecular weight kininogen: localization in the unstimulated and activated platelet and activation by a platelet calpain(s). Blood. 1986;67(1):119-30.
383. Schollmeyer JV, Rao GHR, White JG. An actin-binding protein in human platelets. Interactions with alpha-actinin on gelation of actin and the influence of cytochalasin B. Am J Pathol. 1978;93(2):433-46.
384. Schorer AE, Gerrard JM, White JG, et al. Oral contraceptive use alters the balance

of platelet prostaglandin and thromboxane synthesis. Prostaglandins Med. 1978; 1(1):5-11.

385. Schorer AE, White JG. Interleukin 1 enhances arterial thrombogenicity in vitro. Thromb Res Suppl. 1989;56(4):515-22.

386. Segura D, Monreal L, Perez-Pujol S, et al. Assessment of platelet function in horses: Ultrastructure, flow cytometry, and perfusion techniques. J Vet Intern Med. 2006;20: 581-8.

387. Shah NB, Vercellotti GM, White JG, et al. Blood-Nanoparticle Interactions and in Vivo Biodistribution: Impact of Surface PEG and Ligand Properties. Molecular Pharmaceutics 2012;9:2146-55.

388. Shalev A, Michaud G, Israels SJ, et al. Quantification of a novel dense granule protein (granulophysin) in platelets of patients with dense granule storage pool deficiency. Blood. 1992;80(5):1231-7.

389. Shapiro RS, Gerrard JM, Perry GS, et al. Wiskott-Aldrich syndrome: detection of the carrier state by metabolic stress of platelets. Lancet. 1978;1(8056):121-3.

390. Shapiro RS, Gerrard JM, Ramsay NK, et al. Selective deficiency in collagen-induced platelet aggregation during L-asparaginase therapy. Am J Pediatr Hematol Oncol. 1980; 2(3):207-12.

391. Sharp H, White JG, Krivit W. Histiocytosis X treated with vinblastine sulfate (NSC-49842). Cancer Chemother Reports. 1964; 39:53-9.

392. Sharp HL, Carey JB Jr, White JG, et al. Cholestyramine therapy in patients with a paucity of intrahepatic bile ducts. J Pediatr 1967;71(5): 723-36.

393. Sharp HL, Nesbit ME, White JG, et al. Renal and hepatic pathology following initial remission of acute leukemia induced by prednisone. Cancer. 1967;20(9):1395-402.

394. Shatford RA, Nyberg SL, Meier SJ, et al. Hepatocyte function in a hollow fiber bioreactor: a potential bioartificial liver. J Surg Res. 1992;53(6):549-57.

395. Shencheng Ge, James G. White, and Christy Haynes. Quantal Release of Serotonin from Platelets. Analytical Chemistry. 2009;81(8): 2935-43.

396. Sheppard JR, McSwigan JD, Wehner JM, et al. The adrenergic responsiveness of Down syndrome cells. Prog Clin Biol Res. 1982;97: 307-25.

397. Sheppard JR, Schumacher W, White JG, et al. The alpha adrenergic response of Down's syndrome platelets. J Pharmacol Exp Ther. 1983; 225(3):584-8.

398. Sheppeck RA, Bentz M, Dickson C, et al. Examination of the roles of glycoprotein Ib and glycoprotein IIb/IIIa in platelet deposition on an artificial surface using clinical antiplatelet agents and monoclonal antibody blockade. Blood. 1991;78:673-80.

399. Shoeman DW, White JG, Mannering GH. Cytochrome P-420: tubular aggregated from hepatic mircrosomes. Science. 1969; 165(900):1371-2.

400. Smith CM, Burris SM, Hunninghake DB, et al. Altered platelet deformability in patients with type IIa and type IV hyperlipoproteinemia. Am J Hematol. 1988;27(4):247-52.

401. Smith CM, Burris SM, Rao GHR, et al. Alcohol consumption in the guinea pig is associated with reduced megakaryocyte deformability and platelet size. J Lab Clin Med. 1992;120(5):699-706.

402. Smith CM, Burris SM, Rao GHR, et al. Epinephrine-induced reversal of aspirin effects on platelet deformability. Thromb Res Suppl. 1988;51(1):35-44.

403. Smith CM, Burris SM, Weiss DJ, et al. Comparison of bovine and human platelet deformability, using micropipette elastimetry. Am J Vet Res. 1989;50(1):34-8.

404. Smith CM, Burris SM, White JG. High frequency of elongated platelet forms in guinea pig blood: ultrastructure and resistance to micropipette aspiration. J Lab Clin Med 1990; 115(6):729-37.

405. Smith CM, Burris SM, White JG. Micropipette aspiration of guinea pig megakaryocytes: absence of fragmentation and dependence on maturation stage. Blood. 1989;73(6):1570-5.

406. Smith CM, Burris SM, White JG. Micropipette aspiration of guinea pig megakaryocytes: maturational changes in deformability. Blood. 1989;73:225-7.

407. Smith CM, Hebbel RP, Tukey DP, et al. Pluronic F-68 reduces the endothelial

adherence and improves the rheology of liganded sickle erythrocytes. Blood. 1987;69(6):1631-6.

408. Smith CM, Krivit W, White JG. The irreversibly sickled cell. Am J Ped Hematol Oncol. 1982; 4(3):307-15.
409. Smith CM, Kuettner JF, Tukey DP, et al. Variable deformability of irreversibly sickled erythrocytes. Blood. 1981;58(1):71-7.
410. Smith CM, Tukey DP, Mundshenk D, et al. Filtration deformability of rabbit pulmonary macrophage. J Lab Clin Med. 1982;99(4): 568-79.
411. Smith CM, Williams GC, Krivit W, et al. Micellar properties of 3-alpha, 7 alpha, 12 alpha-trihydroxy-5 beta-cholestan-26-oyl taurine and relationship to in vitro red cell disruption. J Lab Clin Med. 1979;94(4):624-32.
412. Smith DM, Gerrard JM, Juhn SK, et al. Arachidonic acid metabolism in nasal polyps and allergic inflammation. Minn Med. 1981; 64(10):605-10.
413. Smith DM, Gerrard JM, White JG. Comparison of arachidonic acid metabolism in nasal polyps and eosinophils. Int Arch Allergy Appl Immunol. 1987;82(1):83-8.
414. Stark SN, White JG, Langer L, et al. Epsilon amino caproic acid therapy as a cause of intrarenal obstruction in hematuria of hemophiliacs. Scand J Haemat. 1965;2(2):99-107.
415. Statland BE, Heagan BM, White JG. Uptake of calcium by platelet relaxing factor. Nature. 1969;223(205):521-2.
416. Steiger B, White JG, Krivit W. Epsilon-amino-caproic acid for hematuria in hemophilia. Lancet. 1962;82:421-4.
417. Stuart MJ, Gerrard JM, White JG. Effect of cholesterol on production of thromboxane b2 by platelets in vitro. N Engl J Med. 1980;302(1):6-10.
418. Stuart MJ, Gerrard JM, White JG. The influence of albumin and calcium on human platelet arachidonic acid metabolism. Blood. 1980;55(3):418-23.
419. Sullivan PS, Grubbs ST, Olchowy TW, et al. Bleeding diathesis associated with variant von Willebrand factor in a Simmental calf. J Am Vet Med Assoc. 1994;205(12):1763-6.
420. Tate DY, Carlton GT, Nesbit ME, et al. Detection of platelet associated IgG in immune thrombocytopenia: a new assay employing protein A and peroxidase anti-peroxidase (PROA-PAP). Am J Hematol. 1980;9(4): 349-61.
421. Tate DY, Sorenson RL, Gerrard JM, et al. An immunoenzyme histochemical technique for the detection of platelet antibodies from the serum of patients with idiopathic (autoimmune) thrombocytopenia purpura (ITP). Br J Haematol. 1977;37(2):265-75.
422. Thielen N, Huizing M, Krabbe JG, et al. Hermansky-Pudlak syndrome: the importance of molecular subtyping. J Thromb Haemost. 2010;8:1643-5.
423. Tisel WA, Haire RN, White JG, et al. Polyphasic linkage between protein solubility and ligand binding in the hemoglobin-polyethylene glycol system. J Biol Chem. 1980;255(19):8975-8.
424. Velez-Garcia EO, Fradera J, de Lourdes Telmont M, et al. Megakaryoblastic transformation of pH positive chronic granulocytic leukemia. Am J Clin Pathol. 1985;84(2): 228-33.
425. Vincent LM, Adams D, Hess RA, et al. Hermansky-Pudlak Syndrome Type 1 in a patient of Indian descent. Mol. Genet Metab. 2009;97 (3):227-33.
426. Visser MR, Tracy PB, Vercellotti GM, et al. Enhanced thrombin generation and platelet binding on herpes simplex virus-infected endothelium. Proc Natl Acad Sci USA. 1988; 85(21):8227-30.
427. Walsh PN, Mills DC, White JG. Metabolism and function of human platelets washed by albumin density gradient separation. Br J Haematol. 1977;36(2):287-96.
428. Ward PC, Schwartz BS, White JG. Heinz-body anemia: "bite cell" variant—a light and electron microscopic study. Am J Hematol. 1983; 15(2):135-46.
429. Ward PC, Smith CM, White JG. Erythrocytic ecdysis: An unusual morphologic finding in a case of sickle cell anemia with intercurrent cold-agglutinin syndrome. Am J Clin Pathol. 1979;72(3):479-85.
430. Wedemeyer PP, White JG, Nesbit ME, et al. Resection of metastases in Wilm's tumor: a report of three cases cured of pulmonary and hepatic metastases. Pediatrics. 1968; 41(2):446-51.

431. Wei S, Wang H, Zhang G, et al. Platelet I kappa B Kinase-beta Deficiency Increases Mouse Arterial Neointima Formation via Delayed Glycoprotein Ib alpha Shedding. Arterioscler. Thromb. Vasc. Biol. 2013;33:241-8.
432. Weiss DJ, McClay CB, Smith CM, et al. Platelet function in the racing thoroughbred: Implication for exercise-induced pulmonary hemorrhage. Vet Clin Path. 1990;19:35-9.
433. Weiss HJ, Lages B, Vicic W, et al. Heterogeneous abnormalities of platelet dense granule ultrastructure in 20 patients with congenital storage pool deficiency. Br J Haematol. 1993;83(2):282-95.
434. Wells PH, Dreher KL, Burris SM, et al. Concurrent effects of microsieve aspiration and the ionophore A23187 on the morphologic characteristics of the surface of normal erythrocytes. Am J Clin Pathol. 1980;73(6):754-60.
435. Wencel-Drake JD, Dahlback B, White JG, et al. Ultrastructural localization of coagulation factor V in human platelets. Blood. 1986; 68(1):244-9.
436. Westbroek W, Adams D, Huizing M, et al. Cellular Defects in Chediak-Higashi Syndrome Correlate with the Molecular Genotype and Clinical Phenotype. J Invest Dermatol. 2007; 31.
437. White JG, Burris SM. The cytoskeletons of X-linked GATA-1 macrothrombocytes are deficient in talin. Platelets. 2008;19(7):543-50.
438. White JG, Ahlstrand GG. Giant electron dense chains, clusters and granules in megakaryocytes and platelets with normal dense bodies: an inherited thrombocytopenic disorder111Platelet analytical electron microscopy. Platelets. 2003;305-12.
439. White JG, Brunning RD. Neutrophils in the gray platelet syndrome. Platelets. 2004;15: 333-40.
440. White JG, Burris S, Escolar G. Influence of thrombin in suspension, surface activation, and high shear on platelet surface GPIb/IX distribution. J Lab Clin Med. 1999;133(3): 245-52.
441. White JG, Burris S, Smith CM. Relationship of actin filament assembly to clearance of fibrinogen gold, GPIIb-IIIa complexes on spread platelets. Eur J Clin Invest. 1995; 25(4):241-9.
442. White JG, Burris SM, Crowe BS. GATA-1, G208S macrothrombocytes are deficient in talin: Immunofluorescence studies. Platelets. 2009;20(3):216-24.
443. White JG, Burris SM, Hasegawa D, et al. Micropipette aspiration of human blood platelets: a defect in the Bernard-Soulier's syndrome. Blood. 1984;63(5):1249-52.
444. White JG, Burris SM, Tukey D, et al. Micropipette aspiration of human platelets: influence of microtubules and actin filaments on deformability. Blood. 1984;64(1):210-4.
445. White JG, Burris SM. Morphometry of platelet internal contraction. Am J Pathol. 1984; 115(3):412-7.
446. White JG, Clawson CC, Gerrard JM. Platelet ultrastructure. Hemostasis and Thrombosis. AL Bloom and AL Thomas, (Eds), Churchill Livingstone, London. 1981;22-49.
447. White JG, Clawson CC. Blood cells and blood vessels. The Ultrastructure of Normal and Abnormal Skin (Zelickson AS, Ed). New York, Lea and Febiger Co., 1967.
448. White JG, Clawson CC. Chediak-Higashi syndrome: variable cytochemical reactivity of giant inclusions in polymorphonuclear leukocytes. Ultrastruct Pathol. 1980; 1(2):223-36.
449. White JG, Clawson CC. Development of giant granules in platelets during prolonged storage. Am J Pathol. 1980;101(3):635-45.
450. White JG, Clawson CC. Effects of large latex particle uptake on the surface connected canalicular system of blood platelets: a freeze-fracture and cytochemical study. Ultrastruct Pathol. 1981;2(3):277-87.
451. White JG, Clawson CC. Effects of small latex particle uptake on the surface connected canalicular system of blood platelets: a freeze-fracture and cytochemical study. Diagn Histopathol. 1982;5(1):3-10.
452. White JG, Clawson CC. Overview article: biostructure of blood platelets. Ultrastruct Pathol. 1980;1(4):533-58. Review.
453. White JG, Clawson CC. The Chediak-Higashi syndrome: microtubules in monocytes and lymphocytes. Am J Hematol. 1979;7(4): 349-56.

454. White JG, Clawson CC. The Chediak-Higashi syndrome: ring-shaped lysosomes in circulating monocytes. Am J Pathol. 1979;96(3): 781-98.
455. White JG, Clawson CC. The Chediak-Higashi syndrome: Spectrum of giant organelles in peripheral blood cells. Henry Ford Hosp Med J. 1979; 27: 286-99.
456. White JG, Clawson CC. The Chediak-Higashi syndrome; the nature of the giant neutrophil granules and their interactions with cytoplasm and foreign particulates. I. Progressive enlargement of the massive inclusions in immature neutrophils. II. Manifestations of cytoplasmic injury and sequestration. III. Interactions between giant organelles and foreign particuiates. Am J Pathol. 1980; 98(1):151-96.
457. White JG, Clawson CC. The surface-connected canalicular system of blood platelets—a fenestrated membrane system. Am J Pathol. 1980;101(2):353-64.
458. White JG, Cocking-Johnson D, Krumwiede M. Platelet particle processing: an example of surface sorting on single cells. Platelets. 1990;1:205-11.
459. White JG, Conrad WJ. The fine structure of freeze-fractured blood platelets. Am J Pathol. 1973;70(1):45-56.
460. White JG, Davis RB. Alterations of platelet ultrastructure in patients with carcinoid syndrome. Am J Pathol. 1969;56(3):519-31.
461. White JG, de Alarcon P. Platelet spherocytosis: a new bleeding disorder. Am J Hematol. 2002; 70(2):158-66.
462. White JG, Edson JR, Desnick SJ, et al. Studies of platelets in a variant of the Hermansky-Pudlak syndrome. Am J Pathol. 1971;63(2): 319-32.
463. White JG, Escolar G. Current concepts of platelet membrane response to surface activation. Platelets. 1993;4:176-89.
464. White JG, Escolar G. EDTA-induced changes in platelet structure and function: adhesion and spreading. Platelets. 2000;11(1):56-61.
465. White JG, Escolar G. Fate of the GPIb/IX receptor complex following activation of human platelets. Blood Coagul Fibrinolysis. 1996;7(2):262-5.
466. White JG, Escolar G. Fibrinogen receptors do not undergo spontaneous redistribution on surface-activated platelets. Arteriosclerosis. 1990;10(5):738-44.
467. White JG, Escolar G. Function of platelet mobile receptors. Thromb Haemost. 1992; 68(6):779.
468. White JG, Escolar G. Induction of receptor clustering, patching, and capping on surface-activated platelets. Lab Invest. 1990; 63(3): 332-40.
469. White JG, Escolar G. Mobility of GPIIb-IIIa receptors within membranes of surface- and suspension-activated platelets does not depend on assembly and contraction of cytoplasmic actin. Eur J Cell Biol. 1990;52(2): 341-8.
470. White JG, Escolar G. Restoring platelet adhesion function. Br J Haematol. 1994;87(2): 439-42.
471. White JG, Escolar G. The blood platelet open canalicular system: a two-way street. Eur J Cell Biol. 1991;56(2):233-42
472. White JG, Estensen RD. Cytochemical electron microscopic studies of the action of phorbol myristate acetate on platelets. Am J Pathol. 1974;74(3):453-66.
473. White JG, Estensen RD. Degranulation of discoid platelets. Am J Pathol. 1972;68(2): 289-302.
474. White JG, Estensen RD. Selective labilization of specific granules in polymorphonuclear leukocytes by phorbol myristate acetate. Am J Pathol. 1974;75(1):45-60.
475. White JG, Estenson RD. Influence of cytochalasin B (CB) on platelet aggregation. J Lab Clin Med. 1971;78(5):849-50.
476. White JG, Gerrard JM, Rao GHR, et al. Differences in platelet storage pool deficiency (SPD) of Hermansky Pudlak syndrome (HPS) and non-albinos (NA). Thromb Diath Haemorrh. 1975;34(1):360-1.
477. White JG, Gerrard JM, Witkop CJ Jr. Platelet-platelet interaction: A simple test for storage pool deficiency and effective prostaglandin synthesis. Proceedings of the workshop on "The Significance of Platelet Function Tests in the Evaluation of Hemostatic and Thrombotic Tendencies." Platelet Function Testing (HJ Day, J Holmsen and MB Zucker, Eds.), DHEW Pub. No. 78-1087 (NIH). 1978;374-85.
478. White JG, Gerrard JM. Interaction of microtubules and microfilaments in platelet

contractile physiology. Methods Achiev Exp Pathol. 1979;9:1-39. Review.

479. White JG, Gerrard JM. Platelet membranes and membrane systems. Convention of the American Association of Blood Banks, San Francisco, "Membrane Structure and Function of Human Blood Cells". 1976;4:61-79.

480. White JG, Gerrard JM. Platelet morphology and the ultrastructure of regulatory mechanisms involved in platelet activation. Platelets: A Multidisciplinary Approach. 1978; 17-34.

481. White JG, Gerrard JM. Platelet ultrastructure in relation to platelet function. Prog Clin Biol Res. 1978;28:5-23.

482. White JG, Gerrard JM. Prostaglandins and platelet ultrastructure. Presented at the International Symposium on Prostaglandins in Hematology. March 4-5, 1976, Philadelphia PA. (Melvin Silver, JB Smith and J Kocsis, Eds.), New York, Spectrum Publications, Inc. 1977;293-319.

483. White JG, Gerrard JM. Recent advances in platelet structural physiology. Suppl Thromb Haemost. 1978;63:49-60.

484. White JG, Gerrard JM. Section D. Platelet function and its disorders: Anatomy and structural organization of the platelet. Hemostasis and Thrombosis. RW Colman, RW Hirsch, J Marder, CJ Salzman, (Eds), JB Lippincott, 1982;343-63.

485. White JG, Gerrard JM. The Cell Biology of Platelets. Handbook of Inflammation (The Cell Biology of Inflammation). G Weissman (Ed), Elsevier/North Holland, Inc., New York. 1980;83-143.

486. White JG, Gerrard JM. The ultrastructure of defective human platelets. Molec Cell Biochem. 1978;21(2):109-28.

487. White JG, Gerrard JM. Ultrastructural features of abnormal blood platelets. A review. Am J Pathol. 1976;83(3):589-632.

488. White JG, Gerrard JM. Ultrastructural features of abnormal blood platelets. Am. J. Pathol. 1976;83:590-606.

489. White JG, Gunay-Aygun M. The York platelet syndrome: a third case. Platelets. 2011;22(2): 117-34.

490. White JG, Hagert KR, Nipper JH, et al. Functional platelets after storage in vitro for 15-21 days. Am J Pathol. 1980;101(3):613-33.

491. White JG, Heagan B. Gels of normal and sickled hemoglobin: comparative study. J Exp Med. 1970;131(6):1079-92.

492. White JG, Heagan B. The fine structure of hemoglobin polymerization. Sickle Cell Disease: Diagnosis, Management, Education and Research. Saint Louis (CV Mosby Co.). 1973; 104-29.

493. White JG, Heagan B. Tubular polymers of normal human hemoglobin. Am J Pathol. 1970; 59(1):101-14.

494. White JG, Heagan BS. The fine structure of cell-free sickled hemoglobin. Am J Pathol. 1970;58(1):1-17.

495. White JG, Hess RA, Gahl WA, et al. Rapid ultrastructural detection of success or failure after bone marrow transplantation in the Chediak-Higashi Syndrome. Platelets. 24:71-White JG: Platelet Structure. In: Platelets-3rd Edition., 2013 Academic Press, (Ed: Alan Michelson). pp. 117-44.

496. White JG, Hess RA, Gahl WA, et al. Rapid ultrastructural detection of success or failure after bone marrow transplantation in the Chediak-Higashi syndrome. Platelets. 2013;24:71-4.

497. White JG, Keel S, Reyes M, Burris SM. Alpha-Delta platelet storage pool deficiency in three generations. Platelets. 2007;18(1):1-10.

498. White JG, Key NS, King RA, et al. A Touch of the White Platelet Syndrome. Platelets. 2005; 16:346-61.

499. White JG, Key NS, King RA, et al. The white platelet syndrome: A new autosomal dominant platelet disorder. 1. Structural abnormalities. Platelets. 2004;15:173-84.

500. White JG, Krivit W, Vernier R. An ultrastructural investigation of the fibrin clot utilizing ferritin labeled anti-human fibrinogen antibody. Blood. 1964;24:443-50.

501. White JG, Krivit W, Vernier R. The platelet-fibrin relationship in human blood clots: an ultrastructural study utilizing ferritin conjugated anti-human fibrinogen antibody. Blood. 1965;25:241-57.

502. White JG, Krivit W. An ultrastructural basis for the shape changes induced in platelets by chilling. Blood. 1967;30(5):625-35.

503. White JG, Krivit W. Changes in platelet microtubules and granules during early

clot development. Thromb Diath Haemorrh Suppl. 1967;26:29-42.
504. White JG, Krivit W. Fine structural localization of adenosine triphosphates in human platelets and other blood cells. Blood. 1965;26(5):554-68.
505. White JG, Krivit W. Surgical excision of pulmonary metastases. Pediatrics. 1962;29(6): 927-32.
506. White JG, Krivit W. The ultrastructural localization and release of platelet lipids. Blood. 1966;27(2):167-86.
507. White JG, Krumwiede M, Burris SM, et al. Isolation of microtubule coils from platelets after exposure to aggregating agents. Am J Pathol. 1986;125(2):319-26.
508. White JG, Krumwiede M, Sauk JJ. Microtubule reassembly in surface-activated platelets. Blood. 1985;65(6):1494-503.
509. White JG, Krumwiede M. Further studies of the secretory pathway in thrombin-stimulated human platelets. Blood. 1987;69(4): 1196-203.
510. White JG, Krumwiede M. Influence of cytochalasin B on the shape change induced in platelets by cold. Blood. 1973;41(6):823-32.
511. White JG, Krumwiede M. Influence of intracellular chelating agents on formation of spike-like pseudopods by human platelets. Platelets. 1999;10(2-3):159-68.
512. White JG, Krumwiede M. Isolation of microtubule coils from normal human platelets. Blood. 1985;65(4):1028-32.
513. White JG, Krumwiede M. Normal-sized primary lysosomes are present in Chediak-Higashi syndrome neutrophils. Pediatr Res. 1987;22(2):208-15.
514. White JG, Krumwiede MD, Cocking-Johnson D, et al. Induction of GPIb/IX-vWF receptor-ligand translocation on surface-activated platelets. Arterioscler Thromb Vasc Biol. 1995; 15(5):642-54.
515. White JG, Krumwiede MD, Cocking-Johnson D, et al. Influence of combined thrombin stimulation, surface activation, and receptor occupancy on organization of GPIb/IX receptors on human platelets. Br J Haematol. 1994;88(1):137-48.
516. White JG, Krumwiede MD, Cocking-Johnson D, et al. Prelabeled glycoprotein Ib/IX receptors are not cleared from exposed surfaces of thrombin-activated platelets. Am J Pathol. 1996;149(2):629-38.
517. White JG, Krumwiede MD, Cocking-Johnson D, et al. Retention of glycoprotein Ib/IX receptors on external surfaces of thrombin-activated platelets in suspension. Blood. 1995; 86(9):3468-78.
518. White JG, Krumwiede MD, Cocking-Johnson D, et al. Uptake of vWF-anti-vWF complexes by platelets in suspension. Arterioscler Thromb Vasc Biol. 1996;16(7):868-77.
519. White JG, Krumwiede MD, Cocking-Johnson DJ, et al. Dynamic redistribution of glycoprotein Ib/IX on surface-activated platelets. A second look. Am J Pathol. 1995; 147(4):1057-67.
520. White JG, Krumwiede MD, Cocking-Johnson DJ, et al. Influence of cytochalasin B (CB) on GP Ib distribution after thrombin or TRAP and before surface activation. Platelets. 1997; 8(1):53-60.
521. White JG, Krumwiede MD, Cocking-Johnson DK, et al. Redistribution of GPIb/IX and GPIIb/IIIa during spreading of discoid platelets. Br J Haematol. 1995;90(3):633-44.
522. White JG, Krumwiede MD, Escolar G. EDTA induced changes to platelet structure and function: influence on particle uptake. Platelets. 1999;10:327-37.
523. White JG, Krumwiede MD, Escolar G. Glycoprotein Ib is homogenously distributed on external and internal membranes of resting platelets. Am J Pathol. 1999;155(6):2127-34.
524. White JG, Krumwiede MD, Johnson DC, et al. Localization of GPIb/IX and GPIIb/IIIa on discoid platelets. Platelets. 1995;6:233-41.
525. White JG, Krumwiede MD. Some contributions of electron microscopy to knowledge of human platelets. Thromb Haemosta. 2007;98:69-72.
526. White JG, Krumwiede MD. The down-side of platelet interaction with surfaces. Eur J Cell Biol. 1994;65(1):178-88.
527. White JG, Kumar A, Hogan MJ. Gray Platelet Syndrome in a Somalian Family. Platelets. 2006;17(8):519-27.
528. White JG, Leistikow EL, Escolar G. Platelet membrane responses to surface and suspension activation. Blood Cells. 1990; 16(1):43-70; discussion 70-2.

529. White JG, Matlack KL, Mundschenk D, et al. Platelet Studies in a Normal and Bleeder Horse. In: Proceedings of the First International Symposium on Equine Hematology (Kitchen H, Krehbiel JD, Eds) 1975; pp. 209-21.
530. White JG, Mattson JC, Nichols WL, et al. A variant of the Sebastian platelet syndrome with unique neutrophil inclusions. Platelets. 2002;13(2):121-7.
531. White JG, Nichols WL, Steensma DP. Platelet Pathology in Sex-linked GATA-1 Dyserythropoietic Macrothrombocytopenia I. Ultrastructure. Platelets. 2007;18(4): 273-83.
532. White JG, Pakzad K, Meister L. The York platelet syndrome: A fourth case with unusual pathologic features. Platelets 2013; 24:44-50.
533. White JG, Radha E, Krumwiede M. Isolation of circumferential microtubules from platelets without simultaneous fixation. Blood. 1986; 67(4):873-7
534. White JG, Rao GHR, Estensen RD. Investigation of the release reaction in platelets exposed to phorbol myristate acetate. Am J Pathol. 1974;75(2):301-14.
535. White JG, Rao GHR, Gerrard JM. A. Platelet stimulus activation contraction secretion coupling: a frequently fractured chain of events. Proceedings of the International Workshop on Regulation of Coagulation. KG Mann and FB Taylor, (Eds), New York, Elsevier/North-Holland. 1980;363-76.
536. White JG, Rao GHR, Gerrard JM. Effects of nitroblue tetrazolium and vitamin E on platelet ultrastructure, aggregation and secretion. Am J Pathol. 1977;88(2):387-402.
537. White JG, Rao GHR, Gerrard JM. Effects of the ionophore A23187 on blood platelets I. Influence on aggregation and secretion. Am J Pathol. 1974;77(2):135-4.
538. White JG, Rao GHR, Gerrard JM. Prostaglandins in platelet activation. Platelets-Cellular Response Mechanisms and Their Biological Significance. A Rotman, FA Meyer C Gitler and A Silberberg, (Eds), John Wiley & Sons, New York. 1980;201-2.
539. White JG, Rao GHR, Gerrard JM. Vitamin E and platelets: cooperative interactions with nitroblue tetrazolium on inhibition of adhesion, aggregation and secretion. Am J Pediatr Hematol Oncol. 1979;1(2):155-68.
540. White JG, Rao GHR. Aggregated-disaggregated, refractory platelets retain sensitivity to ristocetin. Thromb Res. 1996;84(4):253-66.
541. White JG, Rao GHR. Effects of a microtubule stabilizing agent on the response of platelets to vincristine. Blood. 1982;60(2):474-83.
542. White JG, Rao GHR. Influence of a microtubule stabilizing agent on platelet structural physiology. Am J Pathol. 1983;112:207-17.
543. White JG, Rao GHR. Microtubule coils versus the surface membrane cytoskeleton in maintenance and restoration of platelet discoid shape. Am J Pathol. 1998;152(2): 597-609.
544. White JG, Rao GHR. Thrombin-induced inhibition of platelet agglutination by von Willebrand factor (vWF): Reversal by ionized calcium. Platelets. 1996;7:321-8.
545. White JG, Repine JE. Fine structural alterations induced in erythrocytes by phorbol myristate acetate. Am J Pathol. 1978;91(3): 571-80.
546. White JG, Sauk JJ. Microtubule coils in spread blood platelets. Blood. 1984;64(2):470-8.
547. White JG, Sauk JJ. The organization of microtubules and microtubule coils in giant platelet disorders. Am J Pathol. 1984;116(3): 514-22.
548. White JG, Thomas A. Platelet Structural Pathology in a Patient with the X-linked GATA-1, R216Q Mutation. Platelets. 2009;20: 41-9.
549. White JG, Ward PCJ, Smith CM. Defective hemoglobin, defective membranes. A commentary on: Some cytochemical and cytological features of erythrocytopoiesis in thalassemia by Bo Thorell. Blood Cells. 1984;13:205. Commentary
550. White JG, Witkop CJ Jr, Gerritsen SM. The Hermansky-Pudlak syndrome: inclusions in circulating leucocytes. Brit J Haematol. 1973; 24(6):761-5.
551. White JG, Witkop CJ Jr, Gerritsen SM. The Hermansky-Pudlak syndrome: ultrastructure of bone marrow macrophages. Am J Pathol. 1973;70(3):329-43.
552. White JG, Witkop CJ. Effects of normal and aspirin platelets on defective secondary aggregation in the Hermansky-Pudlak

syndrome. A test for storage pool deficient platelets. Am J Pathol. 1972;68(1):57-66.

553. White JG, Yunis E, Colliander M, et al. Prolonged bleeding time in a patient with plasma thromboplastic antecedent deficiency: observations on correction on the bleeding time by platelet transfusion. J Pediatr. 1963;63(6): 1081-6.

554. White JG, Yunis E, Colliander M, Krivit W. The correction of prolonged bleeding times in two brothers by platelet transfusions despite normal in vitro platelet tests. Pediatrics. 1964;33 (4):579-84.

555. White JG. A biphasic response of platelets to serotonin. Scand J Haematol. 1970;7(3): 145-51.

556. White JG. A comment on the ultrastructure of amoebocytes from the horseshoe crab (limulus Polyphemus). "Workshop on Animal Models of Thrombosis and Hemorrhagic Diseases", March 12-13, 1975, Nat Acad Sci. 1976; 97-101.

557. White JG. A commentary on: megakaryocyte fragments and the microtubule coil. Blood Cells. 1987;12:611-14.

558. White JG. A search for the platelet secretory pathway using electron dense tracers. Am J Pathol. 1970;58(1):31-49.

559. White JG. A simple method for preservation of fine structure of blood cells. Thromb Diath Haemorrh. 1967;18(3-4):745-53.

560. White JG. Albinism-oculocutaneous, Hermansky-Pudlak type. Birth Defects Compendium, 3rd edn. 1984;60.

561. White JG. An overview of platelet structural physiology. Scanning Microsc. 1987;1(4): 1677-700. Review.

562. White JG. Anatomy and structural organization of the platelet. Hemostasis and Thrombosis: Basic Principles and Clinical Practice, 3rd Edn. Colman RW and Salzman EW, (Eds), JB Lippincott. 1990.

563. White JG. Anatomy and structural organization of the platelet. In: Hemostasis and Thrombosis, 2nd edn. Colman RW, Hirsh J, Marder VJ, Salzman EW, (Eds). 1987;537-54.

564. White JG. Arrangements of actin filaments in the cytoskeleton of human platelets. Am J Pathol. 1984;117(2):207-17.

565. White JG. Book Review; Platelets. Michelson AD, (Ed), San Diego, CA: Academic Press, 2003. 704pp. Am J. Clin Path 2003.

566. White JG. Chemical ultrastructure of human platelets. Physiology of Hemostasis and Thrombosis. (Johnson SA and Seegers WA Eds.), Springfield, Charles C. Thomas Co., 1967; pp. 224-46.

567. White JG. Combined nephelometric and electron microscopic study of the platelet release reaction. Platelet Adhesion and Aggregation in Thrombosis: Countermeasures. (Mammen EF, Anderson GH, Barnhart MI, Eds), New York, FG Schathauer Verlag, 73-91. Thromb et Diath Haemorrh Suppl. 1970;42:73-91.

568. White JG. Current concepts of platelet structural physiology and pathology. Hum Path. 1974;5:1-6.

569. White JG. Current concepts of platelet structure. Am J Clin Pathol. 1979;71(4):363-78. Review.

570. White JG. Cytoskeletal changes in aging platelets. Prog Clin Biol Res. 1985;195:49-77.

571. White JG. Delivery of platelets from megakaryocytes. Prog Clin Biol Res. 1990;356: 25-39. Review.

572. White JG. Disorders affecting Megakaryocytes: Inherited conditions. Blood and Bone Marrow Pathology Platelets. (Wickramasinghe SN and McCullough J, Eds.) Churchill Livingston. Elsevier Science Limited. Edinburgh. 2003;493-523.

573. White JG. EDTA induced changes in platelet structure and function: influence on particle uptake. Platelets. 1999;10(5):327-37.

574. White JG. EDTA-induced changes in platelet structure and function: clot retraction. Platelets. 2000;11(1):49-55.

575. White JG. Effects of an ionophore, A23187, on the surface morphology of normal erythrocytes. Am J Pathol. 1974;77(3):507-18.

576. White JG. Effects of atropine on platelet structure and function. Scand J Haematol. 1969;6(4):236-45.

577. White JG. Effects of cationic polypeptides on thrombosthenic and afibrinogenemic blood platelets. Am J Pathol. 1972;68(3):447-60.

578. White JG. Effects of colchicine and Vinca alkaloids on human platelets. I. Influence

on platelet microtubules and contractile function. Am J Pathol. 1968;53(2):281-91.

579. White JG. Effects of colchicine and Vinca alkaloids on human platelets. II. Changes in the dense tubular system and formation of an unusual inclusion in incubated cells. Am J Pathol. 1968;53(3):447-61.

580. White JG. Effects of colchicine and vinca alkaloids on human platelets. III. Influence on primary internal contraction and secondary aggregation. Am J Pathol. 1969; 54(3):467-78.

581. White JG. Effects of ethylenediamine tetracetic acid (EDTA) on platelet fine structure. Scand J Haematol. 1968;5(4):241-54.

582. White JG. Effects of heat on platelet structure and function. Blood. 1968;32(2):324-35.

583. White JG. Effects of hypertonic stress on the fine structure of sickled erythrocytes. Blood. 1970;35(4):437-46.

584. White JG. Effects of inhibitors on platelet structure and function. Platelets, Thrombosis, and Inhibitors. P Didisheim and T Shimamoto, (Eds) FK Schattauer-Verlag, New York, Springer-Verlag. 1974;289-99.

585. White JG. Electron Dense Chains and Clusters in Human Platelets. Platelets. 2002;13(5): 317-25.

586. White JG. Electron microscopic studies of platelet secretion. Prog Haemost Thromb. 1974;2(0):49-98. Review.

587. White JG. Electron microscopic studies on relationships between platelet structure and function. Thromb et Diath Haemorrh Suppl. 1971;46:161-6.

588. White JG. Electron microscopy methods for studying platelet structure and function. In: Methods in Molecular Biology, vol 272: Platelets and Megakaryocytes, vol 1: Functional Assays. (Gibbins M and Makaut-Smith, Eds) Human Press, Inc, Totown, NJ. pp. 47-64.

589. White JG. Electron opaque structures in Human Platelets: Which are or are not dense bodies. Platelets. 2008;19:455-66.

590. White JG. Electron-dense chains and clusters in platelets from patients with storage pool-deficiency disorders. J Thromb. and Haemostasis. 2003;1:74-9.

591. White JG. Exocytosis of secretory organelles from blood platelets incubated with cationic polypeptides. Am J Pathol. 1972;69(1):41-54.

592. White JG. Extended survival of platelets in vitro under alkaline conditions. Plasma Ther Trans Technol. 1982;3:309-15.

593. White JG. Fine structural alterations induced in platelets by adenosine diphosphate. Blood. 1968;31(5):604-22.

594. White JG. Fine structural demonstration of acid phosphatase activity in Auer bodies. Blood. 1967;29(4):Suppl: 667-82.

595. White JG. Function des plaquettes. l'Hematologie de Bernard Dreyfus. Breton-Gorius J, Reyes F, Rochant H, Rosa J, Vernant, JP, (Eds) Medicine-Sciences/Flamarion. Paris. 1992;15:129-37.

596. White JG. Functional architecture of platelet activation. Platelet 1990: Platelet and Arteriosclerosis: Interaction of Platelets and Blood Vessels. H Yamazuki, Aoki N, H Hidaka, A Kuramoto and M Okuma, Eds., Kagaku Hyoronska, Tokyo, 1990.

597. White JG. Functional aspects of the platelet cytoskeleton. Proceedings of Twenty Years with ETRO. Barcelona. 1996;44-55.

598. White JG. Functional significance of mobile receptors on human platelets. Arterioscler Thromb. 1993;13(8):1236-43.

599. White JG. Giant electron dense chains, clusters and granules in megakaryocytes and platelets with normal dense bodies: An inherited thrombocytopenic disorder. I. Megakaryocytes. Platelets. 2003;14:53-60.

600. White JG. Giant electron dense chains, clusters and granules in megakaryocytes and platelets with normal dense bodies: An inherited thrombocytopenic disorder. II. Platelet morphology. Platelets. 2003; 14:109-21.

601. White JG. Giant electron dense chains, clusters and granules in megakaryocytes and platelets with normal dense bodies: An inherited thrombocytopenic disorder. III. Platelet analytical electron microscopy. Platelets. 2003;14: 305-12.

602. White JG. Giant electron dense chains, clusters and granules in megakaryocytes and platelets with normal dense bodies: An inherited thrombocytopenic disorder. IV. Ultrastructural cytochemistry and analytical

electron microscopy. Platelets. 2003;14: 313-24.
603. White JG. Giant organelles containing tubules in Chediak-Higashi lymphocytes. Am J Pathol. 1972;69(2):225-38.
604. White JG. Giant platelet disorders. Haematologica. 2002;87:85-89.
605. White JG. Gray platelet syndrome. Encyclopedic Reference of Molecular Mechanisms of Disease. 2009;758-9.
606. White JG. Identification of platelet secretion in the electron microscope. Ser Haematol. 1973;6(3):429-59.
607. White JG. Induction of patching and its reversal on surface-activated human platelets. Br J Haematol. 1990;76(1):108-15.
608. White JG. Influence of microtubule stabilization on platelet physiology. Trans Assoc Am Physicians. 1982;95:264-71.
609. White JG. Influence of Taxol on the response of platelets to chilling. Am J Pathol. 1982; 108(2):184-95.
610. White JG. Inherited abnormalities of the platelet membrane and secretory granules. Hum Pathol. 1987;18(2):123-39.
611. White JG. Interaction of membrane systems in blood platelets. Am J Pathol. 1972;66(2): 295-312.
612. White JG. Long-term storage of functional platelets in vitro. Vox Sang. 1981;(40 Suppl): 119-22.
613. White JG. Lymphocyte inclusions. Ann Intern Med. 1972;76(6):1042-3.
614. White JG. May-Hegglin anomaly: the classic giant platelet syndrome. Intercom Children and Their Health. 1983;5(2):1-4.
615. White JG. May-Hegglin Anomaly: The Classic Giant platelet Syndrome. Department of Pediatrics Intercom. 1983;5:2-5.
616. White JG. Mechanisms of platelet production. Blood Cells. 1989;15(1):48-57.
617. White JG. Membrane abnormalities in congenital disorders of human blood platelets. Prog Clin Biol Res. 1982;97:351-70.
618. White JG. Membrane defects in inherited disorders of platelet function. Am J Pediatr Hematol Oncol. 1982;4(1):83-94.
619. White JG. Morphological and functional aspects of cellular hemostatic mechanisms. Hämostaseologie. 1996;16:78-87.
620. White JG. Morphological studies of platelets and platelet reactions. Vox Sang. 1981;(40 Suppl):8-17.
621. White JG. Morphology and ultrastructure of platelets. Platelets in Thrombotic and non-thrombotic disorders: Pathophysiology, Pharmacology and Therapeutics. (Gresele P, Page CP, Fruster V, and Vermylen J, Eds.) Cambridge University Press. New York. 2002; 41-69.
622. White JG. Observations on the mechanism of erythrocyte sickling. Pediatr Res. 1969; 3(3):220-7.
623. White JG. Origin and function of platelet dense bodies. Ser Haematol. 1970;3(4): 17-46.
624. White JG. Physico-chemical dissection of platelet structural physiology. Platelets: production, function, transfusion and storage. M Baldini, S Ebbe, (Eds.) 1974;235-52.
625. White JG. Physiology of platelets. In: State of the Art in Idiopathic Thrombocytopenic Purpura (ITP) of Childhood. Del Principe D, Menichelli A, Rossi P, Guazzini S. Proceedings of the Satellite Symposium Annual Meeting of the European Society for Pediatric Research, Padua, September 10, 1987.
626. White JG. Platelet disorders. Curr Sci ISSN 2. 1990;130-3.
627. White JG. Platelet Function and Its Disorders. A. Anatomy and Structural Organization of the Platelet. Hemostasis and Thrombosis, 2nd Ed. R Colman, J Hirsch, V Marder and E Salzman, (Eds), JB Lippincott Co. 1985.
628. White JG. Platelet glycosomes. Platelets. 1999; 10(4):242-6.
629. White JG. Platelet granule disorders. Crit Rev Oncol Hematol. 1986;4(4):337-77. Review.
630. White JG. Platelet interior imaging technologies. Blood. 2010;116:6150-51. Carmona-Rivera C, Golas G, Hess R, Cardillo ND, Martin E, O'Brien K, Tsilou E, Gochuico BR, White JG, Huizing M, Gahl WA. Clinical, molecular and cellular features of non-Puerto Rican Hermansky-Pudlak syndrome patients of Hispanic descent. Journal of Investigative Dermatology. 2011; 131:2394-400.

631. White JG. Platelet membrane interactions. Platelets. 1999;10(6):368-81.
632. White JG. Platelet membrane ultrastructure and its changes during platelet activation. Prog Clin Biol Res. 1988;283:1-32. Review.
633. White JG. Platelet microtubules and giant granules in the Chediak-Higashi syndrome. Am J Med Technol. 1978;44(4):273-8.
634. White JG. Platelet microtubules and microfilaments: effects of cytochalasin B on structure and function. Platelet Aggregation (J Caen, Ed.), Paris, Masson & Cie. 1971;15-52.
635. White JG. Platelet morphology and function. Principles of Hematology. McGraw-Hill. 1972; 1023-39.
636. White JG. Platelet morphology. The Circulating Platelet (SE Johnson, Ed), New York, Academic Press, 1971;45-121.
637. White JG. Platelet pathology in carriers of the X-linked GATA-1 macrothrombocytopenia. Platelets. 2007;18:620-27.
638. White JG. Platelet secretion during clot retraction. Platelets. 2000;11(6):331-43.
639. White JG. Platelet secretory granules and associated proteins. Lab Invest. 1993;68(5): 497-8.
640. White JG. Platelet secretory process. Blood. 1999;93(7):2422-5.
641. White JG. Platelet size: A preamble to the discussion of giant platelets. Intercom (Department of Pediatrics, University of Minnesota) 1982;4:1-4.
642. White JG. Platelet storage lesions. Guest Editorial. Blood Cells. 1992;18:359.
643. White JG. Platelet Storage Pool Deficiency in the Jacobsen syndrome. Platelets. 2007; 18(7): 522-7.
644. White JG. Platelet structural physiology: the ultrastructure of adhesion, secretion and aggregation in arterial thrombosis. Cardiovasc Clin. 1987;18(1):13-33.
645. White JG. Platelet Structure. In: Platelets (Michelson A, ed) II nd edition. 2006 Academic Press, Burlington, Ma, pp. 1343.
646. White JG. Platelet ultrastructure in the chemistry of coagulation. Univ Minn Med Bull. 1965;37:381-4.
647. White JG. Platelet Ultrastructure.pp20-46. In: Haemostasis and Thromb. (Bloom AL, and Thomas, DR, Eds.) Churchill Livingstone London and New York. 1987
648. White JG. Platelets and atherosclerosis. Eur J Clin Invest. 1994;24(Suppl 1):25-9.
649. White JG. Platelets are covercytes, not phagocytes: Uptake of bacteria involves channels of the open canalicular system. Platelets. 2005;16:121-31.
650. White JG. Platelets in perspective (editorial). West J Med. 1981;134:148-9.
651. White JG. Preservation of platelet function after prolonged storage in vitro. Proceedings of the 1980 Conference on Management and Logistics of Blood Banking. RE Huit and RC Hubbell, (Eds), Denver, Colorado. 1981.
652. White JG. Scanning electron microscopy of erythrocyte deformation: the influence of a calcium ionophore, A23187. Semin Hematol. 1976;13(2):121-32.
653. White JG. Self-association of bound fibrinogen on platelet surfaces. J Lab Clin Med. 1997; 129(6):653-5.
654. White JG. Separate and combined interactions of fibrinogen-gold and latex with surface-activated platelets. Am J Pathol. 1990;137(4): 989-98.
655. White JG. Serotonin storage organelles in human megakaryocytes. Am J Pathol. 1971; 63(3):403-10.
656. White JG. Shape change. Platelets, Thrombosis, and Inhibitors. P Didisheim and T Shimamoto (Eds.) FK Schattauer-Verlag, New York, Springer-Verlag). 1974;247-62.
657. White JG. Structural defects in inherited and giant platelet disorders. In: Hariis H and Herschorn KH, eds. Advances in Human Genetics. Plenum Pub. Corp, New York, 1989; pp. 133-234.
658. White JG. Structural defects in inherited and giant platelet disorders. Adv Hum Genet. 1990;19:133-234. Review.
659. White JG. The Chediak-Higashi syndrome. Fine structure of giant inclusions in freeze-fractured neutrophils. Am J Pathol. 1973; 72(3):503-20.
660. White JG. The Chediak-Higashi syndrome: a possible lysosomal disease. Blood. 1966; 28(2):143-56.
661. White JG. The Chediak-Higashi syndrome: cytoplasmic sequestration in circulating leukocytes. Blood. 1967;29(4):435-51.

662. White JG. The cytoskeleton of fresh and stored platelets. Third Joint US-USSR Symposium on Blood Transfusion, 1985.
663. White JG. The cytoskeleton of human blood platelets. Blood Cell Biochemistry, Plenum Pub. Corp. 1990;2:113-48.
664. White JG. The cytoskeleton of human blood platelets. Blood Cell Biochemistry, Megakaryocytes, Platelets, Macrophages and Eosinophils. Plenum Pub. Corp., New York and London. 1991;2:113-48.
665. White JG. The dense bodies of human platelets. Origin of serotonin storage particles from platelet granules. Am J Pathol. 1968;53(5): 791-808.
666. White JG. The dense bodies of human platelets. Platelet Amine Storage Granules, K Myers, (Ed), Academic Press 1992;1-29.
667. White JG. The dense bodies of human platelets: inherent electron opacity of serotonin storage particles. Blood. 1969;33(4):598-606.
668. White JG. The fine structure of sickled hemoglobin in situ. Blood. 1968;31(5):561-79.
669. White JG. The importance of history in the diagnosis of congenital coagulation disorders. Lancet. 1962;82:408-12.
670. White JG. The interplatelet zone. Am J Pathol. 1970;58(1):19-29.
671. White JG. The morphology of platelet function. Methods in Hematology, Series 8L: Measurements of Platelet Function. LA Harker and TS Zimmerman, (Eds), Churchill-Livingstone, New York. 1983;1-25.
672. White JG. The origin of dense bodies in the surface coat of negatively stained platelets. Scand J Haemat. 1968;5(5):371-82.
673. White JG. The secretory pathway of bovine platelets. Blood. 1987;69(3):878-85.
674. White JG. The secretory process in platelets. The Cell Biology of the Secretory Process. M Cantin, (Ed), Karger, New York, NY. 1984; 541-64.
675. White JG. The submembrane filaments of blood platelets. Am J Pathol. 1969;56(2): 267-77.
676. White JG. The substructure of human platelet microtubules. Blood. 1968;32(4):638-48.
677. White JG. The transfer of thorium particles from plasma to platelets and platelet granules. Am J Pathol. 1968;53(4):567-75.
678. White JG. The ultrastructure and regulatory mechanisms of blood platelets. Blood Platelet Function and Medicinal Chemistry. A Lasslo, (Ed), Elsevier/North-Holland Inc. 1984;15-59.
679. White JG. Time-lapse cinemicroscopy and scanning electron microscope of platelet formation by megakaryocytes: a commentary. Blood Cells. 1983;9(3):419-26.
680. White JG. Tubular elements in platelet granules. Blood. 1968;32(1):148-56.
681. White JG. Ultrastructural analysis of platelet contractile apparatus. Methods Enzymol. 1992;215:109-27.
682. White JG. Ultrastructural analysis of the platelet contractile apparatus. Methods in Enzymology. 1992;215:109-27.
683. White JG. Ultrastructural changes in stored platelets. Blood Cells. 1992;18(3):461-75; discussion 476-9. Review.
684. White JG. Ultrastructural defects in congenital disorders of platelet function. Ann NY Acad Sci. 1972;201:205-33.
685. White JG. Ultrastructural features of erythrocyte and hemoglobin sickling. Arch Intern Med. 1974;133(4):545-62.
686. White JG. Ultrastructural lesions of stored platelets. Vox Sang. 1981;(40 Suppl 1):62-8.
687. White JG. Ultrastructural modifications in platelet membranes and cytoskeleton following activation. Blood Cells. 1983;9(2):237-61.
688. White JG. Ultrastructural physiology and cytochemistry of blood platelets. The Platelet. 1971;6:83-115.
689. White JG. Ultrastructural physiology of platelets with randomly dispersed rather than circumferential band microtubules. Am J Pathol. 1983;110(1):55-63.
690. White JG. Ultrastructural studies of the gray platelet syndrome. Am J Pathol. 1979;95(2): 445-62.
691. White JG. Uptake of latex particles by blood platelets: phagocytosis or sequestration? Am J Pathol. 1972;69(3):439-58.
692. White JG. Use of the electron microscope for diagnosis of platelet disorders. Semin. Thromb Hemost. 1998;24(2):163-8. Review.

693. White JG. Views of the platelet cytoskeleton at rest and at work. Ann N Y Acad Sci. 1987;509: 156-76.
694. White JG. Virus-like particles in the peripheral blood cells of two patients with Chediak-Higashi syndrome. Cancer. 1966;19(6): 877-84.
695. White JG. Why Human Platelets Fail to Kill Bacteria. Platelets. 2006;17(3):191-200.
696. White JG: Comments on the blood platelet contractile system. Hemostasis. 1975;4: 186-92.
697. White JG: Effects of inhibitors on platelet structure and function. Platelets, Thrombosis and Inhibitors. Seminar. Schattauer Verlag. New York. 1974.
698. White JG: Platelet size: A preamble to the discussion of giant platelets. Department of Pediatrics Itercom; 1965;4:3-4.
699. White, JG. Golgi complexes in hypogranular platelet disorders. Platelets. 2005;16:51-60.
700. White, JG. Localization of a lysosomal enzyme in platelets from patients with the White platelet syndrome. Platelets. 2006; 17(4):231-49.
701. White, JG. Medich Giant Platelet Disorder: A Unique α-granule deficiency. 1. Structural abnormalities. Platelets. 2004;15:345-53.
702. Wiesner GL, Bendel CM, Olds DP, et al. Hypopigmentation in the Prader-Willi syndrome. Am J Hum Genet. 1987;40(5):431-42.
703. Wildenberg SC, Oetting WS, Almodovar C, et al. A gene causing Hermansky-Pudlak syndrome in a Puerto Rican population maps to chromosome 10q2. Am J Hum Genet 57. 1995;57(4):755-65.
704. Windhorst DA, White JG, Zelickson AS, et al. The Chediak-Higashi anomaly of the Aleutian trait in mink. Homologous defects of lysosomal structure. Ann NY Acad Sci. 1968;155: 818-46.
705. Windhorst DB, White JG, Dent PB, et al. Defective defense associated with genetic disease of subcellular organelles. Birth Defects, Original Article Series. 1968;4: 424-32.
706. Witkop CJ Jr, Bowie EJ, Krumwiede MD, et al. Synergistic effect of storage pool deficient platelets and low plasma von Willebrand factor on the severity of the hemorrhagic diathesis in Hermansky-Pudlak syndrome. Am J Hematol. 1993;44(4):256-9.
707. Witkop CJ Jr, Hill CW, Desnick S, et al. Ophthalmologic, biochemical, platelet and ultrastructural defects in various types of oculocutaneous albinism. J Invest Dermatol. 1973;60(6):443-56.
708. Witkop CJ Jr, Nance WE, Rawls RF, White JG. Autosomal recessive oculocutaneous albinism in man. Evidence for genetic heterogeneity. Am J Hum Genet. 1970;22(1):55-74.
709. Witkop CJ Jr, Niswander JD, Bergsma DR, et al. Tyrosinase positive oculocutaneous albinism among the Zuni and the Brandywine triracial isolate: biochemical and clinical characteristics and fertility. Am J Phys Anthropol. 1972; 36(3):397-405.
710. Witkop CJ Jr, White JG, Gerritsen SM, et al. Hermansky-Pudlak syndrome (HPS): a proposed block in glutathione peroxidase. Oral Surg Oral Med Oral Pathol. 1973;35(6): 790-806.
711. Witkop CJ Jr, White JG, King RA, et al. Hereditary mucoepithelial dysplasia. Am J Hum Genet. 1979;31(4):414-27.
712. Witkop CJ Jr, White JG, King RA. Oculocutaneous albinism: Hereditable disorder of amino acid metabolism. (Nyhan WL, Ed.), John Wiley & Sons, New York. 1973;177-261.
713. Witkop CJ Jr, White JG, Nance WE, et al. Mutations in the melanin pigment system in man resulting in features of oculocutaneous albinism. Pigmentation: Its Genesis and Biological Control. (Vernon Riley, Ed.) Appleton-Century Crofts, New York. 1972;359-77.
714. Witkop CJ Jr, White JG, Sauk JJ Jr, et al. Clinical, histologic, cytologic and ultrastructural characteristics of the oral lesions from hereditary mucoepithelial dysplasia. A disease of gap junction and desmosome formation. Oral Surg Oral Med Oral Pathol. 1978;46(5):645-57.
715. Witkop CJ Jr, White JG, Waring O. Hereditary mucoepithelial dysplasia, a disease of gap junction and desmosome formation. Birth Defects Orig Artic Ser. 1982;18(6):493-511.
716. Witkop CJ Jr, White JG. Albinism: oculocutaneous Hermansky-Pudlak type. Birth

Defects Encyclopedia, New York: Alan R. Liss. 1987.

717. Witkop CJ Jr, Wolfe LS, Cal SX, et al. Elevated urinary dolichol excretion in the Hermansky-Pudlak syndrome. Indicator of lysosomal dysfunction. Am J Med. 1987; 82(3):463-70.
718. Witkop CJ, Babcock MNB, Rao GHR, Gaudier F,Summers CG,Shanahan F,Harmn KR,Townsend D,Sedano HO,King RA,Cal SX,White JG: Albinism and Hermansky Pudlak Syndrome in Puerto Rico. Bol. Asoc. Med. P. Rico. 1990;82:333-9.
719. Witkop CJ, Krumwiede M, Sedano HO, et al. Reliability of absent platelet dense bodies as a diagnostic criterion for Hermansky-Pudlak syndrome. Am J Hematol. 1987;26(4):305-11.
720. Witkop CJ, White JG, Nance WE, et al. Classification of albinism in man. Birth Defects Orig Artic Ser. 1971;7(8):13-25.
721. Witkop CJ, White JG, Townsend D, et al. Ceroid storage disease in Hermansky-Pudlak syndrome: Induction in animal models. Lipofuscin - 1987: State of the Art. Editor I. Zs. Nagy, Akademiai Kiado, Budapest and Elsevier Science Publishers, Amsterdam. 1988;413-36.
722. Woulfe DS, Klimas Lilliendahl J, August S, et al. Serglycin loss produces platelet function defects. Blood. 2008;111(7):3458-67. 1.
723. Yawata Y, Jacob HS, Matsumoto N, et al. A possible role for cyclic nucleotides in the regulation of erythrocyte shape and permeability. J Lab Clin Med. 1976;88:556-62.
724. Young G, Luban N, White JG. Giant platelet disorders in African-American children misdiagnosed as idiopathic thrombocytopenic purpura. J Pediatr. Hematol Oncol. 1999; 21(3):231-6.
725. Young G, Luban NL, White JG. Sebastian syndrome: case report and review of the literature. Am J Hematol. 1999;61(1):62-5. Review.
726. Zarzour W, Kleta R, Frangoul H, et al. Two Novel CHS1 (LYST) mutations: Clinical correlations in an infant with Chediak-Higashi syndrome. Molecular Genetics and Metabolism. 2005;85:125-32.
727. Zelickson AS, Windhorst DB, White JG, et al. The Chediak-Higashi syndrome: formation of giant melanosomes and the basis for hypopigmentation. J Invest Dermatol. 1967;49(6):575-81.
728. Zhang F, White JG, Iadecola C. Nitric oxide donors increase blood flow and reduce brain damage in focal ischemia: evidence that nitric oxide is beneficial in the early stages of cerebral ischemia. J Cereb Blood Flow Metab. 1994;14(2):217-26.

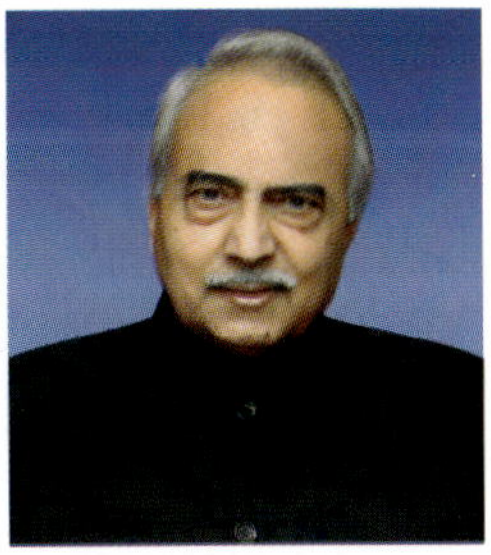

Gundu HR Rao PhD
Emeritus Professor, Laboratory Medicine and Pathology
Director, Thrombosis Research, Lillehei Heart Institute,
University of Minnesota (1970-2012).

Books

1. Rao GHR. Handbook of Platelet Physiology and Pharmacology, Kluwer Academic Publishers, Boston, 1999.
2. Rao GHR, VJ Kakkar. Coronary Artery Disease in South Asians: Epidemiology, Risk Factors, Prevention. Jaypee Medical Publishers, New Delhi, India, 2001.
3. Rao GHR, S Thanikachalam. Coronary Artery Disease: Risk Factors, Pathophysiology and Prevention. Jaypee Medical Publishers, New Delhi, India. 2005.
4. Rao GHR, L Jagannathan, T Eastlund. Handbook of Blood Banking and Transfusion Medicine, Jaypee Medical Publishers, New Delhi, India, 2006.
5. V Mohan, Rao GHR. Diabetes Mellitus (Type-2): Epidemiology, Risk Management and Prevention. Jaypee Medical Publishers, New Delhi, India. 2007.
6. Rao GHR, E Kalidoki, W Leong. J Fareed. Management of Anti-thrombolytic and Thrombolytic Therapy. Kontentworx, India. 2014.
7. Rao GHR, Reddy M. Handbook of Biotechnology, Bioengineering and Biomedical applications. NDRF (DRDO), Institution of Engineers, Bangalore, India. 2015.
8. Rao GHR. Handbook of Coronary Artery Disease. MacMillan Medical Communications, New Delhi, India, 2016.
9. Rao GHR. Morphology, Physiology and Pharmacology of Blood Platelets. Jaypee Medical Publishers, New Delhi, India. 2017.

Journals

1. Afshin A Divani, Nicole D Zantek, Afshin Borgani, et al. Antiplatelet Therapy: Aspirin Resistance and All That Jazz. J Clin Appl Thromb Hemost. 2013;19(1):5-18.
2. Afshin Divani, Gundu H Rao. Past Present and Future of Anti-platelet Therapies (Editorial). J Vasc Interventional Neurol. 2008;1(2):57-60. PMC3317315
3. Authi KS, Rao GHR, Crawford N. Inhibitory action of guanosice 5-0 (2-thiodiphosphat) on thrombin-induced activation in intact and permeabilized platelets. J Cell Biochem Suppl. 1988;12:5503.
4. Authi KS, Rao GHR, Evenden BJ, et al. Action of guanosine-5-0-[2-thidiphosphate] (GDPBS) on thrombin-induced activation and calcium mobilization in saponized and intact human platelets. Biochem J. 1988;255: 885-93.
5. Bano A, Rao GHR, Majumdar SK. Food preference of Sitophilus and Bruchus. In: Proc. of the Second Congress in Zoology. 1962; pp. 393-7.
6. Bonebrake FL, Bertha B, Folts JD, et al. Verapamil combined with aspirin for inhibiting epinephrine-stimulated platelet thrombus formation in stenosed canine coronary arteries. Cor Art Dis. 1991;2:487-92.
7. Brandy KR, Meyer RM, Luo S Rao GHR, et al. Evaluation of Coagulation profile among oral and vaginal combined hormonal contraceptive users using sonoclot coagulation analyzer. Clin and Appl Thromb Hemost. 2012;18 (6):576-81.
8. Burris SM, Smith CM, Rao GHR, et al. Aspirin treatment reduces platelet resistance to deformation. Blood. 1985;66:1089A.

9. Burris SM, Smith CM, Rao GHR. Aspirin treatment reduces platelet resistance to deformation. Arteriosclerosis 1987;7:385-8.
10. Butler AM, Gerrard JM, Peller J, et al. Vitamin E inhibits the release of calcium from a platelet membrane fraction in vitro. Prostaglandins and Medicine 1979;2:203-16.
11. Chandy T, Das GS, Rao GHR. 5 Fluorouracil-loaded chitosan coated polylactic acid microspheres as biodegradable drug carriers for cerebral tumors. J Microencapsulation. 2000;17:625-38.
12. Chandy T, Das GS, Wilson RF, et al. Surface immobilized biomolecules on albumin modified porcine pericardium for preventing thrombosis and calcification. Intern J Artif Organs. 1999;22:547-58.
13. Chandy T, Mooradian DL, Rao GHR. Chitosan/polyethylene glycol-alginate microcapsules for oral delivery of hirudin. J Applied Polymer Sci. 1998;70:2143-53.
14. Chandy T, Mooradian DL, Rao GHR. Evaluation of modified alginate-PEG microcapsules for cell encapsulation. Artif Organs. 1999;23:894-903.
15. Chandy T, Mooradian DL, Rao GHR. Platelet adhesion and spreading on protein coated surfaces. Variations in behavior in washed cells, PRP and whole blood. J Biomat Appl. 1998;13:46-65.
16. Chandy T, Rao GHR, Wilson RF, et al. The development of porous Alginate/PEG/ Composite for Cardiovascular Engineering. J Biomaterial Applications. 2003;17:287-363.
17. Chandy T, Rao GHR. Platelet biomaterial interactions. In: Platelet Physiology and Pharmacology (Rao GHR, Ed.), Kluwer Academic Publishers, USA, 1999.
18. Chandy T, Rao GHR. Preparation of Surface-Engineered Elastin/Laminin Nerve Guide Tubes of Polylactic acid, Polyethylene vinyl acetate. J. Bioacitve & Comp Polymers. 2002; 17:183-195.
19. Chandy T, Vasudev SC, Rao GHR, et al. Pericardial calcification: Changes due to antiplatelet agents. Cardiovasc Eng. 1998;3: 79-85.
20. Chandy T, Vasudev SC, Rao GHR. Changes in pericardial calcification due to anti-platelet agents: in vitro studies. Art Org. 1998; 22:666-71.
21. Chandy T, Wilson RF, Rao GHR, et al. Changes in Cisplatin Delivery Due to Surface-Coated Poly (Lactic Acid) /Poly (e-Carpolactone) Microspheres. J Biomat Appl. 2002;16:275-92.
22. Clawson CC, Rao GHR, White JG. Platelet interaction with bacteria. IV. Stimulation of the release reaction. Am J Pathol. 1975;81: 411-20.
23. Cox AC, Carroll RC, White JG, et al. Recycling of platelet phosphorylation and cytoskeletal assembly. J Cell Biol. 1984;98:8-15.
24. Cox AC, Rao GHR, Gerrard JM, et al. The influence of vitamin E Quinone on platelet structure, function and biochemistry. Blood 1980;55:907-16.
25. Cox AC, Rao GHR, Gerrard JM, et al. Vitamin Quinone: A phospholipase A2 inhibitor and more potent antagonist of platelet function than Vitamin E. XI the International Congress of Biochemistry, 1979.
26. Cox CA, Carrol RC, White JG, et al. Recycling of platelet phosphorylation and cytoskeletal assembly. Circ. 1982;66:16A.
27. Craig A, Einzig S, Castanedo-Zuniga W, et al. Altered vessel wall arachidonate metabolism after angioplasty: Possible mediators of post-angioplasty vasospasm. Am J Cardiol. 1983;51:1441-5.
28. Divani A, Luft AR, Flaherty JD, et al. Direct Diagnosis is superior to risk factor prediction tools for management of Vessel Wall Disease. Frontiers in Neurology. 2012; 1:31-4.
29. Divani AA, Rasmussen K, Vanzquez G, et al. Effect of Blood soluble Clotting Factors on Coagulation Profile. Clin Appl Thromb Hemost. 2010;16(4):475-9.
30. Einzig S, Borgwardt B, Noren GR, 1985. Arachidonic metabolism in thrombocytes and vascular tissues of turkeys. Prostaglandins 1985;30:999-18.
31. Einzig S, Craig A, Rao GHR, et al. Vasospasm and angioplasty. Circulation 1982;66:703A.
32. Einzig S, Rao GHR, Pierpont ME, et al. Acute effects of amrinone on regional myocardial and systemic blood flow distribution in the dog. Can J Physiol. 1982;60:811-18.
33. Einzig S, Rao GHR, White JG. Differential sensitivity of regional vascular beds in the

dog to low dose prostacyclin infusion. Can J Physiol Pharmacol. 1980;58:940-46.

34. Einzig S, Sotomora R, Rao GHR, et al. Prostacyclin does not increase blood flow in acute ischemic canine myocardium. Prost. Med. 1980;5:209-21.

35. Escolar G, Lozano M, Diaz-Ricart M, et al. Modifications in accessibility of membrane glycoproteins binding specific ligands and coagulation factors V during the activation of platelets in blood emerging from bleeding time wounds. Am J Hematol. 1999;60:260-7.

36. Escolar G, Rao GHR, Nieuwenhuis K, et al. Ultrastructure expression of p-selectin on surface activated platelets. Platelets 1996;7: 297-301.

37. Folts JD, Rowe GG, Rao GHR. Problem with aspirin as anti-thrombotic agent in coronary artery disease. Lancet. 1988;1:937.

38. Gandhi PG, Rao GHR. Detection of neuropathy using a SudoMotor test in type-2 diabetes. Degenerative Neurological and Neuromuscular Disease. 2015;5:1-7.

39. Gandhi PG, Rao GHR. The Spectral analysis of photoplethysmography to evaluate an independent cardiovascular risk factor. Int J Gen Med. 2014;7:539-47.

40. Gerard JM, White JG, Rao GHR, et al. Labile aggregation stimulating substance (LASS) in the interaction of Hermansky-Pudalk (HP) and aspirin-treated platelets. Circ. 1974;50: 290.

41. Gerrard JM, Peterson DA, Rao GHR, et al. Some recent advances in understanding the tangle of biochemical events involved in thromboxane-dependent and-independent aggregation. In: The Regulation of Coagulation. Elsevier/North Holland Inc. 1980; pp. 399-408.

42. Gerrard JM, Phillips DR Rao GHR, et al The role of alpha granules and their constituents in platelet function. Studies with the gray platelet syndrome, a selective deficiency of fused organelles. Blood 54, 670A, 1979.

43. Gerrard JM, Phillips DR, Rao GHR, et al. Biochemical studies of two patients with the grey platelet syndrome: Selective deficiency of platelet alpha granules. J Clin Invest. 1980;66:102-9.

44. Gerrard JM, Rao GHR, Stuart MJ, et al. Alterations in the balance of thromboxane and prostacyclin synthesis in platelet and the vessel wall in a diabetic model. In: The Effects of Platelet Active Drugs on the Cardiovascular System (Hirsch J, Steele PP and Vernier RL, Eds.), University of Colorado Press, 1981; pp. 207-23.

45. Gerrard JM, Rao GHR, White JG. The influence of reserpine and ethylenediaminetetra-acetic acid (EDTA) on serotonin storage organelles of blood platelets. Am J Pathol. 1977;87: 633-46.

46. Gerrard JM, Stoddard SF, Shapiro RS, et al. Platelet storage pool deficiency and prostaglandin synthesis in chronic granulocytic leukaemia. Br J Haematol. 1978;40:597-607.

47. Gerrard JM, Stuart MJ, Rao GHR, et al. Alteration in the balance of prostaglandin and thromboxane synthesis in diabetes. J Lab Clin Med. 1980;95:950-7.

48. Gerrard JM, White JG, Rao GHR, et al. Labile aggregation stimulating substance (LASS): The factor from storage pool deficient platelets correcting defective aggregation and release of aspirin-treated normal platelets. Brit. J Haematology. 1975;29:411-20.

49. Gerrard JM, White JG, Rao GHR, et al. Localization of platelet prostaglandin production in the platelet dense tubular system. Am J Pathol. 1976;83:283-99.

50. Gerrard JM, White JG, Rao GHR. Effects of the ionophore, A23187, on blood platelets. II. Influence on aggregation and secretion. Am J Pathol. 1974;77:151-60.

51. Grouse LH, Rao GHR, Weiss DJ, et al. Surface- activated, bovine platelets, do not spread, they unfold. Am J Pathol. 1990;136: 399-408.

52. Guettier J, Georgopoulos A, Tsai M, et al. Polymorphisms in the FABP2 and APOC3 genes are associated with the metabolic syndrome in a South Indian Population. J Clin Endocrinol Metabolism Dec. 2004.

53. Harein PK, Rao GHR. Dichlorvos and Gardona as protectants for stored wheat against granary weevil infestations in laboratory studies. J Econ Entomol. 1972;65:1402-6.

54. Hill TD, White JG, Rao GHR. Platelet hypersensitivity induced by 1-chloro-2,

4-dinitro-benzene, hydroperoxides and inhibition of lipoxygenase. Thromb Res. 1989;53:447-57.

55. Hill TD, White JG, Rao GHR. Role of glutathione and glutathione peroxidase in human platelet arachidonic acid metabolism. Prostaglandins 1989;38:21-32.
56. Hill TD, White JG, Rao GHR. The influence of glutathione depleting agents on human platelet function. Thromb Res. 1989;53:457-67.
57. Horns DJ, Gerrard JM, Rao GHR, et al. Smoking and labile platelet aggregation stimulating substance (LASS) synthesizing activity. Thromb Res. 1976;9:661-8.
58. Johnson GH, Rao GHR, Leis LA, et al. Effects of agents which alter cyclic AMP on arachidonic-induced platelet aggregation in the dog. Blood. 1980;55:722-9.
59. Johnson GJ, Leis LA, Rao GHR, et al. Arachidonate-induced platelet aggregation in the dog. Thromb Res. 1979;14:147-54.
60. Johnson GJ, Rao GHR, White JG. Platelet dysfunction induced by parenteral carbenicillin and Ticarcillin: Studies of the dose-response relationship and mechanism of action in dogs. Am J Pathol. 1978;91:85-166.
61. Johnson GJ, Rao GHR, White JG. Thromboxane A2 -stimulated platelet aggregation is potentiated by epinephrine acting via alpha-adrenergic receptors. Thromb Haemost. 1981;46:1344A.
62. Johnson GJ, Rao GHR, White LG. Epinephrine potentiation of arachidonate-induced dog platelet aggregation. Effect of agents, which alter cAMP. Am Fed Clin Res. 1979.
63. Johnson GJ, Sharda A, Rao GHR. Measurement of Shear-Activated Platelet Aggregate Formation: Utility in Evaluation of Clopidogrel-Aspirin-Induced Platelet Function Inhibition. J Appl Clin Thromb Hemost. 2012;18(2):140-9.
64. Johnson GR, Rao GHR, White JG. Epinephrine potentiation of thromboxane stimulated platelet aggregation. Circ. 1980; 62:050A.
65. Kahmann RD, Donohue JM, Bradford DS, et al. Platelet function in adolescent idiopathic scoliosis. Spine 1992;17:145-8.
66. Kapil N, Datta TH, Alakbarova N, et al. Antiplatelet and anticoagulant therapies for prevention of ischemic stroke. Clin App Thromb Hemost. 2017.
67. Karnicki K, St Cyr J, Ericson D, et al. Preservation of in vitro platelet concentrates with Via Cyte. Vox sangui. 2003;85:262-6.
68. Keeley LL, Rao GHR, Hazal LG. Isolation and purification of Heliothis nuclear polyhedra and virions by density-gradient techniques. Agri Expt Stn Bull. PR-2704, Texas A & M University, College Station, Texas, 1969.
69. Kohler AS, Parks PJ, Mooradian DL, et al. Platelet adhesion to novel phospholipid materials: modified phosphatidylcholine covalently immobilized to silica, polypropylene and PTFE materials. J Biomed Mater Res. 1996;32:237-42.
70. Krishnamurthi S, Wheeler-Jones CPD, Patel Y, et al. Nitroprusside inhibits platelet function primarily by inhibiting calcium mobilization. Biochem Soc Trans. 1990;18:468-70.
71. Kuettner JF, Dreher KL, Rao GHR, et al. Influence of the ionophore, A23187, on the plastic behaviour of normal erythrocytes. Am J Pathol. 1977;88:81-94.
72. Maarek AA, Gandhi PG, Rao GHR. Identifying Autonomic Neuropathy and Endothelial Dysfunction in Type II Diabetic Patients. EC Neuropathy. 2015;2(2):63-78.
73. MacFarlane GD, Herzberg MC, Zhao QI, et al. The role of dense granule secretate and arachidonic acid metabolites in Streptococcus sanguis-induced platelet aggregation. Blood 1992;80:2774-80.
74. Majumdar SK, Rao GHR. Possible use of food preferences of an insect as a factor for its control in stored commodities. Curr Sci. 1962;31: 238-9.
75. Marina Y Zukharova, Rachel Meyer, Kyle Brandy, et al. Risk Factors for Heart Attack and Stroke Associated with Hormonal Contraceptive use. J Clin Appl Thromb Hemost. 2011;7(4):323-31.
76. Murthy M, Rao GHR, Reddy S. 1, 3-dioctanoyl glycerol (1, 3-diC8) is as effective as 1, 2-diC8 in priming phospholipase A2 activation in human platelets and neutrophils. Biochem. Med Met Biol. 1994;52:89-96.

77. Murthy M, Rao GHR, Robinson P, et al. Influx of extracellular calcium and agonist-coupling appear essential for the activation of thromboxane A2-dependent phospholipase A2 in human platelets. Prost Leuko Essen Fatty Acids. 1995;53:31-9.
78. Muthu M, Rao GHR, Majumdar SK. A bioassay method for determining the fumigant concentration in air. Int Pest Control 1971;13:11-4.
79. Neeta Raj Sharma, Rao GHR. Diabetes management: Expectations and Limitations. J Diab Metabol. 2016. DOI: 10.4172/2155-6156.1000662.
80. Nipper JHJ, Rao GHR, Gerrard JM. Computer assisted high-pressure liquid chromatographic (HPLC) analysis of platelet adenine nucleotides, 11th International Congress of Biochemistry. Toronto, Canada. 1979.
81. Pardoni E, Alexandre A, Cavalline L, et al. Human platelet activation is inhibited by the occupancy of glycoprotein IIb/IIIa receptor. Arch. Biochem. Biophys. 1996;333:407-13.
82. Paterson DA, Gerrard JM, Rao GHR, et al. Interaction of arachidonic acid heme iron in the synthesis of prostaglandins. Adv Prost Thromboxane Res. 1980;6:157-61.
83. Peterson DA, Gerrard JM, Glover SM, et al. Epinephrine reduction of heme: Implication for understanding the transmission of an agonist stimulus. Science. 1982;215:71-3.
84. Peterson DA, Gerrard JM, Peller J, et al. Interaction of zinc with arachidonic acid. Prost Med. 1981;6:91-9.
85. Peterson DA, Gerrard JM, Rao GHR, et al. Does epinephrine activate platelets by binding to a receptor and then reducing heme in a membrane enzyme to transmit activating signal? Thromb Haemost. 1981;46:0855A.
86. Peterson DA, Gerrard JM, Rao GHR, et al. Epinephrine and other activators of prostaglandin endoperoxide synthetase can reduce Fe3+ heme to Fe2+ heme. Prost Med. 1980;5: 357-65.
87. Peterson DA, Gerrard JM, Rao GHR, et al. Ferrous iron-mediated oxidation of arachidonic acid. Studies employing nitro blue tetrazolium (NBT). Prostaglandins and Medicine 1978;1:304-17.
88. Peterson DA, Gerrard JM, Rao GHR, et al. Inhibition of ferrous iron induced oxidation of arachidonic acid by indomethacin. Prostaglandins and Medicine 1979;2:97-108.
89. Peterson DA, Gerrard JM, Rao GHR, et al. Reduction in ferric heme to ferrous by lipid peroxides: Possible relevance to the role of peroxide tone in the regulation of prostaglandin synthesis. Prostaglandins and Medicine 1980;4:73-9.
90. Peterson DA, Gerrard JM, Rao GHR, et al. Reduction of heme by lipid peroxides and its potential relevance to understanding the control of cyclooxygenase activity. Prog. Lipid Res. 1981;20:299-302.
91. Peterson DA, Gerrard JM, Rao GHR, et al. Salicylic acid inhibition of the irreversible effect of acetylsalicylic acid on prostaglandin synthetase may be due to competition for the enzyme-cationic-binding site. Prost. Med. 1981;6:161-4.
92. Peterson DA, Gerrard JM, Rao GHR. Interaction of arachidonic acid and heme iron in the synthesis of prostaglandins. International Prostaglandin Conference. Washington DC. 1979.
93. Prikryl P, Siegelova J, Cornelissen G, et al. Chronotherapeutic pilot on 6 persons may guide tests on thousands: toward a circadian optimization of prophylactic treatment with daily low-dose aspirin. In: Chronobiology and Chronomedicine, Humans in Time and Cosmos (Otsuka K, Cornelissen G and Halberg F, Eds.), Life Science Publishing Co., 1994; pp. 113-7.
94. Prikyl P, Siegelova J, Comelissen G, et al. Chronotherapeutic treatment daily low-dose aspirin. University of Minnesota-Medtronic Chronobiology Sem. Ser. 1991; 3:1-8.
95. Radha E, Hill TD, Rao GHR, et al. Glutathione levels in human platelets display a circadian rhythm in vitro. Thromb Res. 1985;40: 823-31.
96. Rai GHR, Gerrard JM, Eaton JW, et al. Arachidonic acid peroxidation, prostaglandin synthesis and platelet function. International Conference on Singlet Oxygen and Related Species in Chemistry and Biology, Pinawa, Manitoba, Canada, 1977.

97. Rao GHR, Anders MW. Aflatoxin detection by high-speed liquid chromatography and mass spectrometry. J Chromatography. 1973;84: 402-6.
98. Rao GHR, Anders MW. Inhibition of microsomal drug metabolism by anticholine-esterase, insecticides. Bull Env Cont Toxicol. 1973;9:409.
99. Rao GHR, Authi KS, Crawford N, et al. Variable mechanisms of calcium mobilization in human platelets. FASEB. 1988;12:598A.
100. Rao GHR, Bharathi M. Maternal and Child Nutrition: First Major Step for Prevention of Cardio-Metabolic Disorders. 2016. J. Cardiol. (Original Research Article. ISJN: 5743-8468)
101. Rao GHR, Burris SM, Gerrard JM, et al. Inhibition of prostaglandin (PG) synthesis in sheep vesicular gland microsomes (SVGM) by nitro blue tetrazolium (BT) and vitamin E. Prost Med. 1979;2:203-16.
102. Rao GHR, Chandy. Role of platelets in blood-biomaterial interactions. Bull of Mater Sci. 1999;22:101-7.
103. Rao GHR, Cox AC, Gerrard JM, et al. Effects of 2, 2′-dipyrydil and related compounds on platelet prostaglandin synthesis and platelet function. Biochim Biophys Acta. 1980;628: 468 79.
104. Rao GHR, Cox CA, Gerrard GM, et al. Alpha-tocopherol quinone (TQ): A potent inhibitor of platelet activation. Prog Lipid Res. 1981;20:549-52.
105. Rao GHR, Cox CA, Mahadevappa VG, et al. Influence of GDP (β)S on agonist-induced calcium mobilization and platelet function. In: Biology of Cellular Transducing Signals (Franklin J, Ed.), Plenum Press, 1989; pp. 343-53.
106. Rao GHR, Cox CA, Witkop CH. Influence of UV light (250 nm) on platelet activation. Prostaglandin and Lipid Metabolism in Radiation Injury. Walden TL., Jr, and Hughes HN, (Eds), NY, Plenum Press, 1987; pp. 339-44.
107. Rao GHR, De Las Casas E. Effect of Chaetomium Spp. On Tribolium confusum. In: North Central Meetings, Entomological Society of America, Des Moines, Iowa, 1974.
108. Rao GHR, Doni MG. Influence of nitrovasodilators on platelet function. Thromb. Athero. 1993;4:293-305.
109. Rao GHR, Einzig S, Noren GH, et al. Vascular and thrombocyte arachidonic acid metabolism in the Turkey. Thromb Haemost. 1984;50:0905A.
110. Rao GHR, Einzig S, Reddy KR, et al. Tranylcypromine-induced hypertension is not mediated by the inhibition of prostacyclin synthesis. Prostaglandins and Medicine 1979;3:201-11.
111. Rao GHR, Ericson DG, Weiss DJ, et al. Influence of aspirin and carbacyclin on bovine platelet function. ASAIO J. 1992;38:830-4.
112. Rao GHR, Escolar G, Smith CM, et al. Influence of heat on platelet biochemistry, physiology and function. J Lab Clin Med. 1993;122:455-65.
113. Rao GHR, Escolar G, White JG. Biochemistry, physiology and function of platelets stored as concentrates. Transfusion 1993;33:766-78.
114. Rao GHR, Escolar G, White JG. Epinephrine reverses the inhibitory influence of aspirin on platelet-vessel wall interaction. Thromb Res. 1986;44:65-74.
115. Rao GHR, Escolar G, White JG. Monitoring signal transduction and cytoskeletal alterations by fluorescent imaging and confocal microscopy. Ann NY Acad Sci. 1994;714: 297-300.
116. Rao GHR, Escolar G, White JR, et al. Differential response of human and bovine platelets to bovine von Willebrand factor and vascular sub endothelium. Platelets. 2001;12:150-5.
117. Rao GHR, Escolar G, Zavoral J, et al. Influence of adrenergic receptor blockade on aspirin-induced inhibition of platelet function. Platelets. 1990;1:145.
118. Rao GHR, et al. Potential Thrombogenic Complications of Recombinant Activated Factor V11. J. IACATH 2008.
119. Rao GHR, et al. The immunogenic potential of Generic Versions of LMWHs may not be the same as Branded Products. E-Thrombosis. 2007; PP. 1-3.
120. Rao GHR, Eugenio C, Christensen CM, et al. Survival & reproduction of confused

flour beetles exposed to fungus metabolites. J Econ Entomol. 1971;64:1563-5.

121. Rao GHR, Fareed J, White JG. Influence of heparins on inositol 1, 4, 5-trisphosphate-induced calcium mobilization in permeabilized human platelets. Biochem Med Met Biol. 1991;45:171-80.

122. Rao GHR, Fields CM, White JG, et al. Promotion of human platelet adhesion and aggregation by a synthetic, triple-helical minicollagen. J Biol Chem. 1994;269:13899-903.

123. Rao GHR, Friedland M, Gerrard JM, et al. The influence of metabolites on the assay of platelet serotonin. Thromb Res. 1977;10:791-802.

124. Rao GHR, Gandhi PG, Sharma V. Clinical Complications of Type-2 Diabetes Mellitus: An Overview. J Diab Met. http://dx.org/10.4172/2155-6156.1000420, 2014.

125. Rao GHR, Gandhi PG. Integrative Medicine: Global Perspective. J Homeop Ayurv Med. http://dx.doi.org/10.4172/2167-1206.1000-150. 2014.

126. Rao GHR, Gandhi PG. Need for a non-invasive Diagnostic Platform for Early Detection and Management of Cardio-Metabolic Disorders. J Clin and Prevent Cardiology. 2014;3 (3):93-8.

127. Rao GHR, Gerrard JM, Eaton JW, et al. Detection of arachidonic acid free radical (AAO) formation, an essential step in platelet prostaglandin (PG) biosynthesis. Am. Soc Heamtol Meetings. 1976.

128. Rao GHR, Gerrard JM, Eaton JW, et al. The role of iron in prostaglandin synthesis: Ferrous iron-mediated oxidation of arachidonic acid. Prostaglandins and Medicine. 1978;1: 55-70.

129. Rao GHR, Gerrard JM, Murthy M, et al. Possible mechanisms of epinephrine actions in human platelets that are refractory to arachidonic acid. Biochem. Med Met Biol. 1993;50: 322-37.

130. Rao GHR, Gerrard JM, Witkop CJ, et al. Origin and role of calcium in platelet activation contraction-secretion coupling. Cell Calcium Metabolism. Fiskum G, (Ed), NY, Plenum Publications, 1988; pp. 411-27.

131. Rao GHR, Gerrard JM, Witkop CJ, et al. Platelet aggregation independent of ADP release or prostaglandin synthesis in patients with the Hermansky-Pudlak syndrome. Prost Med. 1981;6:459-72.

132. Rao GHR, Harein PK. Dichlorvos as an inhibitor of Aflatoxin production on wheat, corn, rice and peanuts. J Econ Entomol. 1972;65: 988-9.

133. Rao GHR, Harein PK. Dichlorvos as an inhibitor of aflatoxin protection on wheat, corn, rice and peanuts. In: Ann. Technol. Agri. Wet Harvested Grains, Paris, France. 1973;22:477-81.

134. Rao GHR, Harein PK. Inhibition of aflatoxin and zearalenone biosynthesis with dichlorvos. Bull Env Toxicol. 1974;10:112-5.

135. Rao GHR, Hill TD, John V, et al. Inhibition of platelet aggregation by novel triphenylethylene analogs. Thromb Res. 1986;44:527-38.

136. Rao GHR, Hordinsky M, Witkop CJ, et al. Influence of psoralen and ultraviolet therapy on platelet function and arachidonic acid metabolism in patients with vitilago. Prostaglandins and Lipid Metabolism in Radiation Injury (Walden TL., Jr, and Hughes HN, Eds.), NY, Plenum Press, 1987; pp. 179-84.

137. Rao GHR, J Fareed. Aspirin Prophylaxis for the Prevention of Thrombosis: Expectations and Limitations. Thrombosis: PMC3289854 doi: 10.1155/2102/104707. 2012

138. Rao GHR, Jachimowicz AA, White JG. Rapid separation of tumour-promoting agents, phorbol and phorbol myristate acetate (12-o-tetradecanyl phorbol-13-acetate) by high-pressure liquid chromatography. J Chromatography 1974;96:151-4.

139. Rao GHR, Johnson GJ, Reddy KR, et al. Ibuprofen protects platelet cyclooxygenase from irreversible inhibition by aspirin. Arteriosclerosis. 1983;3:384-8.

140. Rao GHR, Johnson GJ, Reddy KR, et al. Rapid return of cyclooxygenase active platelets in dogs after a single oral dose of aspirin. Prostaglandins. 1981;22:761-72.

141. Rao GHR, Johnson GJ, White JG. Influence of epinephrine on the aggregation response of aspirin-treated platelets. Prost Med. 1980; 5: 45-58.

142. Rao GHR, Johnson GR, White JG. Separation of secretion from prostaglandin synthesis in

Ibuprofen- treated platelets. Blood 1984;62: 965A.
143. Rao GHR, Johnson JM, Einzig S, et al. Effect of amrinone: A cardiotonic drug on hemodynamics and platelet function. Prost Med. 1981;6:75-90.
144. Rao GHR, Kishore NP, Peller JD, et al. Influence of polyenoic acids on arachidonic acid metabolism and platelet function. Cardiovascular Disease (Gallo L, Ed.), NY, Plenum Press, 1987; pp. 495-505.
145. Rao GHR, Kishore NP, White JG. Differential effects of lipoxygenase inhibitors on arachidonic acid metabolism in cell free and intact platelet preparations. Prost Leuko Med. 1987;26:281-90.
146. Rao GHR, Krick TP, White JG. Preparation, separation and characterization of vitamin E Quinone. J Chromatography. 1980;196: 506-11.
147. Rao GHR, Krishanmurthi S, Raij L, et al. Influence of nitric oxide on agonist-mediated calcium mobilization in platelets. Biochem. Med Met Biol. 1990;43:271-5.
148. Rao GHR, Mahadevappa VG, Hill TD, et al. Arachidonic acid oxidation and platelet function (Reddy CC, Hamilton GA and Madyasta KM, Eds.), Biological Oxidation Systems, Academic Press, 1990;770-90.
149. Rao GHR, Majumdar SK. Intergranular space as a limiting factor for growth of pulse beetles, a new principle for pest control. J Econ Entomol. 1964;57:1013-14.
150. Rao GHR, Majumdar SK. Repellency of Kaempferia galanga Linn (Zingiberaceae) to adults of Tribolium castaneum. In: Proceedings Symp. Med Plants Sci and Cult. 1963;32:461-2.
151. Rao GHR, Majumdar SK. Repellency of species, aromatic materials and essential oils to adults of Tribolium castaneum. In: Proc Symp Med Plants, Jammu, India. 1965.
152. Rao GHR, Mohanty D, Rao ASC. Coronary heart disease: risk factors for Indian men and women. Ind J Hematol Blood Trans. 1997;15:3-8.
153. Rao GHR, Nagendra HR. Holistic approach for the management of heart disease and type-2 diabetes. J Preven Cardiol. 2013; 2(1):231-8.
154. Rao GHR, Parthasarathy S. Antioxidants, atherosclerosis and thrombosis. Prost. Leuko Essen Fatty Acids. 1996;54:155-66
155. Rao GHR, Peller JD, Lee JY, et al. Biochemical and functional responses of platelets from patients with Alzheimer's disease. Ind J Physiol Pharmacol. 1996;40:5-14.
156. Rao GHR, Peller JD, Prakash YS, et al. Monitoring signal transduction and cytoskeletal alterations in adherent platelets. Arterioscler Thromb. 1994;5:155-65.
157. Rao GHR, Peller JD, Richards KL, et al. Rapid separation of nucleotides from granulocytes by isocratic, reverse-phase, high performance liquid chromatography. J Chromatography 1982;229:205-10.
158. Rao GHR, Peller JD, Semba CP, et al. Influence of the calcium sensitive fluorophore Quin 2 on platelet function. Blood. 1986;67:354-61.
159. Rao GHR, Peller JD, White JG. Influence of ionized calcium on thrombin-induced down-regulation of GPIb/IX receptors in human platelets. Thromb Res. 1997;85: 23-31.
160. Rao GHR, Peller JD, White JG. Measurement of ionized calcium in blood platelets with a new generation calcium indicator. Biochem. Biophys Res Commun. 1985;132:652-7.
161. Rao GHR, Peller JD, White JG. Rapid separation of platelet nucleotides by reverse-phase, isocratic, high pressure liquid chromatography with a rapidly compressed column. J Chromatography. 1981;226:466-70.
162. Rao GHR, Radha E, Johnson GJ, et al. Enteric-coated aspirin, platelet cyclooxygenase activity and function. Prost Leuko Med. 1984;13: 3-12.
163. Rao GHR, Radha E, White JG. Irreversible platelet aggregation does not depend on lipoxygenase metabolites. Biochem Biophys Res Commun. 1985;131:50-57.
164. Rao GHR, Raij L, Lester B, et al. Inhibition of agonist-induced human platelet activation by nitric oxide. Proc. Royal Society Sym. (Moncada S and Higgs EA, Eds.), Elsevier Publishing Company Inc, NY, 1990; pp. 355-67.
165. Rao GHR, Rao ASC, White JG. Aspirin in ischemic heart disease: An overview. Ind Heart J. 1993;45:73-9.

166. Rao GHR, Rao ASC, White JG. Influence of low-dose enteric coated aspirin on platelet function. Ind Heart J. 1992;44:365-71.
167. Rao GHR, Rao AT. Pharmacology of platelet inhibitory drugs. Ind J Physiol Pharmacol. 1994;38:69-84.
168. Rao GHR, Rao PT, Sheth J. Need for the development of Clinical and Translational Science Institutes (CTSI) in India. J Clin Prevent Cardiology. 2015;4:66-75.
169. Rao GHR, Rao PT. Development of Comprehensive e-Health Platform for the Prevention and Management of Non-Communicable Diseases (NCDs). J Clin Prevent Cardiology. 2015;4:32-41.
170. Rao GHR, Reddy KR, Hagert K, et al. Influence of pH on the prostacyclin (PGI2)-mediated inhibition of platelet function. Prostaglandins and Medicine. 1980;4:263-73.
171. Rao GHR, Reddy KR, White JG. A simple method for the separation of monohydroxy fatty acid metabolites of arachidonic acid metabolism. J Chromatography. 1982;232:176-9.
172. Rao GHR, Reddy KR, White JG. Effect of acetaminophen and salicylate on aspirin-induced inhibition of human platelets cyclooxygenase. Prost Leuko Med. 1982;9:109-15.
173. Rao GHR, Reddy KR, White JG. Influence of Trifluoperazine on platelet aggregation and disaggregation. Prost Med. 1980;5:221-34.
174. Rao GHR, Reddy KR, White JG. Low dose aspirin, platelet function and prostaglandin synthesis: Influence of epinephrine and alpha-adrenergic blockade. Prost Med. 1981;6:485-94.
175. Rao GHR, Reddy KR, White JG. Modification of human platelet response to sodium arachidonate by membrane mediation. Prost Med. 1981;6:75-90.
176. Rao GHR, Reddy KR, White JG. The influence of epinephrine on prostacyclin (PGI2) induced dissociation of ADP aggregated platelets. Prostaglandins and Medicine. 1980;4:385-97.
177. Rao GHR, Schmidt HHO, Reddy KR, et al. Human platelet activation by an alkyl-acetyl analogue of phosphatidylcholine. Biochim Biophys Acta. 1982;715:205-14.
178. Rao GHR, Schmidt HHO, White JG. Epinephrine-induced correction of the response of aspirin treated platelets to arachidonate is not mediated by platelet activating factor. Blood. 1981;58:721A.
179. Rao GHR, Smith CM II, Doni MG, Intracelluar calcium Imaging in adherent human platelets. Arterioscler Thromb. 1994;5:95-105.
180. Rao GHR, Smith CM II, White JG. Influence of calcium antagonists on thrombin-induced calcium mobilization and platelet-vessel wall interactions. Biochem Med Met Biol. 1992;47:226-31.
181. Rao GHR, Suma HN, Reddy LVM. Need for Point-of-Care (POC) Medical Device Development and Testing Platforms in India. In: Handbook of Biotechnology, Bioengineering and Biomedical Applications. 2016. National Design Research Forum (NDRF), Institution of Engineers, Bangalore.
182. Rao GHR, Tate M, Hebbel R, et al. Influence of antioxidants on arachidonic acid metabolism and platelet function. Biochem. Med. Met. Biol. 1994;51:74-9.
183. Rao GHR, Thethi I, Fareed J. Vascular disease: Obesity and Excess Weight as Modulators of Risk. Information Healthcare. 2011;9(4):525-34.
184. Rao GHR, White JG, Cox CA. Influence of a calcium-dependent protease inhibitor on platelet activation and secretion. Thromb. Res. 1987;47:625-37.
185. Rao GHR, White JG, Jachimowicz AA, et al. An improved method for the extraction of endogenous platelet secretion. J Lab Clin Med. 1976;87:129-37.
186. Rao GHR, White JG, Jachimowicz AA, et al. Nucleotide profiles of normal and abnormal platelets by high pressure liquid chromatography. J Lab and Clin Med. 1974;84:839-50.
187. Rao GHR, White JG. An improved method for measuring endogenous serotonin in platelet of patients with Hermansky-Pudlak syndrome. Thromb Res. 1988;51:225-7.
188. Rao GHR, White JG. Arachidonate metabolism and platelet disaggregation-reaggregation. VIII International Congress on Thrombosis and Heamostasis. Toronto, Canada. Thromb Haemsot. 1981;46:856A.

189. Rao GHR, White JG. Aspirin, PGE1 and Quin-2 AM induced platelet dysfunction. Restoration of function by norepinephrine. Prost Leuko Essen Fatty Acids. 1990; 39:141-6.
190. Rao GHR, White JG. Comparative pharmacology of cyclooxygenase inhibitors. Prost Leuko Med. 1985;18:119-31.
191. Rao GHR, White JG. Coronary artery disease: risk factors-an overview. Ind Heart J. 1993;145:143-53.
192. Rao GHR, White JG. Disaggregation and reaggregation of irreversibly aggregated platelets. Circ. 1980;62:1053A.
193. Rao GHR, White JG. Disaggregation and reaggregation of irreversibly aggregated platelets: A method for more complete evaluation of antiplatelet drugs. Agents and Actions 1985;16:425-34.
194. Rao GHR, White JG. Epinephrine and platelet function. J Lab Clin Med. 1997;130:238-9.
195. Rao GHR, White JG. Epinephrine potentiation of arachidonate-induced aggregation of cyclooxygenase deficient platelets. Am J Hematol. 1981;11:355-66.
196. Rao GHR, White JG. Epinephrine-induced membrane modulation restores the response of human platelets to platelet activating factor. Circ. 1982;66:1194A.
197. Rao GHR, White JG. Epinephrine-induced platelet membrane modulation. In: Platelet Amine Storage Granules (Myers, K. Ed.), Academic Press, 1989.
198. Rao GHR, White JG. Epinephrine-induced platelet membrane modulation. In: The Platelet Amine Storage Granule (Meyers KM and Barnes CD, Eds.), CRC Press, Boca Baton, 1992; pp. 117-95.
199. Rao GHR, White JG. Heme-polyenoic acid interaction and prostaglandin synthesis. In: Prostaglandins, Leukotrienes and Lipoxins (Bailey JM, Ed.), Plenum Publications Corporation. 1985; pp. 357-71.
200. Rao GHR, White JG. Influence of calcium antagonists in human platelet activation. Arteriosclerosis. 1990;10:950A.
201. Rao GHR, White JG. Influence of esterase inhibitors on platelet aggregation and release induced by phorbol myristate acetate. Biochem. Pharmacol. 1975;24:293-5.
202. Rao GHR, White JG. Influence of phospholipase A2 on human blood platelet α-adrenergic receptor function. Thromb. Res. 1989;53:427-34.
203. Rao GHR, White JG. Influence of various doses of aspirin (in vivo) on platelet arachidonic acid metabolism (ex vivo) and function. Prost Leuko Essen Fatty Acids. 1994;51:63-9.
204. Rao GHR, White JG. Measurement of platelet serotonin. Fed Proc. 1973;52:3524.
205. Rao GHR, White JG. Mechanisms involved in membrane modulation. Fed Proc. 1983; 42:4297A.
206. Rao GHR, White JG. Membrane modulation corrects the platelet dysfunction caused by Vincristine and Colchicine. Blood. 1983;62: 966A.
207. Rao GHR, White JG. Origin and role of calcium in platelet activation-contraction-secretion coupling. Fed Proc. 1986;45:407A.
208. Rao GHR, White JG. PH influence on prostacyclin-mediated inhibition of platelet function. Blood. 54, 705A, 1979.
209. Rao GHR, White JG. Platelet activating factor (PAF) causes human platelet aggregation through the mechanism of membrane modulation. Prost Leuko Med. 1982;9:459-72.
210. Rao GHR, White JG. Polyenoic acid metabolism and platelet function. Thromb, Haemost. 1985;54:89A.
211. Rao GHR, White JG. Role of arachidonic acid metabolism in human platelet activating and irreversible aggregation. Fifth International Conference on Prostaglandins, Florence, Italy. 1982.
212. Rao GHR, White JG. Role of arachidonic acid metabolism in human platelet activation and irreversible aggregation. Am J Hematol. 1985;19:339-47.
213. Rao GHR, White JG. Thromboxane-independent calcium mobilization in storage pool deficient platelets. Blood 1983;62:967A.
214. Rao GHR, Wilbur DA. Loss of weight in wheat caused by the feeding of lesser grain borer. J Kan Entomol Soc. 1972;45:238-41.
215. Rao GHR, Wilson RF, Singh P, et al: Influence of nitrous compounds on human platelet function. Arteriosclerosis. 1990;10:950A.
216. Rao GHR, Wilson RF, White CW, et al. Influence of thrombolytic agents on human

platelet function. Thromb Res. 1991; 62:319-34.

217. Rao GHR (Editor). Coronary Artery Disease: Risk Promoters, Pathophysiology and Prevention. Jaypee Medical Publishers, New Delhi, India. 2004.

218. Rao GHR. (Press). Signal transduction, second messengers and pathogenesis of cardiovascular disease. Proc Fourth Internat Conf. Health Diseases, India

219. Rao GHR. A tribute to a pioneering Thrombosis Researcher. Obituary J Clin Prevent Cardiol. 2017;6(3):33-5.

220. Rao GHR. Antiplatelet Therapies: An Overview. J Clin Prevent Cardiol. 2016;5:130-37.

221. Rao GHR. Aspirin and coronary artery disease. In: Coronary Artery Disease in South Asians: Epidemiology, Risk Factors and Prevention (Rao GHR, Ed.), 1998.

222. Rao GHR. Aspirin Resistance: A fact or myth? Expt Clin Cardiol. 2005;10:17-20.

223. Rao GHR. Aspirin Resistance: Aspirin Resistance: Need for a Point-of-Care Assay for monitoring anti-platelet and anti-thrombotic therapies. Stroke. 2009;40:2271-2.

224. Rao GHR. Aspirin Resistance: Clinical Significance. J Clin Prevent Cardiol. 2012;1(3): 118-29.

225. Rao GHR. Aspirin Resistance: Does it exist? Post Graduate Medicine Vol XX11, 2008; pp. 223-7.

226. Rao GHR. Aspirin Resistance: Expectations and limitations (Editorial), JAPI. 2008; 56:317-19.

227. Rao GHR. Aspirin Resistance: Expectations and Limitations Recent Adv Hematol. 2011;3(3):110.

228. Rao GHR. Aspirin Resistance: Need for a specific, Rapid, Point of Care Assay. World Heart Journal. 2006;1:63-78.

229. Rao GHR. Aspirin Resistance: Need for a specific, Rapid, Point of Care Assay. In: Frontiers in Atherosclerosis Research (Kepper, KF), Nova Science Publishers, New York, 2007; pp. 191-213.

230. Rao GHR. Bio-wealth and Health Care: Public Health Perspective. Biospectra. 2009.

231. Rao GHR. Circadian variations and coronary artery disease. Chronobiologia 1994; 21: 63-4.

232. Rao GHR. Clinical relevance of platelet research in thrombosis and hemostasis. Int J Cardiovasc Sci. 1996;3:21-4.

233. Rao GHR. Contributions of the South Asian Society on Atherosclerosis and Thrombosis and the Indian Society for Atherosclerosis Research (View Point). J Clin Prevent Cardiol. 2016;5:67-72. DOI: 10. 4103/2250-3528.186501.

234. Rao GHR. Coronary artery disease in South Asians: epidemiology, risk factors and prevention. Jaypee Medical Publishers, New Delhi ISBN #81 7179-811-X (Ed; Gundu H. R. Rao), 2001.

235. Rao GHR. Coronary Artery Disease. MacMillan Medical Publishers, (Springer/ Nature), New Delhi, India. 2016. ISBN #

236. Rao GHR. Effect of exercise on platelet physiology and pharmacology. In: Pharmacology in Exercise and Sports (Somani SM, Ed.), CRC Press, Boca Baton, 1996; pp. 211-34.

237. Rao GHR. Flow Velocity, Fluid dynamics and Vascular Pathology. Sci Pages of Heart. 2016;1:001.

238. Rao GHR. Fungal toxins in foods. Chapter in Current Topics in Applied Microbiology, 1976.

239. Rao GHR. Global risk assessment for diabetes and vascular diseases: New guidelines for risk promoters. IN: CAD: Risk Promoters, Pathophysiology and Prevention. JP Med. Publishers, 2004.

240. Rao GHR. Handbook of Platelet Physiology and Pharmacology, Kluwer Academic Publishers. ISBN #0 7923 8538-1 (Ed. Gundu HR Rao) 1999.

241. Rao GHR. Importance of studying disease and disease process. Editorial. Developments in Clin Med Pathol Crimson Publ. 2018;1:1.

242. Rao GHR. Influence of anti-platelet drugs on platelet-vessel wall interactions. Prost. Leuko Med. 1987;30:133-45.

243. Rao GHR. Influence of calmodulin antagonist (stelazine) on agonist-induced calcium mobilization and platelet activation. Biochem. Biophys. Res Commun. 1987;148: 768-75.

244. Rao GHR. Influence of storage on signal transduction pathways and platelet function. Blood Cells 1992;18:383-96.
245. Rao GHR. Integrative approach to health: Challenges and Opportunities. J Ayur Int Med. 2015;6(3):215-19.
246. Rao GHR. Interventions in Obesity and Diabetes: Point of View. Interventions Obes. Diab. 2017;1(1):IOD.000501.
247. Rao GHR. Management of Type-2 Diabetes by Anti-Platelet Therapies: With special reference to aspirin. Front Bioscience (Scholar Edition), 2011;3:1-15.
248. Rao GHR. Manual of Platelet Morphology, Physiology and Pharmacology, JP Medical Publishers, New Delhi, India. 2018.
249. Rao GHR. Measurement of ionized calcium in normal human blood platelets. Anal Biochem. 1988;169:400-8.
250. Rao GHR. Michiels Jan Jaques: Aspirin Resistance: Does it exist? Sem Thromb Hemost. 2007;33:210-14.
251. Rao GHR. Microbial insecticides. Chapter in Current Topics in Applied Microbiology, 1976.
252. Rao GHR. Mind-Body Spirit Society of India: Opportunities and Challenges. Https://www.researchgate.net/publicaions/2016.
253. Rao GHR. Modern Day Cardiology: Expectations and Limitations. J Cardiol. 2018;2(2): 000116.
254. Rao GHR. Need for a National Platform and Action Plans for Primary Prevention and Integrated Treatment of Heart Disease in India. Biospectra. 2007;2:9-13.
255. Rao GHR. Need for a Point-of-care assay for monitoring antiplatelet and antithrombotic therapies. Stroke. 2009;40:2271-2.
256. Rao GHR. Non-traditional approaches to diagnosis and management of type-2 diabetes mellitus: Point of View. J Diab Metabol. 6:489 doi: 10.4172/2155-6156.1000489.
257. Rao GHR. Novel sub-groups of adult onset diabetes and its clinical complications. Editorial. Archives of Endocrinology and Diabetes Care. 2018;1(1):11-2.
258. Rao GHR. Physiology and pharmacology of platelets. Internat. J Prog Cardiovasc. Sci. 1995;2:108-10.
259. Rao GHR. Physiology of blood platelet activation. Ind J Physiol Pharmacol. 1994;37: 263-75.
260. Rao GHR. Platelet Dysfunction in Diabetes. In: Mechanisms of Vascular Diseases in Diabetes. Kartha CC, Ramachandran S, Pillai MR (Eds) Springer International. 2017.
261. Rao GHR. Platelet hypertension as risk for acute coronary syndromes. In: CAD: Risk Promoters, Pathophysiology and Prevention. JP Med. Publishers, 2004.
262. Rao GHR. Platelet Physiology and Pharmacology: An Overview. In: Platelet physiology and Pharmacology (Rao GHR, Ed.), Kluwer Academic Publishers, USA, 1999.
263. Rao GHR. Platelet Physiology and Pharmacology: Expectations and Limitations (https://www.researchgate.net/publication/308313140), 1997.
264. Rao GHR. Platelets as a risk factor for coronary artery disease. In: Coronary artery disease in South Asians: epidemiology, risk factors and prevention (Rao GHR, Ed.), 1998.
265. Rao GHR. Platelets, Prostaglandins and Thrombosis. Med. Update: Assoc Phys Ind. 1988;8:33-38, 1998.
266. Rao GHR. Polyenoic acids and platelet function. Recent Advances in essential fatty acid research (Das UN, Ed.), Academic Press, India. 1987; pp. 36-49.
267. Rao GHR. Prevention of vascular disease and development of affordable health for all: Thinking out of box (Viewpoint). J Clin Prevent Cardiol. 2012;1:31-4.
268. Rao GHR. Prevention or reversal of cardiometabolic diseases. J Clin Prevent Cardiol. 2018;7(1):22-8.
269. Rao GHR. Risk assessment, risk prediction, and effective management of risk factors for cardiovascular diseases. Editorial J Clin & Prevent Cardiology. 2012;1:9-10.
270. Rao GHR. Role of cyclic AMP and cyclic GMP as modulators of platelet cytosolic calcium (Brief Review). J Clin Prevent Cardiol. 2016;5: 99-103.
271. Rao GHR. Role of platelet adhesion and aggregation on thrombus formation. Thromb Haemost. 1998;79:454-5.

272. Rao GHR. Signal transduction, second messengers and platelet function. J Lab Clin Med. 1993;121:18-22.
273. Rao GHR. Signal transduction, second messengers and platelet pharmacology. Pharmacol (Life Sci.) 1994;13:39-44.
274. Rao GHR. Signal transduction, second messengers and platelet pharmacology. In: Environ. Physiol. (Mallick BN and Singh R, Eds.), Narosa Publishing House, Delhi. 1994.
275. Rao GHR. The role membrane lipid in the platelet storage lesion. Commentary. Blood Cells. 1992;18:498-500.
276. Rao GHR. Type-2 Diabetes, a Global Epidemic. J. Endocrinology and Thyroid Res. (JETR) MS ID: 555552, 2017. JETR 2017; 1(1):555552.
277. Rao GHR. World Health Organization (WHO) should follow the rotary model for disseminating knowledge, distributing funds and providing funds. CV Network. 2005;4:11-3.
278. Rao SG, Bhat P, Nagesh KS, et al. Bone Regeneration in Extraction Sockets with Autologous Platelet Rich Fibrin Gel. J. Maxillofacial and Oral Surg. 2013;12(1):11-6.
279. Rao, GHR, Radha E, White JG. Effect of Docosahexaenoic acid (DHA) on arachidonic metabolism and platelet function. Biochem. Biophys. Res Commun. 1983;117:549-56.
280. Rao, GHR. Risk assessment, risk prediction, and effective management of risk factors for cardiovascular diseases. J Clin Prevent Cardiol. (Editorial) 2012;1:9-10.
281. Reddy S, Bose R, Rao GHR, et al. Phospholipase A2 activation in human neutrophils requires influx of extracellular calcium and leukotriene B4. Am J Physiol. 1995;268: C138-C146.
282. Reddy S, Rao GHR, Murthy. Differential effects of phorbol 12-myristate 13-acetate and diacylglycerols on thromboxane A2-dependent phospholipase A2 in collagen-stimulated human platelets. Biochem Med Met Biol. 1994;51:118-28.
283. Repine JE, Rao GHR, Beall GD, et al. Inhibition of human neutrophil oxidative metabolism and degranulation in vitro by nitro blue tetrazolium and vitamin E. Am J Pathol. 1978;90:659-74.
284. Richards KL, White JG, Rao GHR, et al. Nucleotide and cyclic nucleotide levels of fresh and stored granulocytes. Transfusion 1982;22:428A.
285. Sahu S, Roy PS, Datta K, et al. Can gene therapy fight your obesity? Obesity Reviews. 2017;23(4):301-18.
286. Schollmeyer JV, Rao GHR, White JG. An actin-binding protein in human platelets: Interaction with actin on gelatin of actin and the influence of cytochalasin BA, J Pathol. 1978;93:443-6.
287. Schorer AE, Kaplan ME, Rao GHR, et al. Interleukin 1 stimulated endothelial cell tissue factor production and expression by a prostaglandin-independent mechanism. Thromb Haemost. 1989;56:256-9.
288. Schorer AF, Moldow CF, Rao GHR, et al. Interleukin (IL-1) promotes tissue factor expression in human endothelial cells. Blood. 1984;64:989A.
289. Smith CM II, Burris SM, Rao GHR, et al. Detergent-resistant cytoskeleton of the surface activated platelet differs from the suspension-activated platelet cytoskeleton. Blood. 1992;80:2774-80.
290. Smith CM, Burris SM, Rao GHR, et al. Epinephrine-induced reversal of aspirin effects on platelet deformability. Thromb Res. 1988; 51:35-44.
291. Song CW, Kim GE, Lynos JC, et al. (In Press). Thermo sensitization by increasing intracellular acidity with amiloride and its analogs. Int. J Radiation Oncol Biol Phys.
292. Sugihara T, Rao GHR, Hebbel RP. Diphenylamine: An unusual antioxidant. Free Rad J. 1993;14:381-7.
293. Tenbit Emiru, Eric M Bershad, Nicole D Zantek, et al. Intracerebral Hemorrhage: A Review of Coagulation Function J. Clin Appl Thromb Hemost. 2013;19(6):652-62.
294. Weiss DJ, McClay CB, Smith CM II, et al. Platelet function in the racing through-bred. Implications for exercise-induced haemorrhage. Vet Clin Pathol. 1990;19:35-9.
295. White JG, Goldberg ND, Estensen RD, et al. Rapid increase in platelet 3', 5-huanosine monophosphate (cGMP) levels in association with irreversible aggregation, degranulation and secretion. J Clin Invest. 1973;52:89.

296. White JG, Hagert K, Nipper JHJ, et al. Functional platelets after storage in vitro for fifteen to twenty days. Am J Pathol. 1980;101: 613-34.
297. White JG, Krumweide MD, Cocking-Johnson DJ, et al. Influence of cytochalasin B (CB) on GPIb distribution after thrombin or TRAP and before surface activation. Platelets 1997;8: 53-60.
298. White JG, Krumwiede MD, Cocking-Johnson D, et al. Retention of GPIb/IX receptors on external surfaces of thrombin-activated platelets in suspension. Blood. 1995;86: 3468-78.1.
299. White JG, Matlack C, Mundschenk D, et al. Platelet disorders in normal and a bleeder horse. First International Symposium on Equine Hematology. 1975; pp. 209-21.
300. White JG, Rao GHR, Estensen RD. Investigation of the release reaction in platelets exposed to phorbol myristate acetate. Am J Pathol. 1974;75:301-14.
301. White JG, Rao GHR, Gerrard JM. Effects of nitro blue tetrazolium and vitamin E on platelet ultrastructure, aggregation and secretion. Am J Pathol. 1977;88:387-402.
302. White JG, Rao GHR, Gerrard JM. Effects of the ionophore, A23187, on blood platelets. I. Influence on aggregation and secretion. Am J Pathol. 1974;77:135-49.
303. White JG, Rao GHR, Gerrard JM. Platelet stimulus activation contraction secretion coupling: A frequently fractured chain of events. In: The Regulation of Coagulation (Mann,Taylor, Eds.), Elsevier/North Holland Inc. 1980; pp. 363-76.
304. White JG, Rao GHR, Gerrard JM. Prostaglandins in platelet activation. In: Platelets-Cellular Response Mechanisms and Their Biological Significance (Rothman AN, Meyers FA, Gitler C and Silberg A, Eds.), John Wiley & Sons Ltd., 1980; pp. 201-11.
305. White JG, Rao GHR, Gerrard JM. Vitamin E and platelets: Cooperative interactions with nitro blue tetrazolium on the inhibition of adhesion, aggregation and secretion. Seminars in Hematology. Am J Ped Hem/Onc. 1979;1:155-68.
306. White JG, Rao GHR, Mundschenk DD. Effects of a calcium ionophore, A23187, on the surface morphology of normal erythrocytes. Amer Soc Hematol. 1975.
307. White JG, Rao GHR. Aggregated-disaggregated, refractory platelets retain sensitivity to ristocetin. Thromb Res. 1996;84:253-6.
308. White JG, Rao GHR. Effects of microtubule stabilizing agent on the response of platelets to vincristine. Blood. 1983;60:474-83.
309. White JG, Rao GHR. Influence of microtubule stabilizing agent on platelet structural physiology. Am J Pathol. 1983;112:217.
310. White JG, Rao GHR. Microtubule coils versus the surface membranc cytoskclcton in maintenance and restoration of platelet discoid shape. Am J Pathol. 1998;152:597-609.
311. White JG, Rao GHR. Thrombin-induced inhibition of platelet agglutination by von Willebrand factor (vWF): Reversal by ionized calcium. Platelets. 1996;7:321-8.
312. White JG, Reddy KR, Rao GHR. Penicillin induced human platelet dysfunction and its reversal by epinephrine. Prost Leuko Med. 1983;11:199-211.
313. Witkop CJ, Babcock MN, Rao GHR, et al. Albinism and Hermansky-Pudlak Syndrome in Puerto Rico Biol Assoc Med Puerto Rico. 1990;82:333-9.

Index

Page numbers followed by *f* refer to figure, *t* refer to table.

R

S

T